ANTIOXIDANT-BASED THERAPIES FOR DISEASE PREVENTION AND MANAGEMENT

ANTIOXIDANT-BASED THERAPIES FOR DISEASE PREVENTION AND MANAGEMENT

Edited by
Pallavi Singh Chauhan, PhD
Sonia Johri, PhD

AAP | APPLE
ACADEMIC
PRESS

First edition published 2022

Apple Academic Press Inc.
1265 Goldenrod Circle, NE,
Palm Bay, FL 32905 USA

4164 Lakeshore Road, Burlington,
ON, L7L 1A4 Canada

CRC Press
6000 Broken Sound Parkway NW,
Suite 300, Boca Raton, FL 33487-2742 USA

2 Park Square, Milton Park,
Abingdon, Oxon, OX14 4RN UK

Library and Archives Canada Cataloguing in Publication

Title: Antioxidant-based therapies for disease prevention and management / edited by Pallavi Singh Chauhan, PhD, Sonia Johri, PhD.

Names: Chauhan, Pallavi Singh, editor. | Johri, Sonia, editor.

Description: First edition. | Includes bibliographical references and index.

Identifiers: Canadiana (print) 20210242795 | Canadiana (ebook) 20210242884 | ISBN 9781771889643 (hardcover) | ISBN 9781774639092 (softcover) | ISBN 9781003129585 (ebook)

Subjects: LCSH: Antioxidants—Therapeutic use.

Classification: LCC RB170 .A55 2022 | DDC 616.07—dc23

Library of Congress Cataloging-in-Publication Data

Names: Chauhan, Pallavi Singh, 1989- editor. | Johri, Sonia, 1971- editor.

Title: Antioxidant-based therapies for disease prevention and management / edited by Pallavi Singh Chauhan, PhD, Sonia Johri, PhD.

Description: First edition. | Palm Bay, FL : Apple Academic Press, 2022. | Includes bibliographical references and index. | Summary: "This volume, Antioxidant-Based Therapies for Disease Prevention and Management, presents a valuable overview of the therapeutic aspects as well as applications of antioxidants. This informative book discusses the basic mechanisms of therapy-based oxidative damage and categorization of nutritional antioxidants. It covers the sources of antioxidants as well as their extraction and quantification. The volume considers the controversies of the usefulness or disadvantages of antioxidant supplementation in relation to adaptation and performance and also looks at the effectiveness of bioactives and antioxidant-based therapies for specific health issues, such as anemia, infectious diseases, urinary tract infections, Parkinson's diseases, and diabetes. The book also discusses the sensing of oxidative stress and the effectiveness of antioxidant treatment, followed by an introduction to several biomarkers to estimate the bioefficacy of dietary/supplemental antioxidants in various forms. Also discussed are free radicals that can cause oxidative stress, a process that can trigger cell damage, and how antioxidant molecules have been shown to counteract oxidative stress in laboratory experiments (for example, in cells or animal studies). Several authors present studies that highlight that high-dose antioxidant supplements may be harmful in some cases. For example, the results of some studies have linked the use of high-dose beta-carotene supplements to an increased risk of lung cancer in smokers and use of high-dose vitamin E supplements to increased risks of hemorrhagic stroke (a type of stroke caused by bleeding in the brain) and prostate cancer. With this book, sports nutrition scientists, nutritionists, food biochemists, advisors, physiologists, students, and research scholars as well as faculty will find factual information on antioxidative therapies"-- Provided by publisher.

Identifiers: LCCN 2021028092 (print) | LCCN 2021028093 (ebook) | ISBN 9781771889643 (hardback) | ISBN 9781774639092 (paperback) | ISBN 9781003129585 (ebook)

Subjects: LCSH: Antioxidants--Therapeutic use.

Classification: LCC RB170 .A56 2022 (print) | LCC RB170 (ebook) | DDC 613.2/86--dc23

LC record available at https://lccn.loc.gov/2021028092

LC ebook record available at https://lccn.loc.gov/2021028093

ISBN: 978-1-77188-964-3 (hbk)
ISBN: 978-1-77463-909-2 (pbk)
ISBN: 978-1-00312-958-5 (ebk)

About the Editors

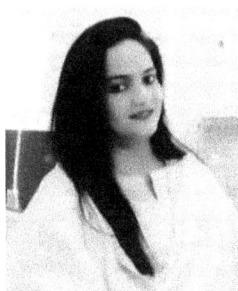

Pallavi Singh Chauhan, PhD

Pallavi Singh Chauhan, PhD, is Assistant Professor at the Amity Institute of Biotechnology, Amity University Madhya Pradesh, Gwalior, India, as well as a researcher. Her research focuses on the synthesis, characterization, and multiple biomedical application of nanoparticles. The major fields of science that are relevant to Dr. Chauhan's work include nanotechnology, nanobioscience, biomedical application of nanotechnology, nanotoxicity, magnetic nanostructures, nanocatalysts, and nanoparticle systems of metals and metal oxides.

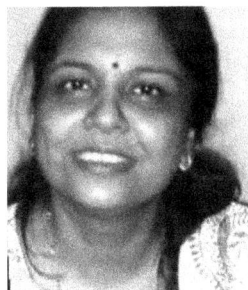

Sonia Johri, PhD

Sonia Johri, PhD, is Dean of Academics and an Associate Professor in the Department of Life Sciences at ITM University, Gwalior, Madhya Pradesh, India. She has over 40 papers to her credit in journals of national and international repute. She is an external member of the Board of Studies in Biochemistry at Jiwaji University. She is also a member of the Institutional Animal Ethical Committee at ITM University, Gwalior. She has authored a book entitled *Practical Biochemistry*, and she is a reviewer for various national and international journals. She is a life member of the Indian Science Congress Association. Dr. Johri has 23 years of research experience and has worked extensively in the diversified fields of metal toxicity, anemia, hepatoprotection, oxidative stress, and biofuels. Though there is vast diversification in her field, she holds expertise in toxicological evaluation of metal toxicants and their therapy in rat models, phytomedicine, oxidative stress, physicochemical characterization of natural products as well as *in vitro and in vivo* biochemical characterization. She has also worked on bioethanol production from agro-wastes. Her field of specialization is diagnostic enzymology. She has attended and presented her work at various international conferences held at Munich, Germany, and Quebec City, Canada. Dr. Johri is a postgraduate in Biochemistry and was awarded her doctoral degree from Jiwaji University, Gwalior, India. Her postdoctoral research was sponsored by the Council of Scientific and Industrial Research, New Delhi, India.

Contents

Contributors

Surbhi Antarkar
Department of Life Sciences, ITM University, Gwalior, Madhya Pradesh, India

Neha Chauhan
Department of Life Sciences, ITM University, Gwalior, India

Pallavi Singh Chauhan
Department of Life Sciences, ITM University, Gwalior, Madhya Pradesh, India

Prachi Dixit
School of Sciences, ITM University Gwalior, Gwalior, Madhya Pradesh, India

Anuj Dubey
Department of Chemistry, ITM University, Gwalior, Madhya Pradesh, India

Rupali Dutt
School of Studies in Biochemistry, Jiwaji University, Gwalior, India

Namrata Jha
School of Life Sciences, ITM University, Gwalior, Madhya Pradesh, India

Sonia Johri
Department of Life Sciences, ITM University, Gwalior, India

Ekta Khare
School of Pharmacy, ITM University, Gwalior, Madhya Pradesh, India

Lalita Kushwah
School of Studies in Biochemistry, Jiwaji University, Gwalior, India

Madhu Parmar
Department of Life Sciences ITM University Gwalior M.P. India

GBKS Prasad
Centre for Translational Research, School of studies in Biochemistry, Jiwaji University, Gwalior, Madhya Pradesh, India

Hradesh Rajput
Department of Food Technology, ITM University, Gwalior, India

Sakshi Talwar
Translational Health Science and Technology Institute, Faridabad, India

Shivam Tayal
School of Pharmacy, ITM University, Gwalior, Madhya Pradesh, India

D. K. Sharma
Department of Zoology, Government Model Science College, Gwalior

Minerva Sharma
Department of Botany, St. John's College, Agra, Uttar Pradesh, India

Portia Sharma
Department of Botany, St. John's College, Agra, Uttar Pradesh, India

Rita Sharma
Department of Life Sciences, ITM University, Gwalior, India

Kavita Singh
Centre for Translational Research, School of studies in Biochemistry, Jiwaji University, Gwalior, Madhya Pradesh, India

Pratistha Srivastava
Department of Food Technology, ITM University, Gwalior, India

Udita Tiwari
Department of Biochemistry, School of Life Sciences, Khandari Campus, Dr. B. R. Ambedkar University, Agra 282004, Uttar Pradesh, India

Manitosh Pandey
Translational Health Science and Technology Institute, Faridabad, India
Department of Life Sciences, ITM University, Gwalior, Madhya Pradesh, India

Aarshi Vashistha
Health Centre, Jiwaji University, Gwalior 474011, MP), India

Renu Yadav
Department of Botany, St. John's College, Agra, Uttar Pradesh, India

Abbreviations

Aβ	amyloid beta
AChE	acetylcholinesterase
AD	Alzheimer's disease
DHA	docosahexaenoic acid
GSH	glutathione
NP	nanoparticle
Sp.	species
ROS	reactive oxygen species
TiO_2	titanium oxide
SiO_2	silica oxide
ZnO	zinc oxide
CdSe	cadmium selenide
CdTe	cadmium telluride
InP	indium phosphide
InAs	indium arsenide
ZnS	zinc sulfide
NIR	near-infrared spectroscopy
PLGA	poly(lactic-*co*-glycolic acid)
SOD	superoxide dismutase
iNOS	inducible nitric oxide synthase
CeO	cerium oxide
GSSG	reduced glutathione
GSHP	glutathione peroxidase

Foreword

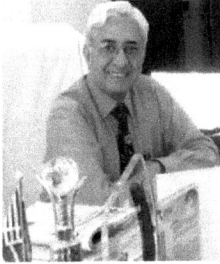

This book serves as a comprehensive overview of the current scientific knowledge on the health effects of dietary and supplemental antioxidants (such as vitamins C and E). Chapters integrate information from basic research and animal studies, epidemiologic studies, and clinical intervention trials. The popular media has taken great interest in antioxidants, with numerous articles emphasizing their role in preventing disease and the possible slowing of the aging process. These antioxidant vitamins may be important in preventing not only acute deficiency symptoms, but also chronic disorders such as heart disease and certain types of cancer. This book, therefore, is not only for scientists and doctors, but also for health writers, journalists, and informed lay people. The text focuses on several human conditions for which there is now good scientific evidence that oxidation is an important etiological component. Specifically, antioxidants may prevent or slow down the progression of cancer, cardiovascular disease, immune system disorders, cataracts, neurological disorders, and degeneration due to the aging process.

—**Dr. Kamal Kant Dwivedi**
Vice Chancellor, ITM University Gwalior, M.P., India

Preface

Up to now, there has been no book on recent advancement in antioxidant therapies. It is an honor that we are editing the book in this field, and it was exciting for me and my colleague that so many renowned researchers in the field accepted to send a chapter. Many, many thanks to you all!

Originally, I intended to title this book "Multiple Antioxidant Therapies," but considerations with regard to attracting as many readers as possible led us to title it as "Recent Advances in Antioxidant Therapies." Although in some respects it is not absolutely appropriate, we perceived the term "antioxidant" as very suitable as it polarizes and fosters discussions. Polarization and discussion are engines to stimulate research in a specific field.

This book consists of 12 scientifically based chapters with regard to the basic mechanisms of therapy-based oxidative damage and categorization of nutritional antioxidants. It covers the antioxidant supply in various forms and discusses the controversies of the usefulness or disadvantages of antioxidant supplementation. Many chapters refer to antioxidants and/or bioactives and their effectiveness, and a few chapters cover nanocomposite-based antioxidative therapies. This book will open new arenas of research and will prove to be very interesting for the readers as it provides chapters that discuss antioxidant supplementation in relation to adaptation and performance as well as the relation between supplementation with advanced antioxidant compounds and/or supplements and the immune system. Last but not least, few chapters discuss sensing of oxidative stress and the effectiveness of antioxidant treatment, followed by introduction to several biomarkers to estimate the bioefficacy of dietary/supplemental antioxidants in various forms.

With this book, sport nutrition scientists, nutritionists, food biochemists, advisors, physiologists, students, and research scholars in related fields as well as faculties working in educational institutes will find actual information and relevant antioxidative therapies. Hope that our efforts may prove to be a useful tool for further research strategies. Have a good time with it!

Introduction

The book highlights manmade or natural substances that may prevent or delay some types of cell damage. Diets high in vegetables and fruits, which are good sources of antioxidants, have been found to be healthy; however, research has not shown antioxidant supplements to be beneficial in preventing diseases. Examples of antioxidants include vitamins C and E, selenium, and carotenoids, such as beta-carotene, lycopene, lutein, and zeaxanthin. Thus, this book provides the basic information about antioxidants and conceptualizes what the science says about antioxidants and health and suggests sources for additional information.

Few discussions in the book suggest that free radicals are highly unstable molecules that are naturally formed when you exercise and when your body converts food into energy. Your body can also be exposed to free radicals from a variety of environmental sources, such as cigarette smoke, air pollution, and sunlight. Free radicals can cause "oxidative stress," a process that can trigger cell damage. Oxidative stress is thought to play a role in a variety of diseases, including cancer, cardiovascular diseases, diabetes, Alzheimer's disease, Parkinson's disease, and eye diseases such as cataracts and age-related macular degeneration.

Some of the chapters in the book have highlighted that antioxidant molecules have been shown to counteract oxidative stress in laboratory experiments (e.g., in cells or animal studies). However, there is debate as to whether consuming large amounts of antioxidants in supplement form actually benefits the health of the individual. There is also some concern that consuming antioxidant supplements in excessive doses may be harmful.

The authors have highlighted that high-dose antioxidant supplements may be harmful in some cases. For example, the results of some studies have linked the use of high-dose beta-carotene supplements to an increased risk of lung cancer in smokers and use of high-dose vitamin E supplements to increased risks of hemorrhagic stroke (a type of stroke caused by bleeding in the brain) and prostate cancer.

Readers may be benefited by knowing the facts that in order to consider a dietary supplement, one should be thoroughly informed on it from reliable sources. It is emphasized that dietary supplements may interact with medications. The book presents a brief overview of some of the diseases that are associated with free radicals and discusses the roles of some of dietary antioxidants in disease prevention, with particular reference to the findings of latest clinical trials.

Acknowledgment

A work can never exist and thrive in solitude. Research work is never the work of an individual. It is more the combination of views, suggestions, contributions, and work involving many individuals. This book also bears the imprint of many people. Thus, one of the pleasant parts of writing this book is the opportunity to thank all those who motivated us in writing of this book. We avail this opportunity to thank the Almighty and our parents who are the most treasured gift to us. We feel at a loss of words to express the magnitude of boundless love and tireless sacrifice and affection showed by them. This book is dedicated to those novel souls. We convey our wholehearted thanks to many of our well-wishers and other friends and request their forgiveness for not mentioning them here by name.

CHAPTER 1

Nano-Antioxidants, A Next-Generation Therapeutic Strategy

PALLAVI SINGH CHAUHAN[1*], SHIVAM TAYAL[2], and NAMRATA JHA[3]

[1]*Department of Life Sciences, ITM University, Gwalior, Madhya Pradesh, India*

[2]*School of Pharmacy, ITM University, Gwalior, Madhya Pradesh, India*

[3]*School of Life Sciences, ITM University, Gwalior, Madhya Pradesh, India*

Corresponding author. E-mail: pallavi.chauhan97@gmail.com

ABSTRACT

For the treatment of oxidative-stress related disorders, cellular uptake of dietary antioxidants is an important setback. Neurodegenerative disease such as Alzheimer's and Parkinson disease is still an unsolved challenge. Nanotechnology can be an alternative therapeutic strategy for eradicating the problem of bioabsorption, targeted effect, and it may act as a delivery system for protecting antioxidants. This chapter is thus focused on nano-medicine-based therapy for treating oxidative stress as well as oxidative damage.

1.1 INTRODUCTION

In recent years, nanotechnology has major contribution to the field of medicine. The application of nanotechnology in medicinal field is known to be as nanomedicine. Nanoparticles (NPs) have various biomedical applications (Burduşel et al., 2018). The major drawback of using NPs in biomedical applications is their cellular toxicity, thus ultimately limiting their usage for clinical use (Patra et al., 2018). The present study will highlight mainly two aspects. The first aspect comprises the NPs type depending on their characteristics, where the second one is focused on the biomedical applications of NPs with special reference to oxidative stress (Zhang et al., 2016). Oxidative stress parameters are associated with reduction in nitric oxide (NO) level. The NO level is associated with regulation of vascular tone along with endothelial dysfunctioning (Gaynullina et al., 2019). The endothelial dysfunctioning is considered to be as a primary stage in the origin of cardiovascular diseases (Marchio et al., 2019). Moreover, the antioxidative property of NPs makes them more compatible with the improvisation of vascular dysfunctioning. Vascular dysfunctioning has major consequences such as atherosclerosis and hypertension (Yao et al., 2019).

The potential applications of nanotechnology made them more suitable to use in the field of biomedical science, biomedical engineering, biosensors, biodiagnosis, and molecular and cell biology (Ramos et al., 2017). The nanomedicines have unique properties such as high surface-to-volume ratio that makes them more suitable to use as theranostic agents. This unique property also allows the NPs to increase the absorption of drugs and ultimately accelerates male easy spread of the drug of interest to bloodstream (Rizvi et al., 2018). Along with absorption, this unique property of the NPs also influences its other characteristics (Fig. 1.1).

The antioxidative properties of NPs are seeking attention of various researchers in order to treat multiple diseases developed as a consequence of enhanced oxidative stress (Mauricio et al., 2018). The development of reactive oxygen species (ROS) in the biological system emerges as a result of increase in various cardiovascular risk factors (Vona et al., 2019). Atherosclerosis, an inflammatory disease, is one of the finest examples of the diseases that occur as a result of oxidative stress (Liguori et al., 2018). Thus it is prerequisite to optimize antioxidative systems to lower the associated risk factors. NPs due to their ease of internalization along antioxidant properties are of major focus.

1.2 NANOMEDICINE

1.2.1 BASIC CHARACTERISTICS

The emergence of the field of nanotechnology and its applications in biological purposes greatly influence the medicinal area. Nanotechnology is an emerging field that allows the synthesis as well as material manipulation at nanoscale level (Pampaloni et al., 2018). Nanotechnology is involved in the development of new multidimensional tools. According to the American Society for Testing and Materials, NPs have various applications in biomedical field such as for the treatment, diagnosis, monitoring, and control of biological systems, referred as nanomedicine (Pelaz et al., 2017).

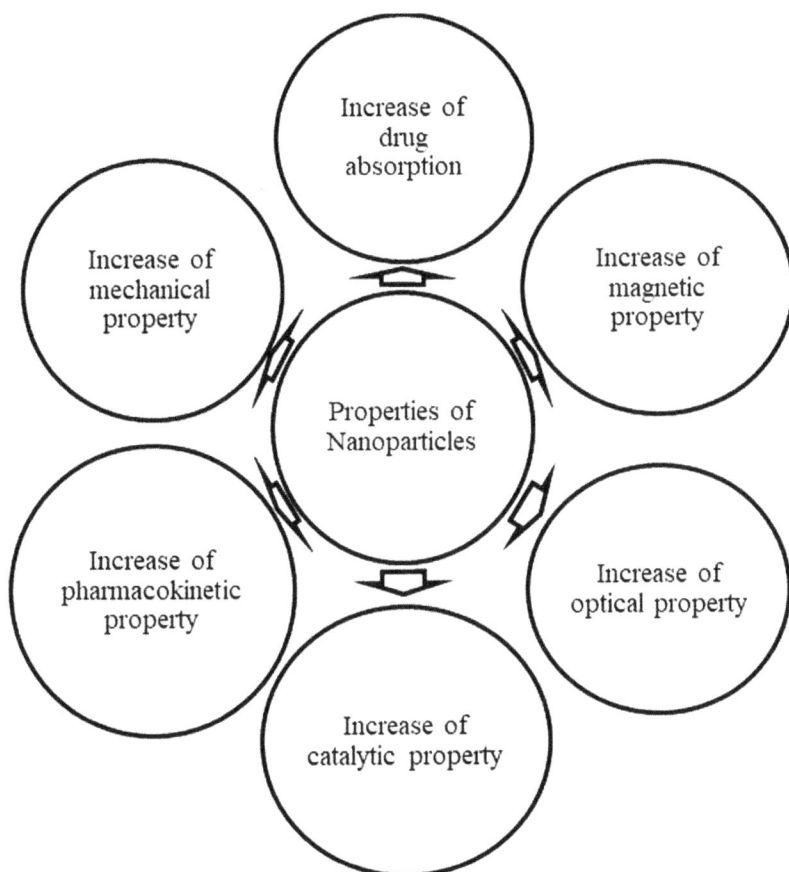

FIGURE 1.1   Diverse applications of nanoparticles.

The physical and chemical properties of NPs are quite different as compared with the bulk materials. Along with having high surface area-to-volume ratio, NPs also have unique quantum size effect. Along with it, it is necessary to synthesize monodispersed NPs in order to facilitate their cellular absorption and minimizing aggregation (Fathi-Achachelouei et al., 2019). The NPs may also have synergistic effect when modified by combination of two or more materials.

1.2.2   TYPES OF NANOPARTICLES

Depending on the nature of the NPs, they can be classified into organic, inorganic, and carbon based (Teleanu et al., 2018). The organic NPs include liposomes and polymers, and inorganic NPs include metals, and quantum dots. (Zottel et al., 2019) (Fig. 1.2).

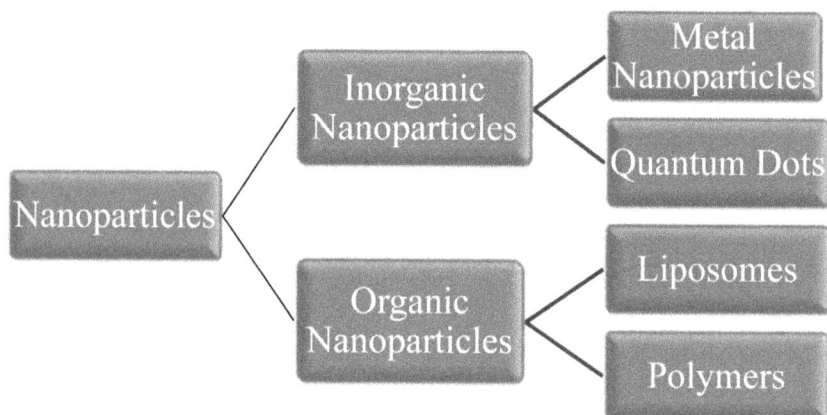

FIGURE 1.2   Classification of nanoparticles.

1.2.2.1   LIPOSOME

The liposomes have lipid bilayer, are spherical vesicles, and also consist of an aqueous substance. For the preparation of liposomes, amphiphilic molecules are used, which have resemblance with the biological membranes (Di Sotto et al., 2018). The liposomes, along with improving the efficiency of the drug, also enhance the drug safety. The drugs contain active compound, and the active components of the drug could be hydrophilic or hydrophobic (Desai et al., 2018). If they are hydrophilic, their location could be aqueous space and if they are hydrophobic, they normally remain in the lipid membrane.

There are few parameters that influence the liposome characteristics, some of which are the physicochemical properties of the entrapped drug along with liposomal compounds, the base medium, the entrapped compound concentration along with its potential toxicity, process used in the fabrication of liposomes, dispersity, shape, size, stability of the liposomes, etc. (Hua et al., 2019). The synthesis of liposomes can be achieved by sonication of a dispersion of amphipathic lipids. Multilamellar liposomes can be created by low shear rates. Instead of using sonication method for the drug encapsulation, few other methods can be used such as extrusion and Mozafari method (Lujan et al., 2019).

Sonication method could alter the properties of the drug entrapped, ultimately making material of no use for human, and thus alternative strategies can be used (Panahi et al., 2017). Reports have also shown that for the preparation of liposomes, any lipid can be utilized rather than using phosphatidylcholine (He et al., 2019). These days liposomes are regularly being used to deliver chemotherapeutic drugs for effective anticancer therapy. They are also used for the delivery of various bioactive materials as well as food ingredients, thus have diverse application areas like nanomedicine, food, and cosmetics industries (Kaul et al., 2018). They have various unique properties as compared to bulk materials like high biocompatibility and biodegradability.

Nanoliposome technology is an emerging area these days, which advances food technologies with special reference to encapsulation, controlled release, stability, and bioavailability (Ganesan et al., 2018). Thus, in order to carry active components, liposomes are of prime concern for the researchers these days.

1.2.2.2 POLYMERIC NANOPARTICLES

Biodegradability and biocompatibility are the basic characteristics of polymeric NPs. They are the mostly used nanocomposites in drug delivery systems, made up of natural polymers, that is, chitosan, PLA, PMMA, and PEG (Vasile et al., 2018). They have added advantages of being getting surface modified, with great pharmacokinetics that can be manipulated during manufacture.

There are various methods of manufacturing polymeric NPs like emulsification-based two-step procedures and precipitation-based one-step procedures (Soh et al., 2019). Characterization of the synthesized nanocomposites can be done using EDS, ζ-potential, SEM, XPS, TEM, FTIR, XRD, etc. (Ahmad et al., 2019). To advance the pharmaceutical application of the synthesized polymeric NPs, improvement of drug-loading efficiency, drug–polymer interaction, and physicochemical properties should be of prime concern.

1.2.2.3 METALLIC NANOPARTICLES

Metal NPs may include metals like gold, copper, zinc, or silver, and NPs with magnetic properties are also included in this category (Sanzari et al., 2019). The advantage of using metal NPs is that they pose unique electronic and optical properties. They are very much biocompatible with modifiable properties, and also they are less toxic with huge biocompatibility. An advanced feature of gold NPs is their surface, which provides it more susceptibility to conjugate ligands (Anderson et al., 2019).

The ligands that can be conjugated to the surface of metal NPs are proteins, oligonucleotides, and antibodies (Markwalter et al., 2018). Mainly the functional groups of such ligands, including phosphines, amines, and mercaptans, bind with greater affinity to the gold surface. Such conjugates offer a wide range of applications in enhancing localized surface plasmon resonance (Wang et al., 2019). The enhanced Surface Plasmon Resonance (SPM) of synthesized NPs can be utilized for various imaging tools and techniques as well as biomedicine along with disease diagnosis like cancer imaging. Cancer imaging technique includes transportation of gold NPs into the nucleus of cancer cell (Peng et al., 2019). The drug regime that researchers include is the gold NP-conjugated peptide along with nuclear localization signal (Jeong et al., 2018).

1.2.2.4 METAL OXIDE NANOPARTICLES

In order to apply NPs in biomedical applications, exploitation of potent properties of NPs was done. The potential properties of NPs may include antioxidant activities, catalytic property, optoelectronic properties, bioavailability, and biocompatibility. Because of the surface biocompatibility, ceria NPs are increasingly being used in the various antioxidant therapies as well as a potential anti-inflammatory agent (Dhall et al., 2018).

Similarly, TiO$_2$ has broad applications in biosensors because of their properties like biocompatibility and optical properties (Xiong et al., 2018). Cerium oxide NPs because of their interchangeable oxidation states make them more prone to use in application of treatment of oxidative stress. The two oxidation states of cerium oxide NPs, that is, cerium (IV) and cerium (III), are interconvertible, resulting in redox coupling and ultimately providing them catalytic potential (Medina et al., 2019). Studies report that this fluctuation in oxidation states may arise due to defects on their surface (Fig. 1.3).

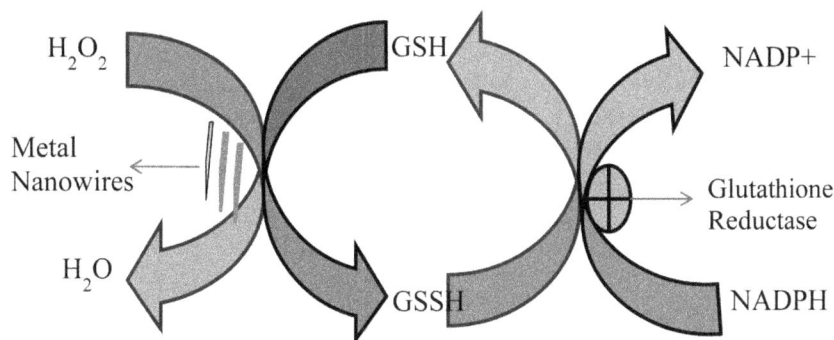

H$_2$O$_2$ GSH   NADP+

Metal
Nanowires   Glutathione
                                              Reductase

H$_2$O
          GSSH   NADPH

FIGURE 1.3   Mechanism of action of metal nanoparticles/nanowires.

Porous silica (SiO$_2$) is another example of NPs endowing catalytic property and thus has wide biomedical applications. The advanced properties of NPs as compared to the bulk material are due to their unique properties such as large surface-area-to-volume ratio, stability, biocompatibility, and bioavailability. Due to the mesoporous behavior of silica NPs, researchers are more focused toward their application in the development of drug delivery systems, to explore it in the area of biomedicine as well as biosensors (Narayan et al., 2018).

Surface-modified zinc oxide NPs were also reported to have applications in drug delivery, biosensors, bioimaging, and fluorescence imaging. Surface modification of such NPs is essential to make their dissolution easy in the biological systems containing water and acidic solutions. Doped ZnO NPs are currently the prime focus of researchers (Ebrahimi et al., 2019).

1.2.2.5   CERAMIC NANOPARTICLES

These days the porous nature of ceramic nanocompounds is used as a drug delivery vehicle. The transportation of the compound they perform may include peptides, enzymes, lipids, or drugs. Drug delivery through ceramic NPs is so effective that they remain unaffected by external parameters such as pH, temperature, and moisture conditions (Saghazadeh et al., 2018). Silica and aluminum are mostly used components in such NPs. These have the advantage of having the core component; however, the core of these NPs is not only limited to a single material, but also it could be a combination of both metal and nonmetallic materials.

For the β-cyclodextrin-based treatment of cancer cells, vehicle system of ceramic NPs capped mesoporous silica NPs has been developed (Watermann et al., 2017). Calcium phosphate, calcium carbonate, etc. are more widely used components in the field of nanomedicine, regeneration of tissue, orthopedy, dentistry, and other biomedical fields (Priyadarsini et al., 2018).

1.2.2.6   QUANTUM DOTS

Quantum dots are known to have fluorescent properties as they basically consist of semiconductor materials, specifically their core component is of prime advantage, for example, CdSe, CdTe, InP, and InAs (Berends et al., 2019). They may also have quantum dots capped with shell, for example, ZnS. The capping may avoid leaking of toxic metals, and thus the property may help these particles to improvise their optoelectronic properties along with other physical properties (Wegner et al., 2019). They have wide applications in the area of bioimaging, biosensing, and biotherapeutical strategies.

For various biomedical and biosensing applications, biocompatibility of quantum dots plays a significant role. There are various methods available for synthesis of biocompatible quantum dots, and the three major routes for their synthesis are biomimetic synthesis, biosynthesis, and chemical synthesis (Ovais et al., 2018). The biomimetic synthesis technique uses various biomolecules such as nucleic acids, peptides, proteins, and enzymes as templates. The biosynthesis technique utilizes live organisms or plants, the quantum dots thus prepared by this technique are toxic as well as less hazardous to the environment, also they do not require stringent protocol and sophisticated conditions for synthesis (Spicer et al., 2018).

1.2.2.7 CARBON-BASED NANOPARTICLES

The carbon-based NPs basically include fullerenes, which are allotropes of carbon (approximately 60 carbon atoms) having polygonal morphology and nanotubes that are synthesized by employing chemical vapor method for deposition of graphite. The carbon nanotubes basically include two classes, that is, single walled and multiwalled (Simon et al., 2019). The multiwalled carbon nanotubes are known to have potential antimicrobial activity, and also due to their unique physical and optical properties, they have multiple biomedical as well as imaging applications (Hasan et al., 2018). To enhance the biodegradability, they need to be surface modified to avoid aggregation.

Optical transitions of carbon nanotubes occur within the near-infrared region, that is, low scattering, high resolution, and more penetration, thus having multiple applications in the treatment of biological tissues and cells (Yudasaka et al., 2017). Near-infrared (NIR) fluorescence microscopy and optical coherence tomography are a few of the standard techniques used to visualize cellular as well as tissue level, that is, studying phagocytic cells and various in vivo studies. But there are some disadvantages as far as biomedical applications of carbon nanotubes are concerned, such as cytotoxicity with special reference to incomplete removal of impurities from nanocomposites, cellular uptake, and oxidant activity (Bai et al., 2016). The altered properties of carbon nanotubes are due to their varied size, morphology, and charge.

1.3 NANOCOMPOSITES AND OXIDATIVE STRESS TREATMENT

Antioxidants are compounds that inhibit oxidation. Oxidation is the chemical reaction that produces free radicals, leading to the chain reactions that may damage the cells of organisms. Some of the antioxidants terminate the chain formation such as thiols and ascorbic acid. For the balancing of the oxidative stress, plants and animals maintain complex systems of overlaying antioxidants, such as glutathione and enzymes, produced internally or the dietary antioxidants vitamin C and vitamin E. Mostly the antioxidants are used for two different groups of substances. Industrial chemicals are used for the prevention of oxidation of the products, oxidation inhibitors in fuels and naturally occurring compounds that are present in food and tissue.

In nature, there are three types of antioxidants, which include phyto-chemicals, vitamins, and enzymes. The most powerful antioxidants naturally found in the plants, including the fact that they are exposed to ultra-violet (UV) lights, generate a large amount of free radical, and due to the prevention system present in them, they did not get harm through those free radicals. Antioxidant enzymes come into the body through the proteins and minerals that we intake along with the food we eat. Some of these enzymes are also produced inside the human body, which are super-oxide dismutase (SOD), glutathione peroxidase, glutathione reductase, and catalases. The human body does not produce antioxidant vitamins so we have to intake through food and common vitamins such as vitamins A, C, E, folic acid, and beta carotene. Phytochemical are those antioxidants that are naturally used by the plants to protect themselves against radia-tion. Phytochemicals are broken down into different forms, carotenoids, flavonoids, allyl sulfides, and polyphenols. Studies have revealed the role of free radicals and oxidative stress that contributes to the large number of decrease of events leading to dopamine cell degeneration in Parkin-son's disease. In general, the in-built protective mechanisms consist of enzymatic and nonenzymatic antioxidants in the central nervous system of humans play decisive roles in preventing neuronal cell loss that can occur due to free radicals. With an increase in age, the ability of producing antioxidant decreases. Therefore, the therapy of the antioxidant alone or in combination with current treatment methods represents an attractive strategy for treating or we can say in preventing the neurodegeneration as seen in Parkinson's disease. Therefore, antioxidants might be one of the ideal agents to prevent free radical–mediated tissue destruction and inhibit some of the early degenerative events trafficking in the central nervous system that lead to neurodegeneration in Parkinson's disease and its experimental models. Antioxidants are widely discussed in both the lay press and the scientific literature as health-promoting agents that may protect against various age-related diseases. Antioxidants are exogenous or endogenous molecules that act against any form of oxidative stress and its associated ill effects on cellular systems. The state of oxidative imbalance found during neurodegenerative processes is triggered by one or more factors such as brain aging, genetic predisposition, mitochondrial dysfunction, free radical production, and environmental toxins. Treatment of Parkinson's disease with the drug of choice, L-dopa, is limited only to the relief of symptoms, and long-term use may further add to the oxidative load by producing free radicals during normal metabolism and play a role in disease progression. Major factors responsible for nonphysiological ROS production and their importance in Parkinson's disease are transitional metals, including iron. In vitro utilization of various toxin-induced cell lines such as PC12, SH-SY5Y, and MN9D mimic many aspects of dopaminergic neuron death observed in Parkinson's disease. The in vivo classical animal models of Parkinson's disease rely on the systemic or intracerebral administration of neurotoxins such as reserpine, haloperidol, 1-methyl-4-phenyl-1,2,3,6-tetrahydropyridine (MPTP), 6-OHDA, and, more recently, the pesticides rotenone, maneb, and paraquat, which have the ability to generate ROS in neurons and induce oxidative damage in the nigrostriatal dopaminergic system. *N*-Acetyl-L-cysteine is a pharmaceutical drug and nutritional supplement, which has been used primarily as a mucolytic agent and in the management of paracetamol overdose. Researchers have hypothesized that *N*-acetyl-L-cysteine supplementation in drinking water (40 mM) protects against SNCA toxicity. Oxidative stress may increase the accumulation of toxic forms of SNCA in a DA-dependent manner. The neuroprotective effects were present due to the presence of its antioxidant effects, which is caused by induction of pathways that is known to be regulated through the Nrf2/antioxidant response element (ARE) signaling pathway. It is indicated that NP7 could be used in the prevention or protection from neuroprotecting agent against oxidative stress in Parkinson's disease (PD).

Oxidative stress is the only one of the major risk factors that is present in the body and could initiate or promote degeneration of dopamine neurons. Antioxidant therapy could prevent or help in the reduction the rate of increasing of this disease nowadays that is emerging too fast. It has been studied that antioxidant compounds are able to protect neuronal cells by scavenging free radicals or activating the antioxidant mechanisms and also for reducing the effect of the ROS inside the body. Numerous in vitro and in vivo animal studies reported during the last 5 years centered on oxidative stress and ROS-mediated mechanisms such as radical scavenging, metal chelating, and/or regulation of antioxidant enzymes. The compounds studied not only properly work for the reduction of these effects of disease but also provide a support for its reduction. The combination therapy along with antioxidants and existing drugs is more beneficial and enhances the efficiency of standard therapy in the treatment of Parkinson's disease.

Clinical applications such as diagnosis, medicines, drug delivery, and therapy have benefited by utilization of NPs. Other essential benefits due to their small surface-to-volume ration may include easy cellular uptake, targeted delivery, absorption, and controlled drug release. The abovementioned benefits make them more suitable for therapeutic perspective of treating oxidative stress (Hua et al., 2019).

Recently, exogenous antioxidants such as vitamins, C E, β-carotene have been utilized in regular practice to treat reactive oxygenic species (Kurutas et al., 2015). But they have minor disadvantages of not getting easily internalized by the cells, and also the results obtained may vary. Thus there is a prime requisite to synthesize other modified exogenous substances that may have advanced antioxidant properties. Various metal nanocomposites like cerium oxide, carbon-based NP, that is, fullerenes and yttrium oxide, have gained the attention of researchers due to their advanced properties like radical-quenching of ROS and catalysis, etc. Thus they can be used as a novel therapy for treating oxidative stress (Ghaznavi et al., 2015).

NPs are known to have various advances over other natural and synthetic antioxidants, which are reported to have disadvantages such as poor solubility, less bioavailability, reduced bioabsorption, and specificity, also they are reported to have prooxidant properties that can be compensated by usage of biodegradable carrier molecules, that is, albumin or poly(lactic-co-glycolic acid) (PLGA) (Caellano et al., 2019). Polymeric NPs thus can be utilized to protect small active natural antioxidants molecules from degradation by encapsulating them. Also, they provide added advantages to active natural antioxidant molecules in order to give them protection from degradation, increased solubility, surface functionalization, and promote targeted distribution (Jampilek et al., 2019).

NPs like SOD-containing NPs play role as antioxidants carrier, thus ultimately promoting free radicals scavenging activity during oxidative stress, along with prolonged specificity, permeability, etc. (Tan et al., 2018). Catalytic ROS scavengers have added advantage that even as low concentration, there is a rare possibility of getting depleted during scavenging mechanism and can eliminate as more as ROS molecules by neutralizing oxide and H_2O_2 to oxygen (He et al., 2017).

Under oxidative stress conditions, for performing potent cellular delivery and avoidance of degradation by enzymes present in serum, engineered nanocomposites could be prepared having NPs with SOD conjugation (Lee et al., 2018). The permeability of blood–brain barrier could be enhanced by this conjugation, which may advances applications of treating ischemia with sustainable SOD release and other associated brain disorders. By internalization of the NPs in the cells through endocytosis, they perform catalysis of oxide (Teleanu et al., 2019).

The infarct size can be limited to a certain range by providing treatment based on SOD NPs. Copper or zinc SOD having histidine tag is recombined with silica NPs thus allowing them to provide an ease for sustainable transmembrane delivery (Zhou et al., 2018). Platinum NPs have recently been reported to provide biomedical applications, such as their usages as a chemotherapeutic agent have taken them to next level in the therapeutic aspect (Ahmedova et al., 2018). Cisplatin is already been known to have catalytic property such as they are able to perform hydrogenation and oxidation reactions with great efficacy (Esposito et al., 2019). They have been used for treatment of oxidative stress-related diseases as they have potential of converting oxide radicals to hydrogen peroxide and then conversion the same to water or free oxygen (Collin et al., 2019).

Cerium NPs play a significant role in catalyzing the conversion of hydrogen peroxide to water and oxygen, and it is also involved in the generation of Ce^{3+} from Ce^{4+} and then after reacting with HO•, reverting it to Ce^{4+}. Ceria through their diverse antioxidant properties is reported to have potential to degrade hydrogen peroxide (Zafar et al., 2019).

Ceria nanocomposites decrease macrophagial NO production by downregulating iNOS and ultimately lowers inflammation. Also, ceria nanocomposites are reported to scavenge a reactive nitrogen species, that is, ONOO− (Ferreira et al., 2018). But still, there are few conflicts, as they are reported to have various toxic effects on various cell lines possibly because of the size of the ceria particles. Ceria nanocomposites have greater biosorption property but they are known to have greater aggregation tendency that affects their antioxidant properties and limits their usage (Muthu et al., 2017).

Anything within a tissue-specific way enhances scavenging of ROS, and ultimately enhancing the antioxidant efficacy. Keeping this in mind, a conjugate was prepared, which itself gets degraded when exposed to ROS. The conjugate consists of copolyoxalate-containing vanillyl alcohol (PVAX) particle having peroxalate ester linkages (Afinjuomo et al., 2019). The whole scenario leads to downregulation of COX-2 and iNOS. PH-sensitive NPs are reported to have various biomedical applications

(Ahmed Hamidu et al., 2019). Nitroxyls like TEMPO are known to be compounds that are themselves radically stable but could generate various nonradical species. Because of their self-regeneration capacity, they are also reported to mimic SOD (Valgimigli et al., 2018).

Reports have shown that in order to protect nitroxyl compounds in vivo, micelle NPs in association with 4-amino-TEMPO have been a prime concern of researchers. In the case of acute cerebrovascular I/R injury in animals, they are known to cause decline in infarct size in an animal model (Tong et al., 2019). As compared to TEMPO, TEMPOL causes alteration/lowering of blood pressure and is known to have shorter half-life. Thus it can be said that TEMPO is better therapeutic agent as compared to TEMPOL. At lower pH levels, many NPs are known to have controlled releasing potential, for example, pH-sensitive radical-containing NP micelles. This potential could be explored in opting therapeutic strategy for treating chronic neurodegenerative diseases (Babic et al., 2019).

Diamond NPs could be synthesized by explosive detonation, followed by purification. In hepatoma cell lines, for scavenging ROS, HO-DNP-supported Au/Pt NPs are known to have efficient antioxidant activity, more biocompatibility, peroxidase activity, and radical training activity (Torres Sangiao et al., 2019). Few reports have shown that during measuring cellular viability in two cell lines, that is, Hep3B and HeLa, ceria-supported gold NPs showed radical training activity with enhanced biocompatibility. As compared to glutathione, various reports have shown that as compared to cytoantioxidants, Au/CeO (2) has potential antioxidant activity (Adeoye et al., 2018). The reports have somehow confirmed that gold as a catalyst has more biocompatibility as far as cellular biology is concerned.

ROS production and oxidative stress and mitochondrial dysfunction are inversely proportional to each other. Thus mitochondrial targeting of various antioxidants may result in lowering level of ROS and proper cell functioning. Triphenylphosphonium is the finest example of a molecule, which is capable of crossing barriers of cell membranes, due to its lipophilic nature and then ultimately targeting mitochondria (Zielonka et al., 2017). In order to enhance activity of triphenylphosphonium or to provide a targeted delivery, a conjugated compound was made by conjugating T with PLGA-*b*-poly NPs (Palma et al., 2018). Forwarding it to the next-level conjugation of this compound was made with curcumin in order to treat human neuroblastoma cells. At last, it can be said that NPs may act as a potential antioxidant therapeutic agent, in the form of carriers itself or as an antioxidant agent itself.

1.4   CONCLUSION

The efficacy, cellular uptake, and specific transport of dietary antioxidants to target organs, tissues, and cells remain the most important setback for their application in the treatment of oxidative stress–related disorders and in particular in neurodegenerative diseases, as brain targeting remains a still unsolved challenge. Nanotechnology-based delivery systems can be a solution for the abovementioned problems, specifically in the case of targeting dietary antioxidants with neuroprotective activity. Nanotechnology-based delivery systems can protect antioxidants from degradation, improve their physicochemical drug-like properties and in turn their bioavailability. The impact of nanomedicine in the improvement of the performance of dietary antioxidants, as protective agents in oxidative-stress events, specifically through the use of drug delivery systems, is highlighted in this review as well as the type of nanomaterials regularly used for drug delivery purposes. From the data, one can conclude that the research combining (dietary) antioxidants and nanotechnology, namely, as a therapeutic solution for neurodegenerative diseases, is still in a very early stage. So, a huge research area remains to be explored that hopefully will yield new and effective neuroprotective therapeutic agents in a foreseeable future.

KEYWORDS

- **nanotechnology**
- **nanomedicine**
- **drug delivery**
- **drug targeting**
- **oxidative stress**

REFERENCES

Adeoye, O.; Olawumi, J.; Opeyemi, A.; Christiania, O. Review on the Role of Glutathione on Oxidative Stress and Infertility. *JBRA Assisted Reprod.* **2018,** *22* (1), 61.

Afinjuomo, F.; Barclay, T. G.; Parikh, A.; Song, Y.; Chung, R.; Wang, L.; Garg, S. Design and Characterization of Inulin Conjugate for Improved Intracellular and Targeted Delivery of Pyrazinoic Acid to Monocytes. *Pharmaceutics* **2019,** *11* (5), 243.

Ahmad, S.; Munir, S.; Zeb, N.; Ullah, A.; Khan, B.; Ali, J.; Ali, S. Green Nanotechnology, A Review on Green Synthesis of Silver Nanoparticles—An Ecofriendly Approach. *Int. J. Nanomed.* **2019,** *14,* 5087.

Ahmed Hamidu, A. M.; Mansor, R.; Razak, I. S. A.; Danmaigoro, A.; Jaji, A. Z.; Bakar, Z. A. Modified Methods of Nanoparticles Synthesis in pH-Sensitive Nano-Carriers Production for Doxorubicin Delivery on MCF-7 Breast Cancer Cell Line. *Int. J. Nanomed.* **2019,** *14,* 3615.

Ahmedova, A. Biomedical Applications of Metallosupramolecular Assemblies—Structural Aspects of the Anticancer Activity. *Front. Chem.* **2018,** *6,* 620.

Anderson, S. D.; Gwenin, V. V.; Gwenin, C. D. Magnetic Functionalized Nanoparticles for Biomedical, Drug Delivery and Imaging Applications. *Nanoscale Res. Lett.* **2019,** *14* (1), 1–16.

Babić, N.; Peyrot, F. Molecular Probes for Evaluation of Oxidative Stress by In Vivo EPR Spectroscopy and Imaging, State-of-the-Art and Limitations. *Magnetochemistry* **2019,** *5* (1), 13.

Bai, W.; Wu, Z.; Mitra, S.; Brown, J. M. Effects of Multiwalled Carbon Nanotube Surface Modification and Purification on Bovine Serum Albumin Binding and Biological Responses. *J. Nanomater.* **2016,** *4,* 2016.

Berends, A. C.; Mangnus, M. J.; Xia, C.; Rabouw, F. T.; de Mello Donega, C. Optoelectronic Properties of Ternary I–III–VI2 Semiconductor Nanocrystals, Bright Prospects with Elusive Origins. *J. Phys. Chem. Lett.* **2019,** *10* (7), 1600–1616.

Burduşel, A. C.; Gherasim, O.; Grumezescu, A. M.; Mogoantă, L.; Ficai, A.; Andronescu, E. Biomedical Applications of Silver Nanoparticles, An Up-to-Date Overview. *Nanomaterials* **2018,** *8* (9), 681.

Caellano, G.; Comi, C.; Chiocchetti, A.; Dianzani, U. Exploiting PLGA-Based Biocompatible Nanoparticles for Next-Generation Tolerogenic Vaccines Against Autoimmune Disease. *Int. J. Mol. Sci.* **2019,** *20* (1), 204.

Collin, F. Chemical Basis of Reactive Oxygen Species Reactivity and Involvement in Neurodegenerative Diseases. *Int. J. Mol. Sci.* **2019,** *20* (10), 2407.

Desai, D.; Åkerfelt, M.; Prabhakar, N.; Toriseva, M.; Näreoja, T.; Zhang, J.; Rosenholm, J. Factors Affecting Intracellular Delivery and Release of Hydrophilic Versus Hydrophobic Cargo from Mesoporous Silica Nanoparticles on 2D and 3D Cell Cultures. *Pharmaceutics* **2018,** *10* (4), 237.

Dhall, A.; Self, W. Cerium Oxide Nanoparticles, a Brief Review of Their Synthesis Methods and Biomedical Applications. *Antioxidants* **2018,** *7* (8), 97.

Di Sotto, A.; Paolicelli, P.; Nardoni, M.; Abete, L.; Garzoli, S.; Di Giacomo, S.; Petralito, S. SPC Liposomes as Possible Delivery Systems for Improving Bioavailability of the Natural Sesquiterpene β-Caryophyllene, Lamellarity and Drug-Loading as Key Features for a Rational Drug Delivery Design. *Pharmaceutics* **2018,** *10* (4), 274.

Ebrahimi, R.; Hossienzadeh, K.; Maleki, A.; Ghanbari, R.; Rezaee, R.; Safari, M.; ... Puttaiah, S. H. Effects of Doping Zinc Oxide Nanoparticles with Transition Metals (Ag, Cu, Mn) on Photocatalytic Degradation of Direct Blue 15 Dye under UV and Visible Light Irradiation. *J. Environ. Health Sci. Eng.* **2019,** *17* (1), 1–14.

Esposito, S. "Traditional" Sol-Gel Chemistry as a Powerful Tool for the Preparation of Supported Metal and Metal Oxide Catalysts. *Materials* **2019**, *12* (4), 668.

Fathi-Achachelouei, M.; Knopf-Marques, H.; Riberio de Silva, C. E.; Barthès, J. G. D.; Bat, E.; Tezcaner, A.; Vrana, N. E. Use of Nanoparticles in Tissue Engineering and Regenerative Medicine. *Front. Bioeng. Biotechnol.* **2019**, *7*, 113.

Ferreira, C. A.; Ni, D.; Rosenkrans, Z. T.; Cai, W. Scavenging of Reactive Oxygen and Nitrogen Species with Nanomaterials. *Nano Res.* **2018**, *11* (10), 4955–4984.

Ganesan, P.; Karthivashan, G.; Park, S. Y.; Kim, J.; Choi, D. K. Microfluidization Trends in the Development of Nanodelivery Systems and Applications in Chronic Disease Treatments. *Int. J. Nanomed.* **2018**, *13*, 6109.

Gaynullina, D. K.; Schubert, R.; Tarasova, O. S. Changes in Endothelial Nitric Oxide Production in Systemic Vessels during Early Ontogenesis—A Key Mechanism for the Perinatal Adaptation of the Circulatory System. *Int. J. Mol. Sci.*, **2019**, *20* (6), 1421.

Ghaznavi, H.; Najafi, R.; Mehrzadi, S.; Hosseini, A.; Tekyemaroof, N.; Shakeri-zadeh, A.; Sharifi, A. M. Neuro-Protective Effects of Cerium and Yttrium Oxide Nanoparticles on High Glucose-Induced Oxidative Stress and Apoptosis in Undifferentiated PC12 Cells. *Neurol. Res.* **2015**, *37* (7), 624–632.

Hasan, A.; Morshed, M.; Memic, A.; Hassan, S.; Webster, T. J.; Marei, H. E. S. Nanoparticles in Tissue Engineering, Applications, Challenges and Prospects. *Int. J. Nanomed.* **2018**, *13*, 5637.

He, H.; Lu, Y.; Qi, J.; Zhu, Q.; Chen, Z.; Wu, W. Adapting Liposomes for Oral Drug Delivery. *Acta Pharm. Sin. B* **2019**, *9* (1), 36–48.

He, L.; He, T.; Farrar, S.; Ji, L.; Liu, T.; Ma, X. Antioxidants Maintain Cellular Redox Homeostasis by Elimination of Reactive Oxygen Species. *Cell. Physiol. Biochem.* **2017**, *44* (2), 532–553.

Hua, S. Physiological and Pharmaceutical Considerations for Rectal Drug Formulations. *Front. Pharmacol.* **2019**, *10*, 1196.

Hua, S.; Vaughan, B. In Vitro Comparison of Liposomal Drug Delivery Systems Targeting the Oxytocin Receptor, a Potential Novel Treatment for Obstetric Complications. *Int. J. Nanomed.* **2019**, *14*, 2191.

Jampilek, J.; Kos, J.; Kralova, K. Potential of Nanomaterial Applications in Dietary Sulements and Foods for Special Medical Purposes. *Nanomaterials* **2019**, *9* (2), 296.

Jeong, W. J.; Bu, J.; Kubiatowicz, L. J.; Chen, S. S.; Kim, Y.; Hong, S. Peptide–Nanoparticle Conjugates, A Next Generation of Diagnostic and Therapeutic Platforms? *Nano Convergence* **2018**, *5* (1), 38.

Kaul, S.; Gulati, N.; Verma, D.; Mukherjee, S.; Nagaich, U. Role of Nanotechnology in Cosmeceuticals, A Review of Recent Advances. *J. Pharm.* **2018**.

Kurutas, E. B. The Importance of Antioxidants which Play the Role in Cellular Response against Oxidative/Nitrosative Stress, Current State. *Nutr. J.* **2015**, *15* (1), 71.

Lee, M. S.; Kim, N. W.; Lee, J. E.; Kim, M. G.; Yin, Y.; Kim, S. Y.; Lim, D. W. Targeted Cellular Delivery of Robust Enzyme Nanoparticles for the Treatment of Drug-Induced Hepatotoxicity and Liver Injury. *Acta Biomater.* **2018**, *81*, 231–241.

Liguori, I.; Russo, G.; Curcio, F.; Bulli, G.; Aran, L.; Della-Morte, D.; Abete, P. Oxidative Stress, Aging, and Diseases. *Clin. Interventions Aging* **2018**, *13*, 757.

Lujan, H.; Griffin, W. C.; Taube, J. H.; Sayes, C. M. Synthesis and Characterization of Nanometer-Sized Liposomes for Encapsulation and MicroRNA Transfer to Breast Cancer Cells. *Int. J. Nanomed.* **2019**, *14*, 5159.

Marchio, P.; Guerra-Ojeda, S.; Vila, J. M.; Aldasoro, M.; Victor, V. M.; Mauricio, M. D. Targeting Early Atherosclerosis, a Focus on Oxidative Stress and Inflammation. *Oxidative Med. Cell. Longevity* **2019**.

Markwalter, C. F.; Kantor, A. G.; Moore, C. P.; Richardson, K. A.; Wright, D. W. Inorganic Complexes and Metal-Based Nanomaterials for Infectious Disease Diagnostics. *Chem. Rev.* **2018,** *119* (2), 1456–1518.

Mauricio, M. D.; Guerra-Ojeda, S.; Marchio, P.; Valles, S. L.; Aldasoro, M.; Escribano-Lopez, I.; Victor, V. M. Nanoparticles in Medicine, a Focus on Vascular Oxidative Stress. *Oxidative Med. Cell. Longevity **2018***.

Medina, O. E.; Gallego, J.; Restrepo, L. G.; Cortés, F. B.; Franco, C. A. Influence of the Ce^{4+}/Ce^{3+} Redox-Couple on the Cyclic Regeneration for Adsorptive and Catalytic Performance of NiO-PdO/$CeO^{2\pm\delta}$ Nanoparticles for n-C7 Asphaltene Steam Gasification. *Nanomaterials* **2019,** *9* (5), 734.

Muthu, M.; Wu, H. F.; Gopal, J.; Sivanesan, I.; Chun, S. Exploiting Microbial Polysaccharides for Biosorption of Trace Elements in Aqueous Environments—Scope for Expansion via Nanomaterial Intervention. *Polymers* **2017,** *9* (12), 721.

Narayan, R.; Nayak, U. Y.; Raichur, A. M.; Garg, S. Mesoporous Silica Nanoparticles, A Comprehensive Review on Synthesis and Recent Advances. *Pharmaceutics* **2018,** *10* (3), 118.

Ovais, M.; Khalil, A. T.; Ayaz, M.; Ahmad, I.; Nethi, S. K.; Mukherjee, S. Biosynthesis of Metal Nanoparticles via Microbial Enzymes, A Mechanistic Approach. *Int. J. Mol. Sci.* **2018,** *19* (12), 4100.

Palma, E.; Pasqua, A.; Gagliardi, A.; Britti, D.; Fresta, M.; Cosco, D. Antileishmanial Activity of Amphotericin B-Loaded-PLGA Nanoparticles, An Overview. *Materials* **2018,** *11* (7), 1167.

Pampaloni, N. P.; Giugliano, M.; Scaini, D.; Ballerini, L.; Rauti, R. Advances in Nano Neuroscience, From Nanomaterials to Nanotools. *Front. Neurosci.* **2018,** *12,* 953.

Panahi, Y.; Farshbaf, M.; Mohammadhosseini, M.; Mirahadi, M.; Khalilov, R.; Saghfi, S.; Akbarzadeh, A. Recent Advances on Liposomal Nanoparticles, Synthesis, Characterization and Biomedical Applications. *Artif. Cells Nanomed. Biotechnol.* **2017,** *45* (4), 788–799.

Patra, J. K.; Das, G.; Fraceto, L. F.; Campos, E. V. R.; del Pilar Rodriguez-Torres, M.; Acosta-Torres, L. S.; Habtemariam, S. Nano Based Drug Delivery Systems, Recent Developments and Future Prospects. *J. Nanobiotechnol.* **2018,** *16* (1), 71.

Pelaz, B.; Alexiou, C.; Alvarez-Puebla, R. A.; Alves, F.; Andrews, A. M.; Ashraf, S.; Bosi, S. Diverse Applications of Nanomedicine. *ACS Nano* **2017**.

Peng, J.; Liang, X. Progress in Research on Gold Nanoparticles in Cancer Management. *Medicine* **2019,** *98* (18).

Priyadarsini, S.; Mukherjee, S.; Mishra, M. Nanoparticles Used in Dentistry, A Review. *J. Oral Biol. Craniofac. Res.* **2018,** *8* (1), 58–67.

Ramos, A. P.; Cruz, M. A.; Tovani, C. B.; Ciancaglini, P. Biomedical Applications of Nanotechnology. *Biophys. Rev.* **2017,** *9* (2), 79–89.

Rizvi, S. A.; Saleh, A. M. Applications of Nanoparticle Systems in Drug Delivery Technology. *Saudi Pharm. J.* **2018,** *26* (1), 64–70.

Saghazadeh, S.; Rinoldi, C.; Schot, M.; Kashaf, S. S.; Sharifi, F.; Jalilian, E.; Yue, K. Drug Delivery Systems and Materials for Wound Healing Applications. *Adv. Drug Deliv. Rev.* **2018,** *127,* 138–166.

Sanzari, I.; Leone, A.; Ambrosone, A. Nanotechnology in Plant Science, to Make a Long Story Short. *Front. Bioeng. Biotechnol.* **2019,** *7,* 120.

Simon, J.; Flahaut, E.; Golzio, M. Overview of Carbon Nanotubes for Biomedical Applications. *Materials* **2019,** *12* (4), 624.

Soh, S. H.; Lee, L. Y. Microencapsulation and Nanoencapsulation Using Supercritical Fluid (SCF) Techniques. *Pharmaceutics* **2019,** *11* (1), 21.

Spicer, C. D.; Pashuck, E. T.; Stevens, M. M. Achieving Controlled Biomolecule–Biomaterial Conjugation. *Chem. Rev.* **2018,** *118* (16), 7702–7743.

Tan, B. L.; Norhaizan, M. E.; Winnie-Pui-Pui Liew, H. S. Antioxidant and Oxidative Stress, A Mutual Interplay in Age-Related Diseases. *Front. Pharmacol.* **2018,** *9.*

Teleanu, D. M.; Chircov, C.; Grumezescu, A. M.; Teleanu, R. I. Neuronanomedicine, An Up-to-Date Overview. *Pharmaceutics* **2019,** *11* (3), 101.

Teleanu, D. M.; Chircov, C.; Grumezescu, A. M.; Volceanov, A.; Teleanu, R. I. Impact of Nanoparticles on Brain Health, An Up to Date Overview. *J. Clin. Med.* **2018,** *7* (12), 490.

Tong, Q.; Zhu, P. C.; Zhuang, Z.; Deng, L. H.; Wang, Z. H.; Zeng, H.; Wang, Y. Notoginsenoside R1 for Organs Ischemia/Reperfusion Injury, A Preclinical Systematic Review. *Front. Pharmacol.* **2019,** *10.*

Torres Sangiao, E.; Holban, A. M.; Gestal, M. C. Applications of Nanodiamonds in the Detection and Therapy of Infectious Diseases. *Materials* **2019,** *12* (10), 1639.

Valgimigli, L.; Baschieri, A.; Amorati, R. Antioxidant Activity of Nanomaterials. *J. Mater. Chem. B* **2018,** *6* (14), 2036–2051.

Vasile, C. Polymeric Nanocomposites and Nanocoatings for Food Packaging, A Review. *Materials* **2018,** *11* (10), 1834.

Vona, R.; Gambardella, L.; Cittadini, C.; Straface, E.; Pietraforte, D. Biomarkers of Oxidative Stress in Metabolic Syndrome and Associated Diseases. *Oxidative Med. Cell. Longevity* **2019.**

Wang, D.; Loo, J. F. C.; Chen, J.; Yam, Y.; Chen, S. C.; He, H.; Ho, H. P. Recent Advances in Surface Plasmon Resonance Imaging Sensors. *Sensors* **2019,** *19* (6), 1266.

Watermann, A.; Brieger, J. Mesoporous Silica Nanoparticles as Drug Delivery Vehicles in Cancer. *Nanomaterials* **2017,** *7* (7), 189.

Wegner, K. D.; Dussert, F.; Truffier-Boutry, D.; Benayad, A.; Beal, D.; Mattera, L.; Reiss, P. Influence of the Core/Shell Structure of Indium Phosphide Based Quantum Dots on Their Photostability and Cytotoxicity. *Front. Chem.* **2019,** *7,* 466.

Xiong, S.; Deng, Y.; Zhou, Y.; Gong, D.; Xu, Y.; Yang, L.; Deng, X. Current Progress in Biosensors for Organophosphorus Pesticides Based on Enzyme Functionalized Nanostructures, A Review. *Anal. Methods* **2018,** *10* (46), 5468–5479.

Yao, B. C.; Meng, L. B.; Hao, M. L.; Zhang, Y. M.; Gong, T.; Guo, Z. G. Chronic Stress, A Critical Risk Factor for Atherosclerosis. *J. Int. Med. Res.* **2019,** *47* (4), 1429–1440.

Yudasaka, M.; Yomogida, Y.; Zhang, M.; Tanaka, T.; Nakahara, M.; Kobayashi, N.; Kataura, H. Near-Infrared Photoluminescent Carbon Nanotubes for Imaging of Brown Fat. *Sci. Rep.* **2017,** *7,* 44760.

Zafar, M. S.; Quarta, A.; Marradi, M.; Ragusa, A. Recent Developments in the Reduction of Oxidative Stress through Antioxidant Polymeric Formulations. *Pharmaceutics* **2019,** *11* (10), 505.

Zhang, X. F.; Liu, Z. G.; Shen, W.; Gurunathan, S. Silver Nanoparticles, Synthesis, Characterization, Properties, Applications, and Therapeutic Approaches. *Int. J. Mol. Sci.* **2016,** *17* (9), 1534.

Zhou, Y.; Yan, D.; Yuan, S.; Chen, Y.; Fletcher, E. E.; Shi, H.; Han, B. Selective Binding, Magnetic Separation and Purification of Histidine-Tagged Protein Using Biopolymer Magnetic Core–Shell Nanoparticles. *Protein Exp. Purif.* **2018,** *144*, 5–11.

Zielonka, J.; Joseph, J.; Sikora, A.; Hardy, M.; Ouari, O.; Vasquez-Vivar, J.; Kalyanaraman, B. Mitochondria-Targeted Triphenylphosphonium-Based Compounds, Syntheses, Mechanisms of Action, and Therapeutic and Diagnostic Applications. *Chem. Rev.* **2017,** *117* (15), 10043–10120.

Zottel, A.; Videtič Paska, A.; Jovčevska, I. Nanotechnology Meets Oncology, Nanomaterials in Brain Cancer Research, Diagnosis and Therapy. *Materials* **2019,** *12* (10), 1588.

CHAPTER 2

Role of Phytomedicine in the Challenges to Combat Anemia

SONIA JOHRI

Department of Life Sciences, ITM University, Gwalior, India

E-mail: johrisonia@gmail.com

ABSTRACT

Medicinal plants possess healing properties and unlike synthetic drugs, which may cause adverse side effects. A herbal medicine or a phytopharmaceutical preparation can be defined as a medicine derived exclusively from a whole plant or parts of plants and manufactured in a crude form or as a purified pharmaceutical formulation. However, the World Health Organization emphasizes that between 70 and 95% of the population residing in numerous developing countries still rely more on traditional herbal medicines for their primary medication against diseases. Oxidative stress is an imbalance between free radicals and antioxidant molecules that can play an important role in the pathogenesis of iron-deficiency anemia. The plant extract inhibits nitrite formation by directly competing with oxygen in the reaction with nitric oxide. In this study, nitric oxide radical scavenging effect of *Carica papaya* in a concentration of 0.5 mg/ml was found to be more in *n*-butanol extract (74.28%) compared with petroleum ether, ethyl acetate, and aqueous extracts. Antihemolytic activity indicated that *n*-butanol extract of *Triticum aestivum* grass and *Piper betel* leaves and petroleum ether extracts of *C. papaya* showed maximum percent of antihemolysis. The highest hydroxyl (OH) radical scavenging activity had shown 60.3% in *n*-butanol extract of wheatgrass.

2.1   INTRODUCTION

Natural antioxidants originate from plants and have the potential to reduce various antioxidative compounds to counteract reactive oxygen species (ROS). Anemia is one of the major health problems in the present day world. According to the World Health Organization (WHO), about 30% of people throughout the world suffer from anemia. Iron deficiency is the most common cause of anemia; however, generation of ROS has a great potential to cause anemia. ROS in erythrocytes occur either by activation of ROS generation, which cause suppression of antioxidative/redox system. When erythrocytes experience an excessive elevation of ROS, oxidative stress develops. ROS are considered to play a crucial role in the pathogenesis of many disorders of erythrocytes, such as sickle cell anemia, thalassemia, and glucose-6-phosphate dehydrogenase (G6PD) deficiency. Deficiency of antioxidant enzymes such as superoxide dismutase 1 (SOD1) develops oxidative stress in erythrocytes and causes anemia. A number of medicinal plants have been used in ethnomedicine by traditional healers in the management of many diseases. A medicinal plant as defined by the WHO is a plant, one or more parts of which contain substances that can be used for therapeutic purposes or which are precursors for the synthesis of useful drugs (Ogamba et al., 2011). In recent decades, many researchers are interested in medicinal plants for evaluation of antioxidant phytochemicals such as phenols, flavonoids, and tannins, as they have the potential role in the prevention of human disease (Lee et al., 2000).

The use of plant extracts in traditional medicine is a worldwide practice. Medicinal plants form the basis of primary health care for majority of the people living in the rural and remote areas in Nigeria and other third-world countries (Awosika, 1993). The use of plants such as herbs, shrubs, or trees in parts or in a whole in the treatment and management of disease and disorders dates back to prehistoric days (Akindele and Busavo, 2011). Plant extracts have been used in folk medicinal practices for the treatment of various ailments since antiquity. The medicinal value of plants has assumed a more important dimension in the past few decades. Extracts from plants contain not only minerals and primary metabolites but also a diverse array of secondary metabolites with antioxidant potentials (Sofowora, 1993; Okigbo et al., 2009a).

Muhammad et al. (2009) reported that biochemical compounds appear to play a significant role as antioxidants in the protective effect of plant-derived foods (Muhammad et al., 2009). Phenolics have become the focus of current nutritional and therapeutic interest. The antioxidant activity of dietary phenolics is considered to be superior to that of the essential vitamins and is ascribed to its high redox potential that allows them to interrupt free radical–mediated reactions by donating hydrogen from the phenols hydroxyl groups (Chandra, 2003). Furthermore, some plant constituents such as anthocyanin and condensed tannins have also been documented to exhibit various biological activities including anti-inflammatory, antiartherosclerotic, antitumor, antimutagenic, anticarcinogenic, antibacterial, and antiviral activities (Papi et al., 2008; Beevi et al., 2009). However, majority of these plants have not been investigated for their antioxidant potency.

The genus *Asphodelus tenuifolius* Cav. belongs to the Liliaceae family, which comprises 187 genera and 2500 species. This species distributed in North African, Southern Europe, India, and Pakistan. Various species of this genus are used as antiulcer and anti-inflammatory agents, and also as a diuretic and for the prevention of atherosclerosis (Baquar, 1989). The ethnopharmacological and chemotaxonomic importance of the *A. tenuifolius* Cav. prompted us to carry out phytochemical studies on one of its species. It is a small erect annual herb, which commonly grows in different areas of Southeast of Algeria (Muhammad et al., 2009). Literature survey revealed that no phytochemical or pharmacological studies have so far been carried out on this species.

In Asian countries, most of the allelopathic medicinal plants in nature have been used a popular folk and oriental medicine treatments against many diseases such as hypertension, hypercholesterolemia, and gastric ulcer (Paterson, 2006). Natural therapies such as the use of plant-derived products may reduce adverse side effects (Desai et al., 2008). The compounds in plants have protective effects against environmental mutagens, carcinogens, and endogenous mutagens (Mastan et al., 2007). *Aerva lanata* known as polpala (treatment for renal disease) is a prostrate, decumbent, and sometimes erect herb found throughout tropical India as a common weed in fields and wasteland. The plant is useful for curing diabetes. It is anthelmintic, demulcent and is helpful in lithiasis, cough, sore throat, and wounds (Pullaiah and Naidu, 2003). In China for instance, blood diseases such as malformation of blood circulatory system, anemia, varicose veins, and hemorrhages have been treated with plant materials (Richard, 1978).

Any changes in the rate of removal or production leads to the generation of ROS leading to oxidative stress. Oxidative stress is initiated by free radicals. All human cells protect themselves against free radical damage by enzymes such as SOD and catalase, or compounds such as ascorbic acid, tocopherol, and glutathione. Sometimes these protective mechanisms are disrupted by various pathological processes and antioxidant supplements vital to combat oxidative damage. The diseased state stimulates cells to produce ROS, thereby resulting in hemoglobin degradation. Indeed, it produces depressed level of plasma. The effects of antioxidants with oral iron to combat the stress and side effects have been tried in both human (Carier et al., 2002) and animals (Srigiridhar and Nair, 1998). Studies of this kind in children are scanty (Tekin et al., 2001). Commonly used antioxidants are vitamins C and E. Vitamin E is the most potent liposoluble antioxidant and has the potential to improve tolerance of iron supplementation and prevent further tissue damage (Burton et al., 1986). Vitamin C helps in the absorption of iron by reducing nonheme ferric to ferrous iron.

Oxidative stress is shown to play an important role in pathogenesis of iron-deficiency anemia (IDA) (Vives et al., 1995). The results of a recent study confirmed that antioxidant enzymes activity like glutathione peroxidase (GSH-Px) is decreased in children with IDA. These are indicators of increased lipid peroxidation (Tekin et al., 2001). Furthermore, it has been shown that the addition of synthetic antioxidants in the treatment of children with IDA results in decrease of lipid per oxidation, prevention of pathologic progression, and rapid improvement of clinical manifestations (shved et al., 1995). This confirms iron IDA is a state of oxidative stress. Oxidative damage of cells and biomolecules due to oxygen/nitrogen species (ROS/RNS) is reduced by antioxidants (Fiorentino et al., 2008).

Antioxidant compounds can donate electrons to reactive radicals, reducing them into more stable and nonreactive species. Antioxidants can be classified into two major groups, that is, enzymatic and nonenzymatic. The enzymatic antioxidants that are produced endogenously include nitric oxide reductase, SOD, catalase, glutathione peroxidase. The nonenzymatic antioxidants include tocopherols, carotenoids, ascorbic acid, flavonoids, and tannins that are obtained from natural plant sources (Naskar et al., 2010). The effects of antioxidants with oral iron to combat the stress and side effects have been tried in both human subjects (Carier et al., 2002) and animals (Srigiridhar and Nair, 1998). Vitamin E is the most potent liposoluble antioxidant and has the potential to improve tolerance of iron supplementation and prevent further tissue damage (Burton et al., 1986). Vitamin C helps in the absorption of iron by reducing non heme ferric to ferrous iron (Chen et al., 2004; Srigiridhar and Nair, 1998). Iron deficiency is a state of oxidative stress as it is required as a structural and functional component of various compounds (catalase, peroxidase, cytochrome oxidase, NADPH reductase, iron–sulfur complex). It plays a vital role in maintaining the anti-oxidant defense system of our body. In iron deficiency anemia, the enzymes involved in the antioxidant defense system will be functionally defective. So the balance gets tilted toward free radicals triggering oxidative damage. Furthermore, iron-dependent mitochondrial oxidative phosphorylation also gets affected in iron deficiency causing decreased ATP production and ulti-mately leading to loss of structural and functional integrity of cell. Studies (Moriarty et al., 1995; Kumerova et al., 1998) are on par with the fact that antioxidant status is lowered in iron deficiency.

Natural antioxidants, which are ubiquitous in medicinal plants, have received great attention and have been studied extensively. Since they are effective free radical scavengers and are assumed to be less toxic than synthetic antioxidants, such as butylated hydroxyanisole and butylated hydroxyltoluene, they are suspected of being carcinogenic and causing liver damage (Ratnam et al., 2006; Ke-Xue et al., 2011). Natural products have long been used to treat and prevent cancer, and thus, they are good candidates for the development of anticancer drugs (Smith-Warner et al., 2000). Recent epidemiological studies have indicated that diets rich in fruits, vegetables, and those of selected plant compounds are correlated with reduced incidence of cardiovascular and chronic diseases like cancer (Perez-Jimenez and Saura-Calixto, 2005). The phenolic compounds or polyphenols, secondary metabolites, constitute a wide and complex array of phytochemicals that exhibit antioxidant action and consequently a benefi-cial physiological effect (Enayde et al., 2005; Martinez et al., 2000). Their ability to delay lipid oxidation in food stuff and biological membranes, in addition to their propensity to act as a prophylactic agent, has motivated research into food science and biomedicine (Farombi et al., 2000).

Presence of phenolics in a wide range of vegetables, is considered as natural antioxidants and the vegetable source that contains is regarded as functional food. There are over 400 types of anemia, including hemolytic anemia being the most common (Fasidi et al., 2008). More than half of the world's population experience some forms of anemia in their life time (Duff, 2011a). The incidence of anemia is higher in the third world than in developed countries (Ogbe et al., 2010). A study in a rural population of Nigeria reported that 19.7% of the children were anemic (Akinkugbe, 1991). Such prevalence has been attributed to various aggravating factors such as poor nutrition and high prevalence of blood parasites, for example, plasmodium, trypanosome, and helminthes infection (Ogbe et al., 2010). Prolonged uses of nonsteroidal anti-inflammatory drugs as well as exposure to toxic chemicals such as phenyl hydrazine have also been implicated to cause the condition (Sharda et al., 2011; Kumar et al., 2007; Sanni et al., 2005). Due to the high prevalence and possibility of even further increase (Duff, 2011a), there is the need to prevent it or seek for more cost-effective and better treatment strategies. The rural populations in various parts of the world do not have adequate access to high-quality drugs for the treatment of anemia, so they depend heavily on plants and herbal products for the treatment of diseases and anemia. As a result of the fact that anemia is very common and the incidence is likely to increase in future (Duff, 2008b), there is need to prevent it or seek for more cost-effective and better treatment strategies.

Anemia is a serious and widespread public health concern with major consequences for human health as well as social and economic development in both developing and developed countries. It contributes to 20% of all maternal deaths. Poverty, inadequate diet, high incidence of communicable diseases, pregnancy/lactation, and low immunity are the main causes, thereby affecting 20–50% of the world's population. Malaria, HIV/AIDS, hookworm infestation, schistosomiasis, and other infections such as tuberculosis are particularly important factors contributing to the high prevalence of hemolytic anemia in some area (Nair, 2002). Anemia is a condition when the number of red blood cells is lower than normal level in the blood. It is usually measured as a decrease in the amount of hemoglobin (William, 2006). It is caused due to various factors such as deficiency of iron, reduced intake of vitamin B12 or folic acid, destruction of red bone marrow, and hereditary condition (George et al., 2012; Bruner et al., 1996). There are over 400 types of anemia, with hemolytic anemia being the most frequent (Faisidi et al., 2008). Hemolytic anemia has been reported to cause membrane lipid per oxidation and denaturation of cytoskeleton (Jollow and McMillan, 2001). Oxidation of erythrocytes has been used as a model system for oxidative damage of biomembranes. It has been found that most of ROS attack erythrocyte membranes causing oxidation of the lipids and proteins, and they are also involved in some changes in hemoglobin structure resulting in hemolysis of red blood cells (Ogbe et al., 2010). One of the major reasons of development of anemia in malaria seems to be oxidative stress (Kulkarni et al., 2003; Kremsner et al., 2000). Iron deficiency anemia is worldwide nutritional deficiency anemia

(Parischa et al., 2013). Iron is essential for metabolic process in living system (Frnandes et al., 1997). One of the major manifestations of iron deficiency is iron deficiency anemia, which is essential for hemoglobin synthesis (Ponka et al., 1998). It affects 20–50% of the world's population and is common in young children. The numbers are staggering, 2 billion people where over 30% of the world's population is anemic, due to iron deficiency. In India, adolescent girls constitute a vulnerable group of iron deficiency anemia, resulting in a reduced physical work capacity and cognitive function, behavioral disturbances, comorbidity, and delay in the onset of menarche that leads to cephalopelvic disproportion. In developing countries, every second pregnant woman and about 40% of preschool children are estimated to be anemic (Nair, 2002). Iron deficiency anemia is aggravated by worm infections, malaria, and other infectious diseases such as HIV and tuberculosis. The major health consequences include poor pregnancy outcome, impaired physical and cognitive development, and increased risk of morbidity in children and reduced work productivity in adults.

Iron deficiency anemia is a worldwide nutritional deficiency. It occurs in about one-eighth of the world population. The latest world estimate has 42% of pregnant women, 30% of nonpregnant women, 47% of preschool children, and 12.7% of men older being anemic (Ogbe et al., 2010). High prevalence and economic loss due to iron deficiency are more in developing countries (Pasricha et al., 2013). Poverty has been reported to be the likely cause of this high prevalence (Iannotti et al., 2012; Darnton et al., 2005). Among the few verified are *Sorghum bicolor*, *Jatropha tanjorensis*, and *Mangifera indica* L. among others (Oladiji et al., 2007; Nvvinuka et al., 2008). Oxidative stress is shown to play an important role in pathogenesis of IDA (Vives et al., 1995). Reports reveal that antioxidant enzymes activity like GSH-Px is decreased in children with IDA. These are indicators of increased lipid per oxidation (Tekin et al., 2001). Furthermore, Shved et al. (1995) have shown that the addition of synthetic antioxidants in the treatment of children with IDA results in decrease of lipid per oxidation, prevention of pathologic progression and rapid improvement of clinical manifestations, thereby stating iron deficiency anemia a cause of oxidative stress.

One of the common short-term measures to control iron deficiency anemia is oral iron supplementation (Srigiridhar and Nair, 2000). Only 10–15% of orally administered iron gets absorbed in small intestine. There are two forms of iron, namely, heme and nonheme iron. Heme iron gets directly absorbed into the intestinal cells. In the duodenal brush border, Dcytb reduces ferric (trivalent) nonheme iron to the ferrous (divalent) state, which is taken up from the lumen by the "Divalent Metal Transporter 1" (1/4 DMT-1), the expression of which is related to body iron status. The "mucosa block" mechanism reduces iron absorption after a preceding high iron exposure, presumably by diminishing the number of DMT-1 receptors (Chen et al., 2004).

A number of researches have been carried out the study the mechanism of hemolytic actions of several agents on RBCs, and it has been reported that hemolytic injury is associated with oxidative stress within erythrocytes. This concept is supported by the fact that hemolytic damage is accompanied by the generation of ROS, glutathione depletion, hemoglobin oxidation, and Heinz body formation in RBCs (Jollow and McMillan, 2001).

2.2   AIMS AND OBJECTIVES

In the present study, an attempt has been made to provide a therapy for both iron-induced and hemolytic anemia by a phytotherapeutic approach. The present study aims to investigate free radical scavenging and antihemolytic activities of some of the commonly used medicinal plants.

> ➤ To investigate the phytochemical screening.
> ➤ To investigate the antioxidant activities as reducing power, nitric oxide (NO) scavenging activity, DH radical scavenging activity, SOD activity.
> ➤ To investigate antihemolytic activity by hypotonic- and H_2O_2-induced method.

Triticum aestivum (wheat) belongs to Poaceae family. It is maximum edible cereal rich in vitamins, minerals, and proteins as compared to mature cereal plant (Tirgarl et al., 2011). At present, wheatgrass is rapidly becoming one of the most widely used supplemental health foods. It is available in many health food stores as fresh product, tablets, frozen juice, and powder. Wheatgrass provides a concentrated amount of nutrients, including iron, calcium, magnesium, amino acids, and vitamins (A, C, and E) and chlorophyll present in large amounts (70%) (Chia-Che et al., 2013). Some proponents thought wheatgrass as a treatment for cancer (Alitheen et al., 2011), ulcerative colitis (Ben-Arye et al., 2002), and joint pain and also serves as antioxidant (Das et al., 2012). It has been suggested that wheatgrass has a greater nutritional value than several everyday foods, and ingesting wheatgrass is comparable to eating a large amount of vegetables (Handzel et al., 2008). It is usually used as an herbal medicine in a many disease like thalassemia and myelodysplastic syndrome (Marawaha et al., 2004; Mukhopadhyay et al., 2009).

Carica papaya (papaya) is an erect, rapid-growing unbranched tree that is native to Central America but is now being cultivated in many tropical countries (Owoyele et al., 2008). *C. papaya* commonly known as papaya or pawpaw belongs to the genus Carica (Eno et al., 2000). Reports describe that *C. papaya* leaf has a therapeutic effect on dengue and malaria (Ahmad et al., 2011) and has anti-inflammatory effect (Owoyele et al., 2008). Traditionally, its latex is used in the treatment for jaundice, diabetes, food poisoning, and dog bites (Shantabi et al., 2014).

Piper betel called "paan" is green, heart–shaped, and a very famous leaf belonging to the family Piperaceae. *P. betel* leaves are rich in many nutrients like water, protein fats, fiber, calcium, and iron and help in curing various diseases like diabetes, hypertension, brain toxin, halitosis, boils, abscesses, obesity, wound healing, voice problems, conjunctivitis, constipation, itches, ringworm, swelling of gum, rheumatism, abrasion, and cuts and injuries (Singh et al., 2016). *P. betel* leaves contain various biologically active compounds that are responsible for antioxidant activity (Sripradha, 2014). The leaves have an essential oil comprising terpinen-4-ol, safrole, allylpyrocatechol monoacetate, eugenol acetate hydroxychavicol, and eugenol. *P. betel* oil contains cadinene carvacrol, chavicol, *p*-cymene, caryophyllene, chavibetol, cineole, and estragole as the major components (Dwivedi and Tripathi, 2014; Chahal et al., 2011).

2.3 MATERIALS AND METHODS

2.3.1 COLLECTION AND SUCCESSIVE EXTRACTION OF PLANT MATERIAL

2.3.1.1 WHEATGRASS

The grass of *T. aestivum* was cultivated, chopped, dried in shade, and powdered with a mechanical grinder.

2.3.1.2 CARICA PAPAYA

C. papaya leaves were collected from ITM University, Turari Campus, chopped, dried in shade, and powdered with a mechanical grinder.

2.3.1.3 PIPER BETEL

Fresh *P. betel* leaves were collected from village Sandalpur Antri of Gwalior, M.P. Leaves were cut in to small pieces and shade dried. The dried *P. betel* leaves were ground to a fine powder.

An amount of 50 g of powdered leaves were weighed and extracted with Soxhlet apparatus using various solvent according to their polarity, that is, petroleum ether, chloroform, methanol, *n*-butanol, ethyl acetate, and water. After solvent extraction, it was evaporated to obtain a powdered extract for various biochemical analyses.

2.3.2 QUALITATIVE PHYTOCHEMICAL SCREENING

Preliminary phytochemical screening of the extracts was performed for the presence of alkaloids, flavonoids, steroids, tannins, saponin, phenol, and using the standard procedures.

2.3.2.1 ALKALOIDS

To 1 ml of extract, 2–3 drops of Wagner's reagent were added. The appearance of pale or white precipitate indicated the presence of alkaloids (Harborne, 1973).

2.3.2.2 STEROIDS

To 2 ml of extract, 2 ml of chloroform and 2 ml of concentrated sulfuric acid were added. The tubes were shaken and allowed to stand. Formation of red colored chloroform layer indicates the presence of steroids (Kumar et al., 2012).

2.3.2.3   *TANNINS*

An amount of 3 ml of extracts was treated with 1% lead acetate solution. A red or yellow color precipitate was formed, indicating the presence of tannins (Harborne, 1973).

2.3.2.4   *SAPONINS*

To 3 ml of extracts, few drops of sodium bicarbonate were added and shaken vigorously for 3 min. Honey comb froth was formed, showing the presence of saponins (Harborne, 1973).

2.3.2.5   *PHENOLIC*

To 1 ml of extracts, 2 ml of distilled water and few drops of 10% ferric chloride solution were added. Formation of blue or green color indicates the presence of phenols (Harborne, 1973).

2.3.2.6   *FLAVONOIDS*

To 2 ml of each extract, few drops of 20% sodium hydroxide were added, and the formation of dark yellow color is observed, and by adding 70% hydrochloric acid, the yellow color disappeared. Disappearance of yellow color indicates the presence of flavonoids in the extract (Prabhavathi et al., 2016).

2.3.3   *QUANTITATIVE ESTIMATION OF SECONDARY METABOLITES*

2.3.3.1   *TOTAL PHENOLIC CONTENT*

The total phenolics in the extract were determined using Folin–Ciocalteu method as described by Kujala et al. (2000). To each sample solution (1.0 ml) and standard (1.0 ml), 5 ml of Folin–Ciocalteu was added followed by addition of 4 ml sodium carbonate (7% w/v). The solution was kept for 30 min in the dark at room temperature, after which absorbance was measured at 765 nm using a spectrophotometer. The phenolic content was calculated from the standard curve of gallic acid (Habila, 2010).

2.3.3.2   TOTAL FLAVONOID CONTENT

A known volume of extract was placed in a 10 ml volumetric flask add distilled water to make final volume 5 ml followed by adding 0.3 ml $NaNO_2$ (1.20). An amount of 3 ml of $AlCl_3$ (10%) was added 5 min later. After 6 min, 2 ml (1 mol/l) NaOH was added, and the total was made up to 10 ml with distilled water. The solution was mixed well again, and the absorbance was measured against a blank at 510 nm with a UV–visible Perkin Elmer Lambda 23 with Win Lab N6.0 software. The flavonoid content was calculated with quercetin as standard (Zhuang, 1992).

2.3.4   ANTIOXIDANT ACTIVITIES

Different antioxidant activities were performed to determine the antioxidant power of wheatgrass, *C. papaya, and P. betel* in various extracts.

2.3.4.1   REDUCING POWER ASSAY

A total of 2.5 ml phosphate buffer (0.2 M, pH 6.6) and 2.5 ml 1% potassium ferrocyanide were mixed in 1 ml of different fraction of plant extract at various concentration diluted in distilled water. The test tubes were incubated at 50°C in water bath for 10 min followed by addition of 2.5 ml 10% TCA and centrifuge at 3000 rpm for 10 min A total of 2.5 ml of the upper layer was collected, and 2.5 ml distilled water was added followed by 0.5 ml 0.1% $FeCl_3$ (freshly prepared). Increase in absorbance was measured at 700 nm against a suitable blank (Benzie and Strain, 1996).

2.3.4.2   NO RADICAL SCAVENGING ACTIVITY

NO radical scavenging activities of plant extract in different fraction were examined by Royer et al. (2011). To 200 μl sodium nitroprusside (5 mM),

800 µl extracts (0.1–1 mg/ml) were added and dissolved in PBS (25 mM, pH 7.4). The mixture was incubated for 2.5 h at 37°C under normal light and dark incubation for 20 min, and 600 µl Griess reagent (1% sulfanilamide, 0.1% naphthyl ethylene diamine hydrochloride in 2% phosphoric acid) was added and incubated for 40 min at room temperature and absorbance was measured at 540 nm against a suitable blank (2 ml H_2O and 0.6 ml Griess reagent). Control sample (1.6 ml H_2O, 400 µl sodium nitroprusside [SNP], and 600 µl Griess reagent) was prepared and percent of inhibition was calculated by using this equation.

$$\text{Percentage inhibition} = \text{OD of control} - (\text{OD of extract} / \text{OD of control}) \times 100 \tag{2.1}$$

2.3.4.3 DH FREE RADICAL SCAVENGING ACTIVITY

DH free radical scavenging activity of plant extracts in different fraction was examined by Blois method (Esmaeili and Sonboli, 2010) with minor modification. To 2 ml of plant extract taken at various concentration (20–100 µg/ml), 1 ml of DH solution (0.1 mM in methanol) was added, shaken well and incubated at 37°C for 30 min in dark. Decrease in absorbance was measured at 517 nm spectrophotometrically against a suitable blank and control tube containing methanol and DH. The percentage of inhibition was calculated by using eq (2.1).

2.3.4.4 SUPEROXIDE DISMUTASE (SOD) ASSAY

This assay was done by the method of Kakkar et al. (1984). Fresh wheat-grass (0.5 g), were ground with 5.0 ml of sodium phosphate buffer (50 mM, pH 6.4) centrifuged at 2000×*g* for 10 g and supernatant were collected used for the assay.

Assay mixture contained 1.2 ml of sodium pyrophosphate buffer (0.025 M, pH 8.3), 0.1 ml of phenazine methosulfate (186 µM), 0.3 ml of nitro blue tetrazolium (300 µM), 0.2 ml of plant extract at different concentration (20–100 µg/ml), and distilled water in a total volume of 2.8 ml. The reaction was initiated by addition of 0.2 ml NADH (780 µM). The mixture was incubated at 30°C for 90 s. 1 ml glacial acetic acid was added to stop the reaction. Reaction mixture was shaken with 4 ml *n*-butanol and allowed to stand for 10 min. It was centrifuged at 2000×g for 10 min, and butanol layer was collected. The intensity of chromogen n-butanol layer was measured at 560 nm. The percent of inhibition was calculated by using this equation.

$$\text{Percentage inhibition} = \text{OD of control} -$$
$$(\text{OD of extract} / \text{OD of control} \times \text{mg of protein}) \times 100 \qquad (2.1)$$

2.3.4.5 *ANTIHEMOLYTIC ACTIVITY/MEMBRANE STABILIZING ACTIVITY*

The following two methods were used for conducting this in vitro membrane stabilizing assay:

2.3.4.5.1 *Hypotonic Solution–induced Hemolysis*

This method was done by method of Shinde et al. (1999). A total of 5 ml of whole blood of a healthy person in heparinized tube was collected. The blood was centrifuged at 3000×g for 10 min. The supernatant was removed and RBCs were washed three times with sodium chloride isotonic solution (154 mM NaCl) in 10 mM sodium phosphate buffer (pH 7.4) through centrifugation using the same volume as supernatant. Finally, RBCs were resuspended in the same volume of isotonic buffer solution. After that, 0.5 ml of RBCs suspension was mixed with 5 ml of hypotonic solution (50 mM NaCl in 10 mM sodium phosphate buffer pH 7.4) containing 0.5 ml plant extracts (10 mg/ml). The control sample was prepared by 0.5 ml suspension mixed with hypotonic buffered saline. The mixture was incubated for 10 min at room temperature, centrifuged at 3000×g for 10 min, and the optical density of supernatant was measured at 540 nm.

2.3.4.5.2 *H_2O_2-induced Hemolysis*

This method was done by Ebrahimzadeh et al. (2009). An amount of 5 ml whole blood was collected in heparinized tube, centrifuged (10 min at 1500×g) RBCs separated out from plasma, and the buffy coat is washed three times in 10 mM/l PBS. Washed RBCs were diluted in PBS to obtained 4% suspension. To 2 ml RBCs suspension, 1 ml of plant extracts (10 mg/ml) was added and incubated for 5 min at room temperature, 0.5 ml H_2O_2 was added and shaken well and incubated at 37°C for 30 min. Supernatant was collected and taken absorbance at 540 nm. Percentage of inhibition of was calculated by using eq (2.1).

2.3.5   THIN LAYER CHROMATOGRAPHY (TLC)

Thin layer chromatography (TLC) is a chromatographic method that is employed to separate mixtures. It is performed on aluminum or plastic foil, which is covered with a thin layer of adsorbent substance, generally silica gel aluminum oxide, or cellulose. This film of adsorbent is identified as the stationary silica phase. After the sample has been filled on the plate, a solvent or solvent mixture (mobile phase) is drained up the plate via capillary action. Because dissimilar analytes rise in the TLC plate at different rates, finally the mixture was separated (Abdul, 2016).

2.3.6   FOURIER TRANSFORM INFRARED SPECTROSCOPY

Fourier transform infrared spectroscopy (FTIR) spectra for the *P. betel* leaf extracts were analyzed in the present study (Bhaskar and Parthasarathy, 2010; Pednerkar and Bhanu, 2013). FTIR is used as a tool for the characterization and identification of compounds or functional group (chemical bonds) present in an unknown mixture of plant extract. The FTIR from 4000 to 390 cm^{-1} was recorded on Perkin Elmer (spectrum 2) spectrophotometer.

2.4   RESULTS

2.4.1   QUALITATIVE PHYTOCHEMICAL SCREENING

Table 2.1 shows the qualitative preliminary phytochemical screening of *P. betel* in various extract. From the results, we found that the petroleum extract had high phenolics and flavonoids content followed by alkaloids, steroids, and saponins.

Table 2.2 represents the phytochemical screening of *T. aestivum* grass. Results revealed that *n*-butanol and aqueous extracts present high concentration of flavonoids and moderate concentration of alkaloids. Flavonoids, tannins, phenols, saponins, and steroids were observed in low concentration.

Table 2.3 represents phytochemical screening of *C. papaya* leaves alkaloids, tannins, steroids, and saponins are present in *n*-butanol and aqueous extracts and phenols are absent.

TABLE 2.1   Qualitative Phytochemical Screening of Various Extracts of *P. betel* Leaves.

Fractions	Alkaoids	Steroids	Tannins	Saponins	Phenolics	Flavonoids
Petroleum ether	++	++	++	++	+++	+++
Chloroform	+	+	+	+	+	+
Ethyl acetate	+	+	−	+	+	+
Methanol	+	+	+	+	+	+
n-Butanol	+	+++	++	+	+	++
Aqueous	++	+	+	++	++	++

+, low; ++, moderate; +++, high.

TABLE 2.2   Qualitative Phytochemical Screening of Wheatgrass in Four Extracts.

Extract	Alkaloids	Flavonoids	Tannins	Phenols	Saponins	Steroids
Petroleum ether	+	++	+	+	+	+
Ethyl acetate	+	++	+	+	+	+
n-Butanol	++	+++	+	+	+	+
Aqueous	++	+++	+	+	+	+

+, low; ++, moderate; +++, high.

TABLE 2.3   Phytochemical Screening of *Carica papaya* Leaves.

Extract	Alkaloids	Flavonoids	Tannins	Phenols	Saponins	Steroids
Petroleum ether	+	−	−	+	−	+
Ethyl acetate	−	+	−	+	−	−
n-Butanol	+	−	+	−	+	+
Aqueous	+	−	+	−	+	+

+, low; ++, moderate; +++, high; −, absent.

2.4.2   QUANTITATIVE ESTIMATION OF SECONDARY METABOLITES

Table 2.4 depicts quantitative analysis of flavonoids and phenolic content and revealed that highest flavonoid content was found in petroleum ether, chloroform extract followed by aqueous extract. The phenolic content was also high in petroleum ether followed by chloroform and methanol and lower in aqueous extract.

TABLE 2.4   Quantitative Secondary Metabolite Estimations of Various Extract of *Piper betel* Leaves.

Fractions	Flavonoids	Phenolics
Petroleum ether	10.92 mg/g ± 0.9	38.52 mg/g ± 3.5
Chloroform	10.96 mg/g ± 0.87	21.72 mg/g ± 1.9
Ethyl acetate	7.39 mg/g ± 2.1	31.32 mg/g ± 3.8
n-Butanol	10.15 mg/g ± 0.9	45.12 mg/g ± 0.92
Methanol	7.715 mg/g ± 0.7	12.48 mg/g ± 1.2
Aqueous	10.27 mg/g ± 1.1	10.27 mg/g + 1.1

2.4.3   ANTIOXIDANT ACTIVITIES

2.4.3.1   REDUCING POWER

Figure 2.1 illustrates the reducing power of *P. betel* at different concentration in various extracts. It was observed that *n*-butanol fraction had highest reducing power ability followed by ethyl acetate. *N*-butanol exhibited reducing power capability as 3.2 at 1000 µg/ml. The pattern of reducing ability in *P. betel* was concentration dependent.

Figure 2.2 represents the reducing power of wheatgrass in four different extracts. From the results, we found that maximum reducing power was shown by aqueous extracts (1.008) followed by *n*-butanol extracts 0.760 at 240 µg/ml concentration. Petroleum ether has shown minimum reducing abilities.

Reducing power of papaya leaves in four extracts was shown in Figure 2.3. Highest reducing abilities were observed 1.36 in aqueous extract of papaya leaves followed by 0.966 in *n*-butanol extract at 240 µg/ml concentration at 700 nm.

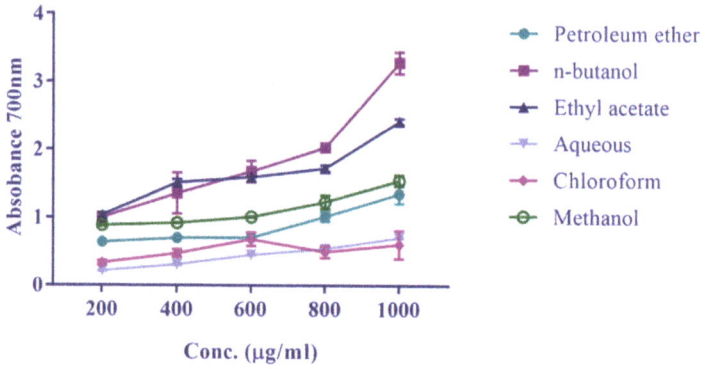

FIGURE 2.1   Reducing power of *Piper betel* leaves in various extracts.

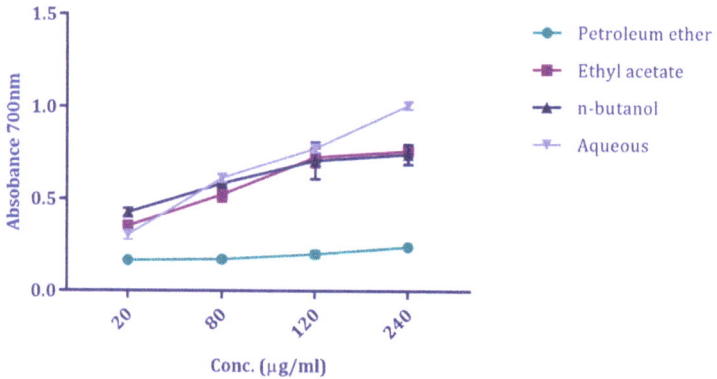

FIGURE 2.2   Reducing power of wheatgrass in four extracts.

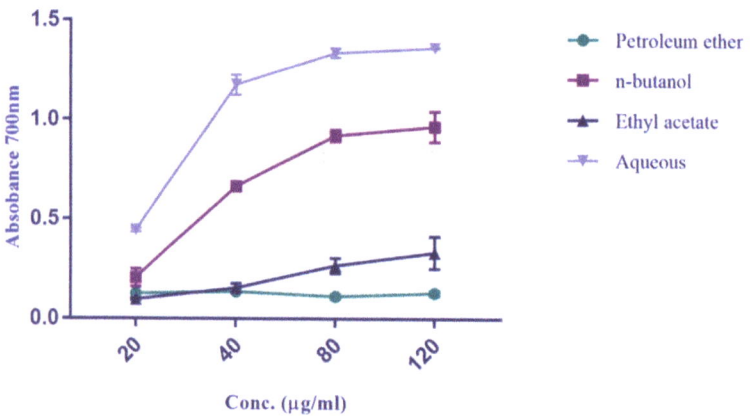

FIGURE 2.3   Reducing power of *Carica papaya* leaves in four extracts.

2.4.3.2 NO SCAVENGING ACTIVITY

Figure 2.4 illustrates the NO scavenging activity of *Piper betel* in four extracts. Highest scavenging activity observed in *n*-butanol was 55.7 and followed by aqueous extract as 51.3 at 1 mg/ml concentration.

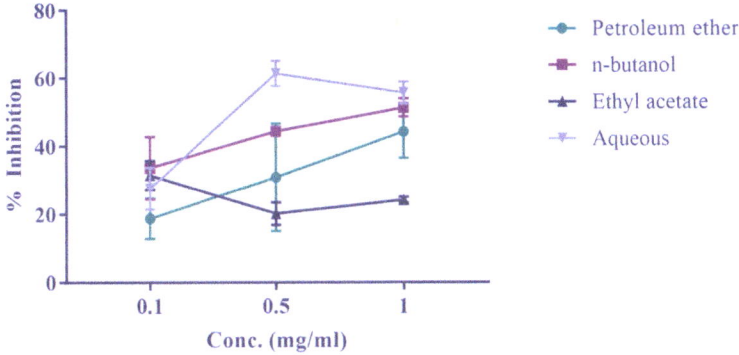

FIGURE 2.4   NO radical scavenging activity of *Piper betel* leaves in four extracts.

Figure 2.5 represents the NO scavenging activity of wheatgrass in four extracts. The maximum scavenging activity in aqueous extract was 60.7 at 1 mg/ml as compared to petroleum ether, ethyl acetate, and *n*-butanol extracts.

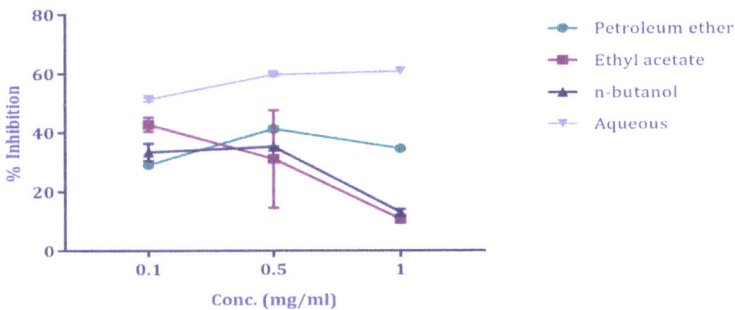

FIGURE 2.5   NO radical scavenging activity of wheatgrass in four extracts.

Figure 2.6 illustrates the NO scavenging activity of papaya leaves in four extracts. The maximum scavenging activity observed in *n*-butanol extracts was 74.28% as compared to others extracts at 0.5 mg/ml concentration.

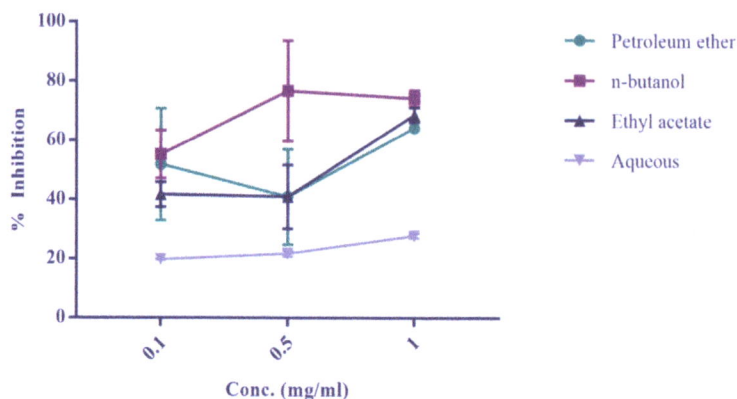

FIGURE 2.6   NO radical scavenging activity of *Carica papaya* leaves in four extracts.

2.4.3.3   DH FREE RADICAL SCAVENGING ACTIVITY

Figure 2.7 shows the DH radical scavenging activity of wheatgrass in four extracts. The highest DH radical scavenging activity was shown in *n*-butanol extract 60.3 at 100 μg/ml followed by ethyl acetate extract as 52.7 at 80 μg/ml.

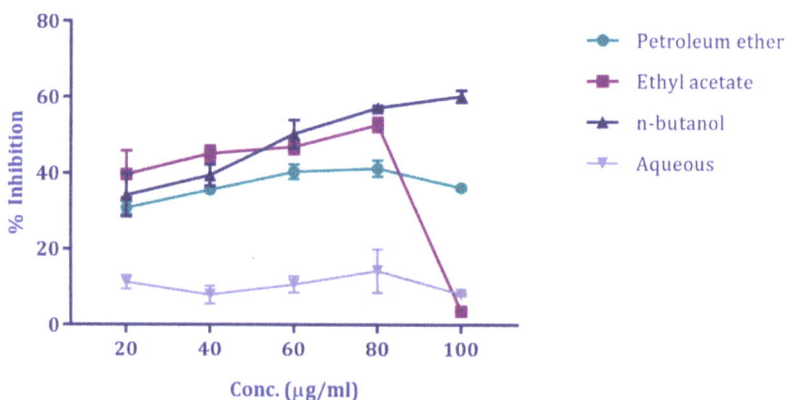

FIGURE 2.7   DH free radical scavenging activity of wheatgrass in four extracts.

Figure 2.8 illustrates the DH radical scavenging activity of *Carica papaya* leaves. In papaya leaves, aqueous extract maximum inhibition was 34.9 followed by *n*-butanol extract as 31.7 at 100 μg/ml.

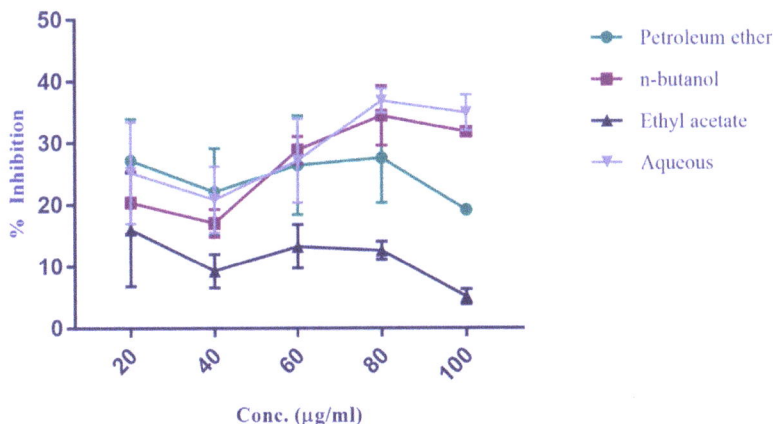

FIGURE 2.8   DH free radical scavenging activity of *Carica papaya* leaves in four extracts.

2.4.3.4   SUPEROXIDE DISMUTASE (SOD) ASSAY

SOD activity was performed from the fresh sample of wheatgrass at various concentration. Table 2.5 represents the SOD activity. Maximum percentage of inhibition was observed at 60–80 µg/ml.

TABLE 2.5   Superoxide Dismutase Activity of Wheatgrass.

S. No.	Concentration (µg/ml)	% Inhibition
1	20	21.9 ± 0.6
2	40	37.1 ± 3.7
3	60	40.9 ± 0.63
4	80	39.3 ± 2.2
5	100	36.5 ± 2.5

Values are expressed as mean± SD (n = 3)

2.4.3.5   ANTIHEMOLYTIC ACTIVITY/MEMBRANE STABILIZING ACTIVITY

Table 2.6 shows the antihemolytic activity of *P. betel*. Control shows 100% hemolysis because it does not contain extract. Petroleum ether extract shows minimum percent of hemolysis as 25.05% followed by *n*-butanol as 55%.

TABLE 2.6   Antihemolytic Activity of *Piper betel* Leaves in Four Extracts.

Sample	% Hemolysis
Control	100
Petroleum ether	25.05
Ethyl acetate	99.6
n-Butanol	55

2.4.3.6 ANTIHEMOLYTIC AND MEMBRANE STABILIZING ACTIVITIES

Antihemolytic and membrane stabilizing activities of wheat are depicted in Table 2.7. In case of hypotonic solution–induced hemolysis, the maximum level of membrane stabilizing activity was observed by *n*-butanol fraction of wheatgrass, which was 75% by H_2O_2-induced hemolysis and 82% by hypotonic solution-induced hemolysis. The minimum antihemolytic activity was exhibited by petroleum ether extract of wheatgrass. The ranges of antihemolytic of all extracts were between 65 and 82%.

TABLE 2.7   Antihemolytic Activity of Wheatgrass in Four Extracts.

Fractions	H_2O_2-induced antihemolysis activity (10 mg/ml) (%)	Hypotonic solution–induced antihemolysis (10 mg/ml) (%)
Control	100	100
Petroleum ether	65	62
Ethyl acetate	68	68
n-Butanol	82	75

Table 2.8 represents the antihemolytic activity of *Carica papaya* leaves in four extracts. Maximum percent antihemolytic activity was observed 42.9% in petroleum ether extracts.

TABLE 2.8   Antihemolytic Activity of *Carica papaya* Leaves in Four Extracts.

Fractions	Hypotonic-induced antihemolysis activity (10 mg/ml) (%)
Control	100
Petroleum ether	42.9
Ethyl acetate	17.9
n-Butanol	23.4

2.4.4 *THIN LAYER CHROMATOGRAPHY (TLC)*

Table 2.9 explains the TLC pattern of various extracts of *P. betel* leaves, the retention factor (RF) of aqueous, *n*-butanol, and petroleu0m ether extract were quite close to quinine standard thus representing high alkaloids content.

TABLE 2.9 Thin-Layer Chromatography (TLC) of Various Extracts of *Piper betel* Leaves for the Presence of Alkaloids.

Sample name	RF values
Quinine standard	0.53
Petroleum ether extract	0.50
Chloroform extract	0.72
Ethyl acetate	0.85
n-Butanol	0.86
Methanolic extract	0.65
Aqueous extract	0.52

2.5 DISCUSSION

Medicinal plants are frequently used as natural antioxidants that present scavenging radicals and inhibiting lipid per oxidation, and preventing oxidative damage in animal tissue or cells oxidative stress imposed by ROS may be direct or indirect cause of tissue damage and many diseases such as aging, cancer, atherosclerosis, cardiac hypertrophy (Paech, 1955). The medicinal properties of plants material are mainly due to the presence of various phytochemical compounds (Lalnundanga et al., 2012). The presence of different phytochemical compounds such as flavonoid, tannin, saponins, alkaloid and glycoside in the phytochemical tests justifies their therapeutic potential (Kavitha et al., 2012; Patel et al., 2012; Ayoola and Adeyeye, 2010). These phytochemical compounds have been reported to have multiple biological effects such as anti-inflammatory, antiallergic, antioxidant, antidiabetic, analgesic, antispasmodic, antibacterial, antiviral, anticancer, and aldose reductase inhibitory activities.

Recent epideomological studies have shown that natural products have been used to prevent and treat many diseases as they are rich in secondary metabolites. The antioxidant activity of dietary phenolics is considered to be superior to that of the essential vitamins and is used as cured to interrupt free radical-mediated reaction by donating hydrogen atom from the phenol hydroxyl group.

Phenolic compounds are known to be a powerful chain breaking antioxidants, and they possess scavenging ability due to their hydroxyl groups (Hatano et al., 2016). Studies have shown that the polyphenols found in dietary and medicinal plants could inhibit oxidative stress by antioxidant method (Manach et al., 2004). In the present study, the antioxidant activity of the petroleum ether extract of *P. betel* leaves as reducing power is possibly due to its high phenolic content.

Flavonoid is one of the main groups of phytochemical compound and widely distributed flavonoid, flavones and flavonols. Many flavonoids and related compounds are reported to possess strong antioxidative characteristics (Dziedzic and Hudson, 1983). In phytochemical screening of wheatgrass and papaya leaves, aqueous and *n*-butanol extracts have high phytochemical content than other extracts.

A comparative study of the phytochemicals in herbs used in treatment of anemia, showed two phytochemicals, saponin, and cardiac glycosides, to be common to all the herbs (Gbadamosi, 2012). The effect of saponin on RBC indices is controversial. While Asif and Wahid (Asif, 2003) reported that saponin in *Fagonia cretica* L.-reduced red blood cell indices, Harikrishnan (2012) reported that saponin increased red blood cell indices. Although some plants containing cardiac glycosides have been report to boost RBC indices (Taheri, 2013; Arhoghro, 2014), unlike saponin, effect of extracted cardiac glycosides from plants on red blood cell indices is yet to be elucidated. Iron, an important factor in the synthesis of hemoglobin, a component of RBC, was reported by Babatunde (2012) to be the highest amount of trace element in the *M. indica* stem bark. Tannins also exhibit various biological activities including anti-inflammatory, antiartherosclerosis, antitumor, anticancer, antibacterial, and antiviral.

Antioxidant activity has become one of the studies on mechanism of the nutraceutical and therapeutical effects of traditional medicines, and there are numerous antioxidant activities (Haung et al., 2005). Due to the complexity of the oxidation–antioxidation processes, it is obvious that no single method is capable of providing a comprehensive depiction of the antioxidant profile of a studied sample.

The reducing ability is generally associated with the presence of reductones, which have been shown to exhibit antioxidant action by breaking the chain reactions and by donating a hydrogen atom. Reductones are also reported to react with certain precursors of peroxide, thus preventing peroxide prevention (Nair et al., 2012).

It is well known that nitric oxide has an important role in various inflammatory processes. Sustained levels of production of this radical are directly toxic to tissues and contribute to the vascular collapse associated with septic shock, whereas chronic expression of nitric oxide radical is associated with various carcinomas and inflammatory conditions, including juvenile diabetes, multiple sclerosis, arthritis, and ulcerative colitis (Hazra et al., 2008). NO released from SNP (sodium nitroprusside) has a strong NO character that can alter the structure and function of many cellular components. The toxicity of NO increases greatly when it reacts with superoxide radical in forming the highly reactive peroxy nitrate anion (ONOO−). The plant extract inhibits nitrite formation by directly competing with oxygen in the reaction with nitric oxide. In this study, nitric oxide radical scavenging effect of *C. papaya* in a concentration of 0.5 mg/ml was found to be more in *n*-butanol extract (74.28%) compared with petroleum ether, ethyl acetate, and aqueous extracts. This results revealed the same that of nitric oxide scavenging effect of *S. pinnata* (Tylor et al., 1997).

The scavenging activity of DH, a stable free radical, is a widely used index and a quick method to evaluate antioxidant activity (Mokbel and Hashinaga, 2006). It is a marker of free radicals originating in lipids (Yasuda et al., 2006). DH is a stable free radical that can accept an electron of hydrogen radical to become a stable diamagnetic molecule (Bijaya and Bikash, 2013). In present study, aqueous extract of *C. papaya* has 34.9% at 100 µg/ml, ethyl acetate extract of *T. aestivum* has 52.7 at 80 µg/ml, *n*-butanol extract of *T. aestivum* has 60.3 at 100 µg/ml concentration. The highest DH radical scavenging activity had shown 60.3% in *n*-butanol extract of wheatgrass. ABTS is an excellent tool for determining antioxidant activity of hydrogen donating antioxidants and of chain breaking antioxidants (Yildirim et al., 2006).

Superoxide anions are the most common free radicals. Their concentrations increase under conditions of oxidative stress and are generated either by autoxidation processes or by enzymes and produce other cell damaging free radicals and oxidizing agents (Liu and Ng, 2000). Super oxide anions damage biomolecules directly or indirectly by forcing H_2O_2, OH, Peroxy nitrate, or singlet oxygen. Super oxide has also been observed to directly initiate lipid per oxidation. In present study, maximum super oxide scavenging activity is 40.9% of fresh wheatgrass at 60 µg/ml. This result is revealed the same by super oxide scavenging of *Cyperus rotundus* (Nagulendran et al., 2007).

Antihemolytic activity of quercetin and the relation between nonchelating activities against oxidative damage to erythrocyte membrane by flavonoid has been reported (Navabi et al., 2012). The results of antihemolytic activity indicated that *n*-butanol extract of *T. aestivum* grass and *P. betel* leaves and petroleum ether extracts of *C. papaya* shown maximum percent of antihemolysis (Tables 2.6–2.8). The increased antihemolytic activity of test sample implies that leaf extract contain flavonoid and glycosides can guard RBC from free radical mediated hemolysis (Dai et al., 2006). Binding of flavonoids to the RBCs membrane inhibits lipid peroxidation and simultaneously enhances their integrity against lysis (Chaudhary et al., 2007).

KEYWORDS

- **anemia**
- **phytomedicine**
- **oxidative stress**
- **SOD**
- **NO**
- **OH radical scavenging**

REFERENCES

Abdul, M.; Shami, M. Isolation and Identification of Alkaloids Extracted from Local Plant in Malaysia. *Ann. Chromatogr. Sep. Tech.* **2016,** *2* (1), 1016.

Alitheen, N. B.; Oon, C. L.; Keong, Y. S.; Chuan, T. K.; Li, H. K.; Yong, H. W. Cytotoxic Effects of Commercial Wheatgrass and Fiber Towards Human Acute Promyelocytic Leukemia Cells (HL60). *Pak. J. Pharm. Sci.* **2011,** *24,* 243–250.

Akinkugbe, O. F. Anaemia, The Perils Plenty. *Clin. Pharm. Herb. Med.* **1991,** *18,* 15–19.

Arhoghro, E. M.; Berezi, E. P.; Prohp, T. P. Phytochemical Constituents and Effect of Combined Ethanolic Leaf Extract of *Costus afer* and Cleome Rutidosperma On Lipid

Profile and Some Haematological Parameters in *Wistar* Rats. *Int. J. Curr. Microbiol. Appl. Sci.* **2014,** *3* (5), 673–679.

Asif, M. S., Sabir, A. W. Effects of *Fagonia cretica* L. Constituents on Various Haematological Parameters in Rabbits. *J. Ethnopharmacol.* **2003,** *85* (2), 195–200.

Ayoola, P. B.; Adeyeye, A. Phytochemical and Nutrient Evaluation of *Carica papaya* (Pawpaw) Leaves. *IJRRAS* **2010,** *5,* 325–328.

Awosika, F. Traditional Medicine as the Solution to Nigeria Health Problems. *Clin. Pharmacol. Herb. Med.* **1993,** *9* (3), 26–31.

Babatunde, A. P. Trace Elements and Major Minerals of *Persea americana, Mangifera indica,* and *Cocos nucifera* Shell Charcoal. *World J. Eng. Pure Appl. Sci.* **2012,** *2* (2), 81–84.

Baquar, S. R. *Medicinal and Poisonous Plants of Pakistan,* 1st ed.; Karachi Printing Press: Karachi, 1989; p 45.

Beevi, S. S.; Mangarnoori, L. N.; Dhand, V.; Siva, R. D. *Foodborne Pathog. Dis.* **2009,** *6,* 129–136.

Ben-Arye, E.; Goldin, E.; Wengrower, D.; Stamper, A.; Kohn, R.; Berry, E. Wheat Grass Juice in the Treatment of Active Distal Ulcerative Colitis. A Randomized Double-Blind Placebo-Controlled Trial. *Scand. J. Gastroenterol.* **2002,** *37,* 444–449.

Benzie, I. F.; Strain, J. J. The Ferric Reducing Ability of Plasma (FRAP) as a Measure of "Antioxidant Power", the FRAP Assay. *Anal. Biochem.* **1996,** *239* (1), 70–76.

Bhaskar, J. S.; Parthasarathy, G. A. Fourier Transform Infrared Spectroscopic Characterization of Kaolinite from Assam and Meghalaya, Northeastern India. *J. Mod. Phys.* **2010,** *1,* 206–210.

Bijaya, I. M.; Bikash, B. Antioxidant Capacity and Phenolics Content of Some Nepalese Medicinal Plants. *Am. J. Plant Sci.* **2013,** *4,* 1660–1667.

Burton, G. W.; Ingold, K. U. Vitamin E, Application of the Principles of Physical; **1986.**

Bruner, A. B.; Joffe, A.; Duggan, A. K.; Casella, J. F.; Brandt, J. *Lancet* **1996,** *348,* 992–996.

Carier, J.; Elaheh, A.; Jim, C.; Johane, P. A. Iron Supplementation Increases Disease Activity and Vitamin E Ameliorates the Effect in Rats with Dextran Sulfate Sodium-Induced Colitis. *J. Nutr.* **2002,** *132,* 3146–3150.

Chahal, J.; Ohlyan, R.; Kandale, A.; Walia, A.; Puri, S. Introduction, Phytochemistry, Traditional Uses and Biological Activity of Genus Piper, A Review. *IJCPR* **2011,** *2* (2), 130–144.

Chandra, S. Y. R. *The Wealth of India, A Dictionary of Indian Raw Materials and Industrial Products*; CSIR-NISCAIR Press: New Delhi, 2003; Vol. I, p 472.

Chaudhuri, S.; Banerjee, A.; Basu, K.; Sengupta, B.; Sengupta, P. K. Interaction of Flavonoid with Red Blood Membrane Lipids and Proteins, Antioxidant and Antihemolytic Activity. *Int. J. Biol. Macromol.* **2007,** *41,* 42–48.

Chen, Q.; Le, G. W.; Shi, Y. H.; Zhang, S. M.; Jin, X. Effect of Iron Supplementation on Intestinal Consequences. *Nutr. J.* **2004,** *3,* 2.

Chia-Che, T.; Chih-Ru, L.; Hsien-Yu, T.; Chia-Jung, C.; Wen-Tai, L.; Hui-Ming, Y., et al. *J. Biol. Chem.* **2013,** *288,* 17689–17697.

Dai, F.; Miao, Q.; Zhou, B.; Yang, L.; Liu, Z. L. Protective Effects of Flavanols and Their Glycosides Against Free Radical-Induced Oxidative Haemolysis of Red Blood Cells. *Life Sci.* **2006,** *78,* 2488–2493.

Darnton-Hill, I.; Webb, P.; Harvey, P. W. J.; Hunt, J. M.; Dalmiya, N.; Chopra, M., et al. Micronutrient Deficiencies and Gender, Social and Economic Costs. *Am. J. Clin. Nutr.* **2005,** *81* (5), 1198–1205.

Das, A.; Raychaudhuri, U.; Chakraborty, R. Effect of Freeze Drying and Oven Drying on Antioxidant Properties of Fresh Wheatgrass. *Int. J. Food Sci. Nutr.* **2012,** *3,* 718–721.

Desai, A. G.; Qazi, G. N.; Ganju, R. K.; EI-Tamer, M.; Singh, J.; Saxena, A. K.; Bedi, Y. S.; Taneja, S. C.; Bhat, H. K. Medicinal Plants and Cancer Chemoprevention. *Curr. Drug Metab.* **2008,** *9,* 581–591.

Dwivedi, V.; Tripathi, S. Review Study on Potential Activity of *Piper betel. J. Pharmacogn. Phytochem.* **2014,** *3* (4), 93–98.

Dziedzic, S. Z.; Hudson, B. J. F. Hydroxyl Isoflavones as Antioxidants for Edible Oils. *Food Chem.* **1983,** *11,* 161–166.

Ebrahimzadeh, M. A.; Nabavi, S. F.; Eslami, B.; Nabavi, S. M. Antioxidant and Antihaemolytic Potentials of Physosperumcornubiense (L.) DC. *Pharmacologyonline* **2009,** *3,* 394–403.

Enayde de, A. M.; Jorge, M. F.; Nonete, B. G. *Lebensm. Wiss. Technol.* **2005,** *11,* 15–19.

Eno, A. E.; Owo, O. I.; Itam, E. H.; Konya, R. S. Blood Pressure Depression by the Fruit Juice of *Carica papaya* [L.] in Renal and DOCA-Induced Hypertension in the Rat. *J. Phytother. Res.* **2000,** *9* (4), 235–239.

Esmaeili, M. A.; Sonboli, A. Antioxidant, Free Radical Scavenging Activities of *Salvia brachyantha* and Its Protective Effect against Oxidative Cardiac Cell Injury. *Food Chem. Toxicol.* **2010,** *48* (3), 8468–8453.

Farombi, E. O.; Briton, G.; Emerole, G. O. *Food Res. Int.* **2000,** *33,* 493–500.

Fernandes, M. I.; Galvao, L. C.; Bortolozzi, M. F.; Oliveira, W. P.; Zucoloto, S.; Bianchi, M. L. Disaccharidase Levels in Normal Epithelium of the Small Intestine of Rats with Iron-Deficiency Anemia. *Braz. J. Med. Biol. Res.* **1997,** *30* (7), 849–854.

Fasidi, D. A.; Gbeassor, M.; Vovor, A.; Eklu-Gadegbeku, K.; Aklikokon, K.; Agbonon, A. Effect of *Tectona grandis* on phenylhydrazine-induced anaemia in rats. *Fitoterapia* **2008,** *79* (5), 332–336.

Florentino, R. F. In *The Burden of Iron Deficiency and an Aemia in Asia, Challenges in Prevention and Control. Nutrition Goals for Asia-Vision 2020,* Proceedings IX Asian Congress of Nutrition, 2003; pp 313–318.

George, A. K.; George, H. S.; Phyllis, E. P. *Res. J. Pharmacol.* **2012,** *6* (2), 20–24.

Gbadamosi, I. T.; Moody, J. O.; Yekini, A. O. Nutritional Composition of Ten Ethnobotanicals Used for the Treatment of Anaemia in Southwest Nigeria. *Eur. J. Med. Plants* **2012,** *2* (2), 140–150.

Habila, J. D.; Bello, I. A.; Dzikwi, A. A.; Musa, H.; Abubakar, N. Total Phenolic and Antioxidant Activity of *Tridax procumbens* Linn. *Afr. J. Pharm. Pharmacol.* **2010,** *4* (3), 123–126.

Handzel, M.; Sibert, J.; Harvey, T.; Deshmukh, H.; Chambers, C. Monitoring the Oxygenation of Blood during Exercise after Ingesting Wheatgrass Juice. *J. Altern. Med.* **2008,** *8,* 1.

Harborne, J. B. *Phytochemical Methods,* 2nd ed.; Chapman and Hall Ltd.: London, 1973; pp 149–188.

Hatano, T.; Edamatzu, R.; Mori, A.; Fujita, Y.; Yasuhara, T.; Yoshida, T.; Okuda, T. Effect of Interaction Tannins with Co-Existing Substances. *Chem. Pharm. Bull.* **1989,** *37,* 2016–2092.

Haung, D. J.; Ou, B. X.; Prior, R. L. The Chemistry behind Antioxidant Capacity Assays. *J. Agric. Food Chem.* **2005**, *53*, 1841–1856.

Hazra, B.; Biswas, S.; Mandal, N. Antioxidant and Free Radical Scavenging Activity of *Spondias pinnata*. *BMC Complement. Altern. Med.* **2008**, *8*, 63–73.

Hatano, T.; Edamatzu, R.; Mori, A.; Fujita, Y.; Yasuhara, T.; Yoshida, T.; Okuda T. Effect of Interaction of Tannins with Co-Existing Substances. *Chem. Pharm. Bull.* **1989**, *37*, 2016–2021.

Iannotti, L. L.; Robles, M.; Pachon, H.; Chiarella, C. Food Prices and Poverty Negatively Affect Micronutrient Intakes in Guatemala, *J. Nutr.* **2012**, *142* (8), 1568–1576.

Kakkar, P.; Das, B.; Viswanathan, P. N. A Modified Spectrophotometric Assay of Superoxide Dismutase. *Ind. J. Biochem. Biophys.* **1984**, *21* (2), 130–132.

Kavitha, T.; Nelson, R.; Thenmozhi, R.; Priya E. Antimicrobial Activity and Phytochemical Analysis of *Anisomeles malabarica* (L) R.BR. *J. Microbiol. Biotech. Res.* **2012**, *2*, 1–5.

Ke-Xue, Z.; Cai-Xia, L.; Xiao-Na, G.; Wei, P.; Hui-Ming, Z. *Food Chem.* **2011**, *126*, 1122–1126.

Kremsner, P. G.; Greve, B.; Lell, B.; Luckner, D.; Schmidt D. Malarial Anaemia in African Children Associated with High Oxygen-Radical Production. *Lancet* **2000**, *355*, 40–41.

Kujala, T. S.; Loponen, J. M.; Klika, K. D.; Pihlaja, K. Phenolics and Betacyanins in Red Beetroot (*Beta vulgaris*) Root, Distribution and Effect of Cold Storage on the Content of Total Phenolics and Three Individual Compounds. *J. Agric. Food Chem.* **2000**, *47*, 3954–3962.

Kulkarni, A. G.; Suryakar, A. N.; Sardeshmukh, A. S.; Rathi, D. B. Studies on Biochemical Changes with Special Reference to Oxidant and Antioxidants in Malaria Patients. *Ind. J. Clin. Biochem.* **2003**, *18* (2), 136–149.

Kumar, S.; Sharma, U. K.; Sharma, A. K.; Pandey, A. K. Protective Efficacy of *Solanum xanthocarpum* root Extract against Free Radical Damage. Phytochemical Analysis and Antioxidant Effect. *Cell. Mol. Biol.* **2012**, *58* (1), 174–181.

Kumar, V.; Abbas, A. K.; Fausto, N.; Aster, J. C. *Robbins and Cotran Pathologic Basis of Disease*, 7th ed.; W.B. Saunders: Philadelphia, 2007; Vol. 2, pp 135–145.

Kumerova, A.; Lece, A.; Skesters, A.; Silova, A.; Petuhovs, V. Anaemia and Antioxidant Defense of the Red Blood Cells. *Mater. Med. Pol.* **1998**, *30*, 12–15.

Lalnundanga, N. L.; Lalrinkima, R. Phytochemical Analysis of the Methanol Extract of Root Bark of *Hiptage benghalensis* (L.) Kurz. *Sci. Vis.* **2012**, *12*, 8–10.

Lee, S.; Suh, S.; Kin, S. Protective Effects of Green Tea Polyphenol (−)− Epigallocatechin Gallate against Hippocampal Neuronal Damage After Transient Global Ischemia in Gerbils. *Neurosci. Lett.* **2000**, *287*, 191–194.

Liu, F.; Ng, T. B. Antioxidative and Free Radical Scavenging Activities of Selected Medicinal Herbs. *Life Sci.* **2000**, *66*, 725–735.

Manach, C.; Scalbert, A.; Morand, C.; Remsey, C.; Jimenez, L. Polyphenols, Food Sources and Bioavailability. *Am. J. Clin. Nutr.* **2004**, *79*, 727–747.

Marawaha, R. K.; Bansal, D.; Kaur, S.; Trehan, A. Wheatgrass Juice Reduces Transfusion Requirement in Patients with Thalassemia Major, A Pilot Study. *Indian Pediatr.* **2004**, *1* (7), 716–720.

Martinez, V. I.; Periago, M. J.; Ros, G. *Arch. Latinnam. Nutr.* **2000**, *50*, 5–18.

Mastan, M.; Prasad, U. V.; Parthasarathy, P. R. Protective Effect of *Bacopa monnieri* L. on Cytarabine Induced Biochemical Changein Chick Embryo. *Indian J. Clin. Biochem.* **2007**, *22*, 122–127.

Mokbel, M. S.; Hashinaga, F. Evaluation of the Antioxidant Activity of Extracts from Buntan (*Citrus grandis* Osbeck) Fruit Tissues. *Food Chem.* **2006**, *64*, 529–534.

Moriarty, P. M.; Picciano, M. F.; Beard, J. L. Classical Selenium Dependent Glutathione Peroxidase Expression is Decreased Secondary to Iron Deficiency in Rats. *J. Nutr.* **1995**, *125*, 293–301.

Mukhopdhyay, S.; Basak, J.; Kar, M.; Mandal, S.; Mukhopdhyay, A. The Role of Iron Chelation Activity of Wheat Grass Juice in Patients with Myelodysplastic Syndrome. *J. Clin. Oncol.* **2009**, *27*, 15.

Muhammad, S.; Muhammad, I.; Rashad, M.; Abdul, M.; Nighat, A.; Lubna, I.; Mehreen, L. *J. Asian Nat. Prod. Res.* **2009**, *11*, 945–950.

Nair, M. Alternate Strategies for Improving Iron Nutrition, Lessons from Recent Modalities. *Croat. Med. J.* **2002**, *43* (1), 16–19.

Srigiridhar, K.; Nair, K. M. Iron-Deficient Intestine is More Susceptible to Peroxidative Damage during Iron Supplementation in Rats. *Free Radic. Biol. Med.* **1998**, *25*, 660–665.

Nair, V. D.; Panneerselvam, R.; Gopi, R. Studies on Methanolic Extract of *Rauvolfia* Species from Southern Western Ghats of India—In Vitro Antioxidant Properties, Characterisation of Nutrients and Phytochemicals. *Ind. Crops Prod.* **2012**, *39*, 17–25.

Nagulendran, K. R.; Velavan, S.; Mahesh, R.; Hazeenabegum, V. In Vitro Antioxidant Activity and Total Poly Phenolic Content of *Cyperus rotundus* Rhizomes. *E-J. Chem.* **2007**, *4*, 440–449.

Navabi, S. M.; Navabi, S. F.; Setzer, W. N.; Alinezhad, H.; Zare, M.; Naqinezhad, A. Interaction of Different Extracts of *Primula heterochroma* Stapf. with Red Blood Cell Membrane Lipids and Proteins, Antioxidant and Antihaemolytic Effects. *J. Diet. Suppl.* **2012**, *9*, 285–292.

Nvvinuka, N. M.; Monanu, M. O.; Nwiloh, B. I. Effects of Aqueous Extract of *Mangifera indica* L. (Mango) Stem Bark on Haematological Parameters of Normal Albino Rats. *Pak. J. Nutr.* **2008**, *7* (5), 663–666.

Ogamba, J. O.; Eze, N. A.; Ogamba, S. E.; Chilaka, K. C. *Trop. J. Med. Res*. **2010**, *142*, 1–6.

Ogbe, R. J.; Adoga, G. I.; Abu, A. H. Antianaemic Potentials of Some Plant Extracts on Phenyl Hydrazine-Induced Anaemia in Rabbits. *J. Med. Plants Res.* **2010**, *4* (8), 680–684.

Okigbo, R. N.; Anuagasi, C. L.; Amadi, J. E. Advances in Selected Medicinal and Aromatic Plants Indigenous to Africa. *J. Med. Plants Res.* **2009**, *3* (2), 086–095.

Oladiji, A. T.; Jacob, T. O.; Yakubu, M. T. Anti-Anaemic Potentials of Aqueous Extract of *Sorghum bicolor* (L.) Moench Stem Bark in Rats. *J. Ethnopharmacol.* **2007**, *3*, 651–656.

Owoyele, B. V.; Adebukola, O. M.; et al. Anti-inflammatory Activities of Ethanolic Extract of *Carica papaya* Leaves. *Inflammopharmacology* **2008**, *16*, 168–173.

Papi, A.; Orlandi, M.; Bartolini, G.; Barillari, J.; Iori, R.; Paolini, M. *J Agric. Food Chem.* **2008**, *56*, 8750–8788.

Paech, D.; Tracey, M. V. *Modern Methods of Plant Analysis*, 4th ed.; Springer Verlag: Wieland, 1955; pp 371–373.

Pasricha, S.-R.; Drakesmith, H.; Black, J.; Hipgrave, D., Biggs, B.-A. Control of Iron Deficiency Anemia in Low-And Middle-Income Countries. *Blood* **2013**, *121* (14), 2607–2617.

Patel, D. K.; Kumar, R.; Kumar, M.; Sairam, K.; Hemalatha, S. Evaluation of Aldose Reductase Inhibitory Potential of Different Fraction of *Hybanthus enneaspermus* Linn F. Muell. *Asian Pac. J. Trop. Biomed.* **2012**, *2*, 134–139.

Paterson, R. R. Ganoderma – A Therapeutic Fungal Biofactory. *Phytochemistry* **2006**, *67*, 1985–2001.

Pednerkar, A.; Bhanu, R. Anti-microbial and Antioxidant Potential with FTIR Analysis of *Ampelocissus latifolia* (Roxb.) Planch. Leaf. *Asian J. Pharm. Clin. Res.* **2013**, *6* (1), 67–73.

Perez-Jimenez, J.; Saura-Calixto, F. *J. Agric. Food Chem.* **2005**, *53*, 5036–5040.

Prabhavathi, R. M.; Prasad, M. P.; Jayaramu, M. Studies on Qualitative and Quantitative Phytochemical Analysis of *Cissus quadrangularis*. *Adv. Appl. Sci. Res.* **2016**, *7* (4), 11–17.

Pullaiah, T.; Naidu, C. K. *Antidiabetic Plants in India and Herbal Based Antidiabetic Research*. Regency Publications: New Delhi, 2003; pp 68–69.

Ratnam, D.; Ankola, D. D.; Bhardwaj, V.; Sahana, D. K.; Kumar, R. M. N. V. *J. Control. Release* **2006**, *113*, 189–207.

Royer, M.; Diouf, P. N.; Stevanovic, T. Polyphenol Contents and Radical Scavenging Capacities of Red Maple (*Acer rubrum* L.) Extracts. *Food Chem. Toxicol.* **2011**, *49* (9), 2180–2188.

Richard, H. Chinese Herbal Medicine: Ancient Art and Modern Science.; Shocker Brook: New York, 1978; 49–52.

Sanni, F. S.; Ibrahim, S.; Esievo, K. A. N.; Sanni, S. Effect of Oral Administration of Aqueous Extract of Khaya Senegalensis Stem Bark on Phenyl Hydrazine-Induced Anaemia in Rats. *Pak. J. Biol. Sci.* **2005**, *8* (2), 255–258.

Shantabi, L., Jagetia, G. C., et al. Phyotchemical Screening of Certain Medicinal Plants of Mizoram, India and their Folklore Use. *Biodivers. Bioprospect. Dev.* **2014**, *2* (1), 1–9.

Sharda, S.; Shukla, A.; Singh, C. S.; Bigoniya, P. A Review on Herbal Anti-anaemia Plants RGI. *Int. J. Appl. Sci. Technol.* **2011**.

Shinde, U. A.; Phadke, A. S.; Nair, A. M.; Mungantiwar, A. A.; Dikshit, V. J. Membrane Stabilizing Activity—A Possible Mechanism of Action for the Anti-inflammatory Activity of *Cedrus deodara* Wood Oil. *Fitoterapia* **1999**, *70*, 251–257.

Shved, M. I.; Palamar, T. O. The Antioxidant Effects of Emoxipin in Patients with Iron Deficiency Anemia. *Lik. Sprava* **1995**, *9*, 72–75.

Singh, E.; Aishwarya, J.; Singh, A.; Tiwari, A. A Review, Nutraceutical Properties of *Piper betel*. *AJPCT* **2016**, *4* (2), 28–49.

Sripradha, S. Betel Leaf – The Green Gold. *J. Pharm. Sci. Res.* **2014**, *6* (1), 36–37.

Sofowora, A. *Medicinal Plants and Medicine in Africa*. Spectrum Books: Ibadan, Nigeria, 1993; pp 120–123.

Taheri, S.; Solati, A.; Moradi, P.; Tavassoly, A.; Yadi, J. Toxic Effects of *Nerium oleander* Aqueous Leaf Extract on Haematological Parameters and Histopathological Changes of the Lungs and Heart in Rabbits. *Comp. Clin. Pathol.* **2013**, *22* (6), 1189–1193.

Tirgarl, P. R.; Thumber, B. L.; Desai, T. R. Isolation Characterization and Biologocical Evaluation of Iron Chelator from *Triticum aestivum* (Wheatgrass). *Int. J. Pharm. Biosci.* **2011**, *2*, 288–296.

Tylor, B. S.; Kion, Y. M.; Wang, Q. I.; Sharpio, R. A.; Billar, T. R.; Geller, D. A. Nitric Oxide Down Regulates Hepatocyte – Inducible Nitric Oxide Synthase Gene Expression. *Arch. Surg.* **1997**, *61*, 400–407.

Vives, C. J. L.; Miguel-Garcia, A.; Pujades, M. A., et al. Increased Susceptibility of Microcytic red Blood Cells to In Vitro Oxidative Stress. *Eur. J. Haematol.* **1995,** *55,* 327–331.

William, M. Idiopathic Autoimmune Hemolytic Anaemia. *J. VeriMed Health Care Netw. Baltimore* **2006,** *15,* 741–449.

Yasuda, T.; Inaba, A.; Ohmori, M.; Endo, T.; Kubo, S.; Ohsawa, K. Urinary Metabolites of Gallic Acid in Rats and their Radical Scavenging Effect on DH. *J. Nat. Prod.* **2000,** *63,* 1444–1446.

Yildirim, A.; Mavi, A.; Kara, A. A. Determination of Antioxidant and Antimicrobial Activities of *Rumex crispus* L. Extracts. *J. Agric. Food Chem.* **2001,** *49,* 4083–4089.

Zhuang, X. P.; Lu, Y. Y.; Yang, G. S. Extraction and Determination of Flavonoid in Ginkgo. *Chin. Herb. Med.* **1992,** *23,* 122–124.

CHAPTER 3

Role of Free Radicals during Infection and the Advancement of Antioxidants to Improve the Treatment of Infectious Diseases

MANITOSH PANDEY[1,2*], SONIA JOHRI[2], and SAKSHI TALWAR[1]

[1]Translational Health Science and Technology Institute, Faridabad, India

[2]Department of Life Sciences, ITM University, Gwalior, Madhya Pradesh, India

Corresponding author. E-mail: manitosh@thsti.res.in

ABSTRACT

Viruses, bacteria, and fungi invade the host cells and activate their machinery to escape from the host defense system. Hostage environment for the foreign particle activates the combat between immune system and microorganism. Adjunct therapy is usually administered along with regular therapy for better clinical outcomes. Since it is known that antioxidants improve immune response against various bacterial and viral infections, antioxidant supplements are often given for their treatment. In HIV-infected people, low concentrations of macro- and micronutrients are associated with increased disease progression and high mortality. Supplementing antiretroviral therapy (HAART) along with multivitamins has been shown to delay the disease progression. The adjunct therapy of vitamins A, C, and E improves T cell-mediated immune response and T-cell proliferation.

3.1 INTRODUCTION

Oxygen is a vital form of life and indispensable element for the survival. Cells utilize the oxygen to generate energy and building blocks of life. Human body maintains the level of oxygen according to the energy requirement. Toxic intermediates are also generated during the energy production process. ROS (reactive oxygen species) and RNS (reactive nitrogen species) are major intermediates that are the bioproducts of oxygen reduction and cellular respiration. Delicately, both the intermediates are maintained by a healthy cell during survival. Inadequate and high level of these intermediates start deteriorating the cell physiology and promote the oxidative burst to eliminate the cell. Several mechanisms have been used by human body to counter these free radicals. Irregular or overproduction of ROS and RNS inside the cell creates a cytotoxic milieu that causes the damage in the tissue or organ. Alcohol intake, smoking, air pollution, and fast food are some external factors that also increase the ROS inside the body. Oxidative stress plays a critical role during chronic infection, cancer metastasis, and in autoimmune disease. Immune system also utilizes oxidative burst as a strategy to eradicate or eliminate the pathogen form the host, while microorganisms modulate the free radical activity through the microbial cytotoxins to escape from the immune system.

Antioxidants work as a free radical scavenger to maintain the balance inside the cell. Cell synthesized the endogenous antioxidants such as SOD—superoxide dismutase, CAT—catalase, GPx—glutathione peroxidase, and GRx—glutathione reductase enzymes to counter the free radicals. Vitamins E and C also work as an antioxidant and help to improve the immunity. Adjunct therapy of antioxidants with the recognized therapy could be an auspicious path for the treatment of several diseases.

3.1.1 FREE RADICALS DURING PATHOGENESIS

Origination and development of a disease is known as pathogenesis. During the span of disease progression, host machinery actively used its defense mechanism to neutralize the active disease progression. Foreign particle or microorganism such as viruses, bacteria, and fungi invades the host cells and tissues and activates their machinery to hide or escape from the host defense system. Hostage environment for the foreign particle activates the combat between immune system and microorganism.

NADPH oxidase 2 (NOX2) starts the production of ROS in response to microbial interaction and starts respiratory burst mechanism to get rid of microbes.[1] Two transmembrane proteins, CYBB and CYBA, formed an enzymatic complex of NADPH oxidase, and their activation brings cytosolic components—NCF-1, NCF-2, NCF-4. Inside the phagosome, O_2^- generated by the transfer of electrons by oxidase transferase to NADPH[2] quickly dismutates into H_2O_2. Fenton reaction converts H_2O_2 into free radical OH^-. Peroxynitrite ($ONOO^-$), a highly reactive reagent, generated after interaction of nitric oxide (NO) and O_2^-.[3] Nitrogen-based free radicals or RNS also contribute to elimination of microorganisms.[4] Conversion of L-arginine and oxygen into L-citrulline and NO is catalyzed by NOS2. Production of NO directly impairs the growth of microbes.[5] The first contact between microorganisms and host is plasma membrane. Through Haber–Weiss reaction, O_2^- and H_2O_2 generate $HO·$, a highly reactive hydroxyl radical. Fenton reaction required iron for the generation of $HO·$ present in broken cells or lysed cells.[6] Cobalt-based radicals could be produced by the Coin cyanocobalamin and healthy cells, which prevent the production of these radicals.[7] A di-heme protein is myeloperoxidase (MPO) composed from two identical heterodimers, and these polypeptide chains are connected to each other via disulfide bonds.[8] MPO is present in neutrophil cytoplasmic granules with a very elevated level. Researchers predicted that MPO–H_2O_2-dependent reaction plays a crucial role during pathogen elimination.[9] Patients with lack of MPO in neutrophils are thought to be immunocompromised[10] and recent experiment done by researchers shows that MPO-deficient mice show susceptibility to various pathogens differentially.[11-13] Cell homeostasis required low level of ROS production to maintain antioxidant response, intermediate level of ROS to activate the NF-kB step in proinflammatory, antiapoptotic response for adaptation and survival, and higher level of ROS production to induce the cell apoptosis and deterioration of cell.[14]

3.1.2 PATHOGENS AND FREE RADICALS, LOVE–HATE RELATIONSHIP

3.1.2.1   INTRACELLULAR

Class of bacteria that evade host system to survive inside the cell is known as intracellular bacteria. They are proficient to grow and replicate inside the host cell by hijacking host machinery. They are divided into faculta-tive and obligate intracellular pathogens. To escape from the host defense machinery, they used several metal ions and masking mechanism to avoid host abuse.

3.1.2.1.1 Salmonella

Despite modern-day sanitation and treatment regimens, *Salmonella enterica* act as facultative intracellular, pathogen causative agent of intestinal and invasive disease. *Salmonella* has property to degrade superoxide through periplasmic SOD, and sodCI is also important for the virulence *Salmonella typhimurium* in phox-competent mice.[15,16] *S. typhimurium* replicates in endosomal compartment in low pH condition.[17] To counter the superoxide diffusing in cytoplasm, its codes SodA and SodB superoxide dismutase.[18] Upregulation of genes sitABCD and manganese transporter system *mntH* leads to degradation of superoxide.[19] Efflux pump MacAB helps to detoxifi-cation of H_2O_2 and also helps *S. typhimurium* to survive and replicate inside the murinemonocytes.[20] DNA repair machinery of *S. typhimurium* lexA, sulA, and recA plays a critical role during ROS tolerance.[21,22] SP1 and SP2 code a type II secretion system involved in translocating effector proteins into host during bacterial host interaction. NF-kB translocation is tackled by SPI1 effector protein AvrA (avirulence protein A), dodged by the expression of cytokines and iNOS in phagocytes.[23] SsrB, response regulator of SPI2, becomes *S*-nitrosylated at cys 203 during NO stress, thus helping bacteria to counter the RNS.[24]

3.1.2.1.2 Mycobacterium tuberculosis

Modulation of plasma membrane is dependent on the microorganism and its path of infection. For example, intracellular pathogen, *Mycobacterium tuberculosis*, exploits the phagocytosis by alveolar macrophages with several factors, lipoarabinomannan (LAM), phenolic glycolipid and phenol phthiocerol diester (PGL-1), trehalose dimycolate (TDM), and protein kinase G (PknG), which help bacteria to protect from host stresses.[25–28] Two NADH dehydrogenases are present in *M. tuberculosis* NDH-1, a multiprotein complex, encoded by operon *nuoABCDEFGHIJKLMN*, NDH-2, essential and required for the growth in vitro and in mouse model.[29] Mutation in *ndh* causes the accumulation of NADH and leads to resistance to isoniazid and ethambutol.[30] Accumulation of NADH also shows resistance to peroxide, acidified nitrite, and ROS.[31,32] TrxR (thioredoxin reductase and thioredoxin) shows disulfide reductase activity and regulates dithiol–disulfide balance to protect *M. tuberculosis* from ROS.[33] Alkyl hydroperoxide subunit C, *AhpC* an alternative peroxidase system, contains three cysteine residues during its active state and detoxify organic peroxide by decreasing into less reactive alcohol derivatives.[34,35] Secreting out the antioxidant enzymes into the host, *M. tuberculosis* controls the abnormal redox situation. KatG is a virulence factor and a key player to provide peroxynitritase, catalase, and peroxide activity during survival inside host.[36] *M. tuberculosis* also contains metalloenzymes such as SodA (FeSOD), a major secretory protein required in homeostatic condition and found to be impart protection against superoxide in vitro. SodC (CuZnSOD) is anchored on the cell wall and protects *M. tuberculosis* from ROS. With the help of DoxX (membrane protein) and SseA (thiol oxidoreductase) forms a membrane-associated oxidoreductase complex that detoxifies the radicals by cytosolic thiol homeostasis. Mycothiol (MSH) is a low-molecular-weight thiol work as a mycobacterial redox buffer in *M. tuberculosis*, which helps bacteria to overcome the oxidative environment in host.[37,38]

3.1.2.1.3 *Plasmodium falciparum*

Plasmodium falciparum invades red blood cells and causes breakdown of hemoglobin. *P. falciparum* is subtle to oxidative stress. Infection induces the generation of hydroxyl radicals in the liver, which cause apoptosis and oxidative stress.[39] Several antioxidant enzymes have been characterized in *P. falciparum*, glutathione synthase that are critical for survival during erythrocytic stage of malaria infection and maintaining reduced intracellular environment to protect oxidative damage.[40] Glutathione reductase plays a central role in antioxidant defense in different phases of infection.[41] SOD is first-line defense against free radicals and *P. falciparum* expresses cytosolic (Fe-SOD) and mitochondrial SOD-2.[42] Glutamate dehydrogenase, GDH, helps to maintain the redox state of the cell and it is a major player for the production of NAD(P)+ in erythrocytes.[43] Glucose 6-phosphate dehydrogenase is a bifunctional enzyme and helps the growth of *P. falciparum* in blood stages.[44] Thioredoxin (Trx) and peroxiredoxins (Prxs) are the part of this system, it maintains reduced environment via thioredoxin reductase

(TrxR), and five thioredoxin systems were identified in *P. falciparum*.[45] α-Tocopherol, known as vitamin, works as a cofactor in different reactions. *P. falciparum* synthesizes vitamin E and works as a potent antioxidant that plays an important role to protect polyunsaturated fatty acids from lipid peroxidation and also helps to maintain ROS levels.[46]

3.1.2.1.4   *Francisella tularensis*

Francisella tularensis is a facultative intracellular pathogen and causative agent of tularemia, a lethal human disease. It infects, macrophages, neutrophils, dendritic cells, and hepatocytes, erythrocytes.[47] *F. tularensis* has a variety of antioxidant enzymatic pathways to tackle the host free radical defense strategy. Major facilitator superfamily-type Emr multidrug efflux pump extracellularly secretes SodB, an iron-containing SOD. SodC is a copper–zinc-containing SOD present in periplasm of *F. tularensis* and protects it from oxidative stress.[48] katG gene encodes a catalase with helps to convert H_2O_2 into H_2O and O_2.[49] *F. tularensis* also encodes Gpx, glutathione peroxidase, MoxR ATpases, Dyp-type peroxidase, GrxA, glutaredoxin A, and methionine sulfoxide reductase (MSR) A, A1, and B.[50,51] OxyR, a highly conserved LysR family regulator, is also present in *F. tularensis*, which regulates the expression of antioxidant enzymes genes, KatG, and alkyl hydroperoxide reductase (ahpC).[52] ahpC belongs to a family of peroxiredoxins and it helps bacteria to scavenge the H_2O_2. AhpC is a crucial antioxidant enzyme in *F. tularensis*, which contributes strong ROS and RNS defense during hostile combat. Deletion of these gene form *F. tularensis* shows attenuation in animal model and showed sensitivity to oxidative and nitrosativestress.[53]

3.1.2.1.5   *Anaplasma phagocytophilum*

To establish an infection in host, *Anaplasma phagocytophilum* induces complex cellular changes, majorly transcriptional alteration and proteomic initiation. Granulocyte and neutrophils conduct the major oxidative defense but *A. phagocytophilum* does not induce ROS as a part of survival inside the host. It reduces the gp91 and p22 subunits of NADPH oxidase in its phagosome membrane.[54] Infection of *A. phagocytophilum* decreases the production of heme-responsive gene 1 protein levels that reduce the heme release into the cytoplasm of midgut cells to decrease the antimicrobial stress caused by ROS.[55] Tick cells decrease MT antioxidants defenses mediated by thioredoxin reductase catalase peroxisomes and glutaredoxin to accumulate ROS, increase the mtROS production limit *A. phagocytophilum* infection. A compensatory mechanism by the host downregulates the AOES to reduce MT antioxidant shield to decrease the ROS levels to protect the cell integrity to limit pathogen infection[56] while pathogen also inhibits alternate pathways of free radical production to intact the cell morphology and fitness. *A. phagocytophilum* uses a common strategy to infect both the host that could be associated with host-specific cell tropism during its life cycle.

3.1.2.1.6   Chlamydia trachomatis

Chlamydia trachomatis is a common sexually transmitted disease causing a gamut disease, urethritis, cervicitis, proctitis, and blinding trachoma. During infection inside the host, ROS is used alternatively as an advantage by stimulating caspase-1.[57] Its triggers activation of oncogenic pathway components Ras–Raf–MEK–ERK and ROS production to promote the growth inside the cell.[57–59] NOX and NLRX1 mediated ROS response promoted by *C. trachomatis*.[57] γH2AX levels and DSB production promoted by the ROS production to increase the growth rate of *C. trachomatis* inside the cell. H, N, K, RAS members of GTPase superfamily activate during infection and known to induce and regulate the production of ROS in cancer cell proliferation.[60,61] Several researchers have shown in their study that C. trachomatis requires ROS production for normal development.[61–63]

3.1.2.1.7   Bacillus anthracis

Bacillus anthracis is a Gram-positive bacterium, causative agent of anthrax, and contains a number of antioxidants enzyme to counter free radicals defense during infection. It contains arginase enzyme that metabolizes L-arginine to L-ornithine and urea to decrease RNS produced by macrophages.[64] Four SODs, SOD15, SODA1, SODC, and SODA2, provide redundant protection from oxidative stress.[65] They have distinct functional activity to protect bacteria from exogenous and endogenous ROS according to their localization in the bacteria. Deletion of SOD15 and SODA1 showed a decrease resistance to oxidative stress but not attenuated in A/J mouse model. Deletion of all four SODs from *B. anthracis* genome showed sensitivity when inoculated intranasally in mice.[65]

3.1.2.2　EXTRACELLULAR

Pathogens that can grow and replicate freely on mucosal surfaces or in the tissue outside host cells of the body to generate infection are known as extracellular pathogens.

3.1.2.2.1　*Burkholderia cenocepacia*

Burkholderia cenocepacia is complex highly pathogenic and intrinsically resistant to multiple stresses and antibiotics. Xanthine oxidase is a key enzyme of purine catabolism pass e⁻ to oxygen to form free ROS and also helps in reduction of nitrite to produce RNS. P47[(phox−/−)] mice show reduced clearance of B. cenocepacia infection compared to wild-type mice,[66] which decipher the role of xanthine oxidase that contribute to generate ROS to clear ROS-sensitive pathogen and play a crucial role in host defense particularly in gastrointestinal tract.[67] Different antibiotics enhance the production of ROS in cells to clear the infection. To avoid antibiotic induced ROS insult, *B. cenocepacia* secretes putrescine protein and helps in generation of resistance against antibiotic induced ROS production.[68]

3.1.2.2.2　*Pseudomonas aeruginosa*

Pseudomonas aeruginosa is an opportunistic pathogen, causative agent of nosocomial infection in immunocompromised patients. *P. aeruginosa* evolved itself to counter immune defense mechanism of host. Antioxidants, enzymes, catalase, *SOD,* alkyl hydroperoxide reductase, and thiol peroxidase degrade ROS toxicity. Methionine sulfoxide reductases are essential during high oxidative damage condition. A tripeptide thiol molecule GSH (glutathione) maintains the cellular homeostasis. GSH is plentifully present inside the cell and provides protection against oxidative stress after interaction with free radicals.[69] Deletion of gshA and gshB genes involved in GSH biosynthesis increased the susceptibility to ROS and RES in *P. aeruginosa*. Loss of GSH genes in *P. aeruginosa* causes severe defect in drosophila model system.[69] ttcA protect bacteria from oxidative stress, lack of ttcA bacteria hypersensitive to H_2O_2 treatment. Deletion of ttcA gene hypersensitive to H_2O_2 treatment and protect for oxidative stress. During infection, oxyR upregulates katA and ttcA expression to enhance catalase activity in response to oxidative stress against host defense mechanism.[70]

3.1.2.2.3   Neisseria gonorrhoeae

Neisseria gonorrhoeae is a Gram-negative diplococcus bacterium causing sexual-transmitted infection known as gonorrhoea. *N. gonorrhoeae* has ability to survive inside the host and evolves its machinery to tackle different stress during infection. SOD was essential for all aerobic bacteria but only SodB is present in *N. gonorrhoeae*. SodB is upregulated during oxidative stress but deletion of SodB will not affect the viability of bacteria but activity of SodB in vitro. Activity of SodB is dependent on iron availability. In contrast, *Neisseria meningitidis* contains SodB and SodC enzymes. SodB in *N. meningitidis* protects from oxidative stress and SodC plays a major role in virulence in a mouse model.[71] *N. gonorrhoeae* accumulates manganese by MntABC transport machinery. mntAB deletion shows severely growth defect even with Mn-supplemented media and mntC has shown severe susceptibility to superoxide and accumulation of Mn also impaired in mntC mutant of *N. gonorrhoeae*.[72,73] Cytoplasmic catalase (KatA) and periplasmic cytochrome c peroxidase (CcP) protect bacteria against H_2O_2 activity in vitro. Deletion of ccp/katA double-knockout strain is more susceptible to in vitro H_2O_2 stress than single katA gene deletion.[71] Methionine sulfoxide reductase (MsrA/B) and (Bfr) bacterioferritin upregulate in response to H_2O_2 stress and also provide a stealthy oxidative defense during oxidative stress.[74] MerR, like transcription regulator NmlR, activates upon exposure to disulfide and redox stress and plays a critical role in defense against RNS. It is a Zn-dependent transcription regulator and deletion of nmlR shows sensitive to hyperoxide, diamide, and nitric oxide compared to wild-type strain.[75]

3.1.2.2.4   Staphylococcus aureus

Staphylococcus species and subspecies represent a wide variety of acute and chronic infection in different hosts. *Staphylococcus* aureus produces carotenoid pigments synthesized from crtPQMN operon quench toxic free radical and plays a crucial role for detoxifying ROS. Crt mutant grows normally but shows sensitivity against ROS, OONO⁻, and HOCl.[76] *S. aureus* possesses two SODs, SodA and SodM. SodA is induced by in vivo stress or internal stress conditions and SodM by exogenous oxidative stress. Both Sods work to maintain cell viability in oxidative stress condition.[77] *S. aureus* has AhpC peroxiredoxin induced during H_2O_2 treatment. Peroxiredoxin detoxifies alkyl hydroperoxides with the help of NADH or NADPH. Mutant strains lacking catalase and AhpC loss inhibit their ability to counter exogenous and endogenous H_2O_2 and show accumulation of H_2O_2.[78] The presence of thioredoxin in *S. aureus* also protects from free radicals and maintains reduced state. *S. aureus* genome also contains paralog of msrA (msrA1, msrA2, MsrA3) and msrB gene to prevent methionine oxidation. Deletion of msrA1 makes bacteria susceptible to oxidative stress. Iron–sulfur cluster proteins also play important during stress conditions in many bacteria.[79,80] Oxidative stress causes severe damage to bacterial proteins and this facilitates by ScdA gene in *S. aureus*. ScdA deletion increased the sensitivity to H_2O_2.[81] PerR is member from Fur family of transcription factor in *S. aureus*. PerR activity depends on the metal ions, presence of high Mn^{2+}, and low Fe^{2+} regulon members repressed during H_2O_2 stress. Deletion of per Rs lightly defected in mouse model. *S. aureus* contains bacterial (bNOS) nitric oxide synthase, and expression of bNOS makes bacteria more resistant to oxidative, neutrophil killing. Nitrite avoids bacterial killing by scavenging HOCL.[82]

3.1.2.2.5   Entamoeba histolytica

Entamoeba histolytica is an enteric protozoan parasite, causative agent of human amoebiasis. It is an anaerobic parasite and maintains intracellular hypoxia during invasion process. During confrontation of several stresses, trophozoites arouse cysteine synthase activity to prevent glycolysis and promote ER-like stress response.[83] Due to the lack of glutathione, this organism has trypanothione, an uncommon form of glutathione. L-Cysteine works as a major thiol in *E. histolytica*.[84] Cultivate amoebas in the absence of L-cysteine ROS levels are higher. Iron–sulfur cluster is vulnerable to oxidative and nitrosative stress. Cysteine plays a crucial role to maintain the integrity of Fe–S cluster. *E. histolytica* has several shielding mechanisms such as thiol-dependent peroxidase (Eh29), SOD, cysteine proteinase 5 (EhCP-5), HSP-70, and peptidylprolyl isomerase from host stresses.[83,85] Overexpression of P-type ATPase/flippase (EhPTPA) and adhesion factor EhSIAF enhanced survival in response to oxidative stress.[86]

3.1.2.2.6 Yersinia pestis

Yersinia pestis is causative agent of bubonic plague and has adaptive response toward H_2O_2 and OCl^-.[87] OxyR transcription factor induces bacterial catalase–peroxidase detoxifying enzymes. O_2^- countered by SoxRS two-component system induces the SOD activity.[88] Flavohemoglobin detoxifies the NO stress in vitro and in macrophages.[87] Yersinia used type III secretion system to translocate effectors for the disruption of phagocytosis and six Yop effectors (YopM, YopT, YopJ/P, YpkA/YopO, YopE, and YopH) which have been identified. YopE is known to be a major player in promoting virulence by inhibiting ROS.[89] These effectors downregulate the signaling path of host defense system for survival in host milieu.

3.2 IMMUNITY AND FREE RADICALS

Free radicals play an important role in natural as well as acquired immune response. Cells like macrophages and neutrophils during cellular processes like respiratory burst result in the production of free radicals such as hypochlorous acid, hydroxyl, peroxynitrite that are bactericidal. Also, oxidative stress can have damaging effects in acquired immunity as it results in NF-Kappa B activation, which in turn induces the expression of cytokines and chemokines and cell adhesion molecules as well.[90]

3.3 INNATE IMMUNITY AND PHAGOCYTOSIS

Neutrophils and macrophages are two of the leukocytes that migrate toward site of infection/inflammation and results in phagocytosis. Phagocytosis mainly involves engulfment of foreign antigen and subsequent killing and digestion.[91] It also involves stimulation of respiratory burst resulting in generation of ROS and nitrogen species. RNS have also shown to be important in certain infectious diseases. Two types of enzymes iNOS (induced-nitric oxide synthase) and cNOS (constitutive) result in generation of RNS from L-arginine. RNS are mainly produced by various cell types, including macrophages, mast cells, neutrophils, vascular smooth muscle cells, and endothelial cells. iNOS is known as killer molecule as it can continuously produce large amount of nitric oxide.[92]

Studies have shown that production of peroxynitrite by macrophages, a form of RNS, happens during *Escherichia coli* infection and its killing is directly proportional to the concentration of RNS.[93] Also, Gregory et al.[94] have demonstrated that overproduction of nitric oxide by mice infected with *Listeria monocytogenes* results in suppression of immune cell proliferation, which in turn suppresses host immunes response. Nitric oxide has been shown to be important in defense against mycobacteria, fungi, helminth, and various protozoan infections.[95,96]

3.4   ANTIOXIDANTS AND THE IMMUNE SYSTEM

Free radicals such as lipoperoxides, aldehydes are also generated by lipid peroxidation, which is an autocatalytic reaction. Lipid peroxidation results in altered immune system because of bilipid cell membrane damage. Intact membrane is necessary for antigen recognition, secretion of cytokines and chemokines, etc. It has been proposed that generation of these ROS and RNS in aging and during various disease conditions also affect that integral membrane function, including cell-mediated immune response.[97,98]

3.5   OXIDATIVE STRESS AND VIRAL INFECTIONS

Not much is known about the role of ROS and RNS in viral infections but it is clear that they play vital role in viral inactivation.[99] Studies have shown that ROS are important in viral infections like influenza, HIV, measles, and hepatitis.[100] It has been shown that deficiency of vitamin A is associated with occurrence of severe measles, pneumonia, and high mortality rate. Deficiency of vitamin E has been shown to be associated with coxsackievirus B3.[100] *N*-Acetylcysteine that is a precursor of anti-oxidant GSH has been shown to attenuated the symptoms of influenza during winters. It has been shown by in vitro studies that enhanced ROS production leads to increased HIV because of activation of TNF-alpha and NF-kB.[101] Mycoplasma, influenza, and paramyxoviruses lead to the production of ROS by directly interacting with macrophages, which in turn increase HIV replication. Patients with HIV infection have been reported to be under chronic oxidative stress.[101]

3.6 ANTIOXIDANTS AND ITS ROLE TO IMPROVE IMMUNITY

Antioxidants are the substances that quench free radicals and maintain health in both humans and animals. All living systems require optimum balance of free radicals in order to prevent the harmful effects of ROS and RNS to immune system. Various dietary micronutrients such as vitamin C, vitamin E, and carotene act as antioxidants. Also, minerals such as manganese, zinc, and copper are required for activity of SOD that is a potent antioxidant. Iron and selenium are required for the activity of catalase and glutathione peroxidase, respectively. Minerals such as folic acid are required for cell-mediated immune response, copper for cytokine response.[102]

Thus, minerals do not directly have antioxidant properties but are required for the activity of antioxidant enzymes.[14,103]

Vitamin A is known as anti-infective vitamin and its deficiency is associated with many diseases. Vitamin A is required for the development and proper functioning of B and T lymphocytes. Thus, decreased vitamin A levels result in decreased cell–mediated immune response and lower and lower antibody production. Also, during inflammation, superoxide radicals are produced that are essential for killing antigen/pathogen. Under these conditions, antioxidants are essential to maintain the level of free radicals. Riboflavin improves humoral immune response, vitamin B6 is required for lymphocyte maturation and differentiation, and vitamin B12 is required for proper neutrophil functioning.[102]

Antioxidants such as vitamins and minerals are absolutely required in order to prevent bacterial and viral infections. A lot of studies have shown the effect of macro- and micronutrients on immune cell function and their impact on protection against infectious microorganisms. Overall, antioxidant supplements also decrease the rate of aging, it results in increased IL-2 levels, increased antibody response to antigen, increased killer activity of NK cells, decreased peroxidation of lipids, increased in number of B and T lymphocytes, etc. Thus antioxidants improve the immune response of humans against various infectious and noninfectious diseases.[104]

3.7   USE OF ANTIOXIDANTS AS AN ADJUNCT THERAPY

Adjunct therapy is usually administered along with regular therapy for better clinical outcomes. Since it is known that antioxidants improve immune response against various bacterial and viral infections, antioxidant supplements are often given for their treatment.

- A number of pathogenic bacteria form biofilm inside human and animal host act as protective barrier for and help in developing persistent infections that are difficult to treat. Studies have shown that the use of NAC (*N*-acetylcysteine) that is a precursor of antioxidant glutathione is effective in both destroying the already developed biofilm and also prevents the formation of biofilm when given in combination with the regular therapy.[105]
- In another study in *B. cenocepacia*, which causes respiratory infections in patients with cystic fibrosis, releases bacterial lipcalin protein BcnA when exposed to antibiotics, making them ineffective and resulting in antimicrobial resistance. It has been shown that the water-soluble and lipid-soluble forms of vitamin E inhibit the binding of BcnA to antibiotics. Thus, vitamin E increases the killing by bactericidal antibiotics through interfering with BcnA binding.[106]
- Zinc is an important micronutrient required for proper functioning of immune system. It is required for development and function of neutrophils, macrophages, NK cells, T and B cells. Cytokine production, phagocytosis, and killing of pathogens are affected by zinc levels. It also functions as antioxidant and stabilizes the membrane thus preventing damage by free radicals produced during inflammation.[107]
- Zinc oral adjunct supplementation has been known to decrease severity and mortality because of diarrhea and pneumonia in children below 5 years of age. In 2004, WHO and UNICEF have recommended the use of zinc adjunct therapy in all childhood episodes of diarrhea.

- Studies, published in Lancet by Bhatnagar et al. have demonstrated the use of zinc as an adjunct therapy along with antibiotics against pneumonia, sepsis, and meningitis in infants showed better clinical outcomes.[108]
- Studies have shown that benign strains of influenza and coxsackieviruses mutate to pathogenic strains under selenium deficiency conditions. Selenium supplement improves their clinical outcomes. Selenium supplementation has been shown to improve the clinical outcomes of HIV and *M. tuberculosis* coinfection. Selenium levels affect both innate and adaptive immune systems. It also helps in differentiation of naïve CD-4 T cells toward T helper cells, thus improving cellular immune response. Also, tissue damage by excessive activation of immune response is prevented by polarizing the macrophages toward M-2 type.[109]
- In *M. tuberculosis*, it has been shown that in guinea pig during infection, there is an increase in the level of oxidative stress during the first 2 weeks of infection as measured by decreased in the blood glutathione levels and increased levels of malondialdehyde within the granulomatous lesions. Treatment of *M. tuberculosis*–infected guinea pigs with *N*-acetylcysteine (NAC) has been shown to restore the blood glutathione levels and decreased bacterial burden in both lung and spleen. Thus, taking a cue from the guinea pig studies, the antioxidants can be tested as adjunct therapy in anti-TB treatment regimen in humans for better clinical outcomes.[110]

Vitamin A has also been used as adjunct therapy in various infections. It improves the immune response when given at the time of immunization. Studies have suggested the role of vitamin A in recovery of children infected with measles. High doses of vitamin A during measles infection reduce the mortality and morbidity rate in children. It has been shown that vitamin A improves antibody titers.

In this regard, vitamin E supplementation may be useful in the treatment of patients with AIDS. Further evidence of the role of oxidative stress comes from an established increased synthesis of interferon-gamma in HIV infections. This cytokine enhances macrophage production of ROS, as well as neopterin and its reduced form, 7,8-dihydroneopterin, and both compounds play significant roles in free radical-mediated processes, which can lead to apoptosis.

In HIV-infected people, low concentrations of macro- and micronutrients are associated with increased disease progression and high mortality. Supplementing antiretroviral therapy (HAART) along with multivitamins has been shown to delay the disease progression. The adjunct therapy includes vitamin A that improves lymphocyte response, vitamin C that improves cell-mediated immune response, and vitamin E improves T cell–mediated immune response and T-cell proliferation.[102]

KEYWORDS

- **antiretroviral therapy**
- **immune response**
- **antioxidants**
- **disease progression**

REFERENCES

1. Nguyen, G. T.; Green, E. R.; Mecsas, J. Neutrophils to the ROScue, Mechanisms of NADPH Oxidase Activation and Bacterial Resistance. *Front. Cell Infect. Microbiol.* **2017,** *7*, 373.
2. Cross, A. R.; Segal, A. W. The NADPH Oxidase of Professional Phagocytes— Prototype of the NOX Electron Transport Chain Systems. *Biochim. Biophys. Acta* **2004,** *1657* (1), 1–22.
3. Samuel, E. L.; Marcano, D. C.; Berka, V.; Bitner, B. R.; Wu, G.; Potter, A.; Fabian, R. H.; Pautler, R. G.; Kent, T. A.; Tsai, A. L.; Tour, J. M. Highly Efficient Conversion of Superoxide to Oxygen using Hydrophilic Carbon Clusters. *Proc. Natl. Acad. Sci. U.S..A.* **2015,** *112* (8), 2343–2348.
4. Weidinger, A.; Kozlov, A. V. Biological Activities of Reactive Oxygen and Nitrogen Species, Oxidative Stress versus Signal Transduction. *Biomolecules* **2015,** *5* (2), 472–484.
5. Forstermann, U.; Sessa, W. C. Nitric Oxide Synthases, Regulation and Function. *Eur. Heart J.* **2012,** *33* (7), 829–837, 837a–837d.
6. Segal, A. W. How Neutrophils Kill Microbes. *Annu. Rev. Immunol.* **2005,** *23*, 197–223.
7. Banerjee, R.; Ragsdale, S. W. The Many Faces of Vitamin B12, Catalysis by Cobalamin-Dependent Enzymes. *Annu. Rev. Biochem.* **2003,** *72*, 209–247.
8. Fiedler, T. J.; Davey, C. A.; Fenna, R. E. X-Ray Crystal Structure and Characterization of Halide-Binding Sites of Human Myeloperoxidase at 1.8 A Resolution. *J. Biol. Chem.* **2000,** *275* (16), 11964–11971.

9. Klebanoff, S. J.; Kettle, A. J.; Rosen, H.; Winterbourn, C. C.; Nauseef, W. M. Myeloperoxidase, A Front-Line Defender against Phagocytosed Microorganisms. *J. Leukoc. Biol.* **2013,** *93* (2), 185–198.

10. Lehrer, R. I.; Hanifin, J.; Cline, M. J. Defective Bactericidal Activity in Myeloperoxidase-Deficient Human Neutrophils. *Nature* **1969,** *223* (5201), 78–79.

11. Aratani, Y.; Koyama, H.; Nyui, S.; Suzuki, K.; Kura, F.; Maeda, N. Severe Impairment in Early Host Defense against *Candida albicans* in Mice Deficient in Myeloperoxidase. *Infect. Immun.* **1999,** *67* (4), 1828–1836.

12. Aratani, Y.; Kura, F.; Watanabe, H.; Akagawa, H.; Takano, Y.; Suzuki, K.; Maeda, N.; Koyama, H. Differential Host Susceptibility to Pulmonary Infections with Bacteria and Fungi in Mice Deficient in Myeloperoxidase. *J. Infect. Dis.* **2000,** *182* (4), 1276–1279.

13. Gaut, J. P.; Yeh, G. C.; Tran, H. D.; Byun, J.; Henderson, J. P.; Richter, G. M.; Brennan, M. L.; Lusis, A. J.; Belaaouaj, A.; Hotchkiss, R. S.; Heinecke, J. W. Neutrophils Employ the Myeloperoxidase System to Generate Antimicrobial Brominating and Chlorinating Oxidants during Sepsis. *Proc. Natl. Acad. Sci. U.S.A.* **2001,** *98* (21), 11961–11966.

14. Kurutas, E. B. The Importance of Antioxidants which Play the Role in Cellular Response against Oxidative/Nitrosative Stress, Current State. *Nutr. J.* **2016,** *15* (1), 71.

15. De Groote, M. A.; Ochsner, U. A.; Shiloh, M. U.; Nathan, C.; McCord, J. M.; Dinauer, M. C.; Libby, S. J.; Vazquez-Torres, A.; Xu, Y.; Fang, F. C. Periplasmic Superoxide Dismutase Protects *Salmonella* from Products of Phagocyte NADPH-Oxidase and Nitric Oxide Synthase. *Proc. Natl. Acad. Sci. U.S.A.* **1997,** *94* (25), 13997–14001.

16. Uzzau, S.; Bossi, L.; Figueroa-Bossi, N. Differential Accumulation of *Salmonella* [Cu, Zn] Superoxide Dismutases SodCI and SodCII in Intracellular Bacteria, Correlation with their Relative Contribution to Pathogenicity. *Mol. Microbiol.* **2002,** *46* (1), 147–156.

17. Allam, U. S.; Krishna, M. G.; Sen, M.; Thomas, R.; Lahiri, A.; Gnanadhas, D. P.; Chakravortty, D. Acidic pH Induced STM1485 Gene is Essential for Intracellular Replication of *Salmonella*. *Virulence* **2012,** *3* (2), 122–135.

18. Najmuldeen, H.; Alghamdi, R.; Alghofaili, F.; Yesilkaya, H. Functional Assessment of Microbial Superoxide Dismutase Isozymes Suggests a Differential Role for Each Isozyme. *Free Radic. Biol. Med.* **2019,** *134,* 215–228.

19. Kroger, C.; Colgan, A.; Srikumar, S.; Handler, K.; Sivasankaran, S. K.; Hammarlof, D. L.; Canals, R.; Grissom, J. E.; Conway, T.; Hokamp, K.; Hinton, J. C. An infection-Relevant Transcriptomic Compendium for *Salmonella enterica* Serovar Typhimurium. *Cell Host Microbe* **2013,** *14* (6), 683–695.

20. Bogomolnaya, L. M.; Andrews, K. D.; Talamantes, M.; Maple, A.; Ragoza, Y.; Vazquez-Torres, A.; Andrews-Polymenis, H. The ABC-Type Efflux Pump MacAB Protects *Salmonella enterica* Serovar Typhimurium from Oxidative Stress. *MBio* **2013,** *4* (6), e00630-13.

21. Humphrey, S.; Macvicar, T.; Stevenson, A.; Roberts, M.; Humphrey, T. J.; Jepson, M. A. SulA-Induced Filamentation in *Salmonella enterica* Serovar Typhimurium, Effects on SPI-1 Expression and Epithelial Infection. *J. Al. Microbiol.* **2011,** *111* (1), 185–196.

22. Buchmeier, N. A.; Libby, S. J.; Xu, Y.; Loewen, P. C.; Switala, J.; Guiney, D. G.; Fang, F. C. DNA Repair is More Important than Catalase for *Salmonella* Virulence in Mice. *J. Clin. Invest.* **1995,** *95* (3), 1047–1053.

23. Srikanth, C. V.; Mercado-Lubo, R.; Hallstrom, K.; McCormick, B. A. *Salmonella* Effector Proteins and Host-Cell Responses. *Cell Mol. Life Sci.* **2011,** *68* (22), 3687–3697.

24. Husain, M.; Jones-Carson, J.; Song, M.; McCollister, B. D.; Bourret, T. J.; Vazquez-Torres, A. Redox Sensor SsrB Cys203 Enhances *Salmonella* Fitness Against Nitric Oxide Generated in the Host Immune Response to Oral Infection. *Proc. Natl. Acad. Sci. U.S.A.* **2010,** *107* (32), 14396–14401.

25. Lee, J. J.; Lee, S. K.; Song, N.; Nathan, T. O.; Swarts, B. M.; Eum, S. Y.; Ehrt, S.; Cho, S. N.; Eoh, H. Transient Drug-Tolerance and Permanent Drug-Resistance Rely on the Trehalose-Catalytic Shift in *Mycobacterium tuberculosis*. *Nat. Commun.* **2019,** *10* (1), 2928.

26. Robinson, N.; Kolter, T.; Wolke, M.; Rybniker, J.; Hartmann, P.; Plum, G. Mycobacterial Phenolic Glycolipid Inhibits Phagosome Maturation and Subverts the Pro-Inflammatory Cytokine Response. *Traffic* **2008,** *9* (11), 1936–1947.

27. Fukuda, T.; Matsumura, T.; Ato, M.; Hamasaki, M.; Nishiuchi, Y.; Murakami, Y.; Maeda, Y.; Yoshimori, T.; Matsumoto, S.; Kobayashi, K.; Kinoshita, T.; Morita, Y. S. Critical Roles for Lipomannan and Lipoarabinomannan in Cell Wall Integrity of Mycobacteria and Pathogenesis of Tuberculosis. *MBio* **2013,** *4* (1), e00472-12.

28. Khan, M. Z.; Bhaskar, A.; Upadhyay, S.; Kumari, P.; Rajmani, R. S.; Jain, P.; Singh, A.; Kumar, D.; Bhavesh, N. S.; Nandicoori, V. K. Protein Kinase G Confers Survival Advantage to *Mycobacterium tuberculosis* During Latency-Like Conditions. *J. Biol. Chem.* **2017,** *292* (39), 16093–16108.

29. Weinstein, E. A.; Yano, T.; Li, L. S.; Avarbock, D.; Avarbock, A.; Helm, D.; McColm, A. A.; Duncan, K.; Lonsdale, J. T.; Rubin, H. Inhibitors of Type II NADH, Menaquinone Oxidoreductase Represent a Class of Antitubercular Drugs. *Proc. Natl. Acad. Sci. U.S.A.* **2005,** *102* (12), 4548–4553.

30. Vilcheze, C.; Weisbrod, T. R.; Chen, B.; Kremer, L.; Hazbon, M. H.; Wang, F.; Alland, D.; Sacchettini, J. C.; Jacobs, W. R.; Jr. Altered NADH/NAD+ Ratio Mediates Coresistance to Isoniazid and Ethionamide in Mycobacteria. *Antimicrob. Agents Chemother.* **2005,** *49* (2), 708–720.

31. Jamaati, H.; Mortaz, E.; Pajouhi, Z.; Folkerts, G.; Movassaghi, M.; Moloudizargari, M.; Adcock, I. M.; Garssen, J. Nitric Oxide in the Pathogenesis and Treatment of Tuberculosis. *Front. Microbiol.* **2017,** *8,* 2008.

32. Firmani, M. A.; Riley, L. W. *Mycobacterium tuberculosis* CDC1551 is Resistant to Reactive Nitrogen and Oxygen Intermediates In Vitro. *Infect. Immun.* **2002,** *70* (7), 3965–3968.

33. Lin, K.; O'Brien, K. M.; Trujillo, C.; Wang, R.; Wallach, J. B.; Schnainger, D.; Ehrt, S. *Mycobacterium tuberculosis* Thioredoxin Reductase Is Essential for Thiol Redox Homeostasis but Plays a Minor Role in Antioxidant Defense. *PLoS Pathog.* **2016,** *12* (6), e1005675.

34. Hillas, P. J.; del Alba, F. S.; Oyarzabal, J.; Wilks, A.; Ortiz De Montellano, P. R.; The AhpC and AhpD Antioxidant Defense System of *Mycobacterium tuberculosis*. *J. Biol. Chem.* **2000,** *275* (25), 18801–18809.

35. Virulence Factors and Pathogenicity of Mycobacterium, **2018**.
36. Master, S.; Zahrt, T. C.; Song, J.; Deretic, V. Mapping of *Mycobacterium tuberculosis* katG Promoters and Their Differential Expression in Infected Macrophages. *J. Bacteriol.* **2001**, *183* (13), 4033–4039.
37. Kumar, A.; Farhana, A.; Guidry, L.; Saini, V.; Hondalus, M.; Steyn, A. J. Redox Homeostasis in Mycobacteria, the key to Tuberculosis Control? *Expert. Rev. Mol. Med.* **2011**, *13*, e39.
38. Sao Emani, C.; Williams, M. J.; Wiid, I. J.; Baker, B. The Functional Interplay of Low Molecular Weight Thiols in *Mycobacterium tuberculosis. J. Biomed. Sci.* **2018**, *25* (1), 55.
39. Percario, S.; Moreira, D. R.; Gomes, B. A.; Ferreira, M. E.; Goncalves, A. C.; Laurindo, P. S.; Vilhena, T. C.; Dolabela, M. F.; Green, M. D. Oxidative Stress in Malaria. *Int. J. Mol. Sci.* **2012**, *13* (12), 16346–16372.
40. Vega-Rodriguez, J.; Franke-Fayard, B.; Dinglasan, R. R.; Janse, C. J.; Pastrana-Mena, R.; Waters, A. P.; Coens, I.; Rodriguez-Orengo, J. F.; Srinivasan, P.; Jacobs-Lorena, M.; Serrano, A. E. The Glutathione Biosynthetic Pathway of Plasmodium is Essential for Mosquito Transmission. *PLoS Pathog.* **2009**, *5* (2), e1000302.
41. Gallo, V.; Schwarzer, E.; Rahlfs, S.; Schirmer, R. H.; van Zwieten, R.; Roos, D.; Arese, P.; Becker, K. Inherited Glutathione Reductase Deficiency and *Plasmodium falciparum* Malaria—A Case Study. *PLoS One* **2009**, *4* (10), e7303.
42. Sienkiewicz, N.; Daher, W.; Dive, D.; Wrenger, C.; Viscogliosi, E.; Wintjens, R.; Jouin, H.; Capron, M.; Muller, S.; Khalife, J. Identification of a Mitochondrial Superoxide Dismutase with an Unusual Targeting Sequence in *Plasmodium falciparum. Mol. Biochem. Parasitol.* **2004**, *137* (1), 121–132.
43. Zocher, K.; Fritz-Wolf, K.; Kehr, S.; Fischer, M.; Rahlfs, S.; Becker, K. Biochemical and Structural Characterization of *Plasmodium falciparum* Glutamate Dehydrogenase 2. *Mol. Biochem. Parasitol.* **2012**, *183* (1), 52–62.
44. Allen, S. M.; Lim, E. E.; Jortzik, E.; Preuss, J.; Chua, H. H.; MacRae, J. I.; Rahlfs, S.; Haeussler, K.; Downton, M. T.; McConville, M. J.; Becker, K.; Ralph, S. A. *Plasmodium falciparum* Glucose-6-Phosphate Dehydrogenase 6-Phosphogluconolactonase is a Potential Drug Target. *FEBS J.* **2015**, *282* (19), 3808–3823.
45. Pannala, V. R.; Dash, R. K. Mechanistic Characterization of the Thioredoxin System in the Removal of Hydrogen Peroxide. *Free Radic. Biol. Med.* **2015**, *78*, 42–55.
46. Sussmann, R. A. C.; Fotoran, W. L.; Kimura, E. A.; Katzin, A. M. *Plasmodium falciparum* Uses Vitamin E to Avoid Oxidative Stress. *Parasit. Vectors* **2017**, *10* (1), 461.
47. Celli, J.; Zahrt, T. C. Mechanisms of *Francisella tularensis* Intracellular Pathogenesis. *Cold Spring Harb. Perspect. Med.* **2013**, *3* (4), a010314.
48. Clemens, D. L.; Horwitz, M. A. Uptake and Intracellular Fate of *Francisella tularensis* in Human Macrophages. *Ann. N. Y. Acad. Sci.* **2007**, *1105*, 160–186.
49. Lindgren, H.; Shen, H.; Zingmark, C.; Golovliov, I.; Conlan, W.; Sjostedt, A. Resistance of *Francisella tularensis* Strains Against Reactive Nitrogen and Oxygen Species with Special Reference to the Role of KatG. *Infect, Immun,* **2007**, *75* (3), 1303–1309.
50. Binesse, J.; Lindgren, H.; Lindgren, L.; Conlan, W.; Sjostedt, A. Roles of Reactive Oxygen Species-Degrading Enzymes of *Francisella tularensis* SCHU S4. *Infect. Immun.* **2015**, *83* (6), 2255–2263.

51. Saha, S. S.; Hashino, M.; Suzuki, J.; Uda, A.; Watanabe, K.; Shimizu, T.; Watarai, M. Contribution of Methionine Sulfoxide Reductase B (MsrB) to *Francisella tularensis* Infection in Mice. *FEMS Microbiol. Lett.* **2017**, *364* (2), 51.

52. Ma, Z.; Russo, V. C.; Rabadi, S. M.; Jen, Y.; Catlett, S. V.; Bakshi, C. S.; Malik, M. Elucidation of a Mechanism of Oxidative Stress Regulation in *Francisella tularensis* Live Vaccine Strain. *Mol. Microbiol.* **2016**, *101* (5), 856–878.

53. Alharbi, A.; Rabadi, S. M.; Alqahtani, M.; Marghani, D.; Worden, M.; Ma, Z.; Malik, M.; Bakshi, C. S. Role of Peroxiredoxin of the AhpC/TSA Family in Antioxidant Defense Mechanisms of *Francisella tularensis*. *PLoS One* **2019**, *14* (3), e0213699.

54. JW, I. J.; Mueller, A. C. Neutrophil NADPH Oxidase is Reduced at the *Anaplasma phagocytophilum* Phagosome. *Infect. Immun.* **2004**, *72* (9), 5392–5401.

55. Villar, M.; Lopez, V.; Ayllon, N.; Cabezas-Cruz, A.; Lopez, J. A.; Vazquez, J.; Alberdi, P.; de la Fuente, J. The Intracellular Bacterium *Anaplasma phagocytophilum* Selectively Manipulates the Levels of Vertebrate Host Proteins in the Tick Vector *Ixodes scapularis*. *Parasit. Vectors* **2016**, *9*, 467.

56. Alberdi, P.; Cabezas-Cruz, A.; Prados, P. E.; Rayo, M. V.; Artigas-Jeronimo, S.; de la Fuente, J. The Redox Metabolic Pathways Function to Limit *Anaplasma phagocytophilum* Infection and Multiplication While Preserving Fitness in Tick Vector Cells. *Sci. Rep.* **2019**, *9* (1), 13236.

57. Abdul-Sater, A. A.; Said-Sadier, N.; Lam, V. M.; Singh, B.; Pettengill, M. A.; Soares, F.; Tattoli, I.; Lipinski, S.; Girardin, S. E.; Rosenstiel, P.; Ojcius, D. M. Enhancement of Reactive Oxygen Species Production and Chlamydial Infection by the Mitochondrial Nod-Like Family Member NLRX1. *J. Biol. Chem.* **2010**, *285* (53), 41637–41645.

58. Gurumurthy, R. K.; Maurer, A. P.; Machuy, N.; Hess, S.; Pleissner, K. P.; Schuchhardt, J.; Rudel, T.; Meyer, T. F. A Loss-of-Function Screen Reveals Ras- and Raf-Independent MEK-ERK Signaling During *Chlamydia trachomatis* Infection. *Sci. Signal.* **2010**, *3* (113), ra21.

59. Vignola, M. J.; Kashatus, D. F.; Taylor, G. A.; Counter, C. M.; Valdivia, R. H. cPLA2 Regulates the Expression of Type I Interferons and Intracellular Immunity to *Chlamydia trachomatis*. *J. Biol. Chem.* **2010**, *285* (28), 21625–21635.

60. Ferro, E.; Goitre, L.; Retta, S. F.; Trabalzini, L.; The Interplay between ROS and Ras GTPases, Physiological and Pathological Implications. *J. Signal. Transduct.* **2012**, *2012*, 365769.

61. Chumduri, C.; Gurumurthy, R. K.; Zadora, P. K.; Mi, Y.; Meyer, T. F.; Chlamydia Infection Promotes Host DNA Damage and Proliferation but Impairs the DNA Damage Response. *Cell Host Microbe* **2013**, *13* (6), 746–758.

62. Siegl, C.; Prusty, B. K.; Karunakaran, K.; Wischhusen, J.; Rudel, T. Tumor Suppressor p53 Alters Host Cell Metabolism to Limit *Chlamydia trachomatis* Infection. *Cell Rep.* **2014**, *9* (3), 918–929.

63. Boncompain, G.; Schneider, B.; Delevoye, C.; Kellermann, O.; Dautry-Varsat, A.; Subtil, A. Production of Reactive Oxygen Species is Turned on and Rapidly Shut Down in Epithelial Cells Infected with *Chlamydia trachomatis*. *Infect. Immun.* **2010**, *78* (1), 80–87.

64. Tonello, F.; Zornetta, I. *Bacillus anthracis* Factors for Phagosomal Escape. *Toxins (Basel)* **2012**, *4* (7), 536–553.

65. Cybulski, R. J., Jr.; Sanz, P.; Alem, F.; Stibitz, S.; Bull, R. L.; O'Brien, A. D. Four Superoxide Dismutases Contribute to *Bacillus anthracis* Virulence and Provide Spores with Redundant Protection From Oxidative Stress. *Infect. Immun.* **2009,** *77* (1), 274–285.

66. Segal, B. H.; Sakamoto, N.; Patel, M.; Maemura, K.; Klein, A. S.; Holland, S. M.; Bulkley, G. B. Xanthine Oxidase Contributes to Host Defense against *Burkholderia cepacia* in the p47(phox-/-) Mouse Model of Chronic Granulomatous Disease. *Infect. Immun.* **2000,** *68* (4), 2374–2378.

67. Vatansever, F.; de Melo, W. C.; Avci, P.; Vecchio, D.; Sadasivam, M.; Gupta, A.; Chandran, R.; Karimi, M.; Parizotto, N. A.; Yin, R.; Tegos, G. P.; Hamblin, M. R. Antimicrobial Strategies Centered Around Reactive Oxygen Species—Bactericidal Antibiotics, Photodynamic Therapy, and Beyond. *FEMS Microbiol. Rev.* **2013,** *37* (6), 955–989.

68. El-Halfawy, O. M.; Valvano, M. A. Putrescine Reduces Antibiotic-Induced Oxidative Stress as a Mechanism of Modulation of Antibiotic Resistance in *Burkholderia cenocepacia*. *Antimicrob. Agents Chemother.* **2014,** *58* (7), 4162–4171.

69. Wongsaroj, L.; Saninjuk, K.; Romsang, A.; Duang-Nkern, J.; Trinachartvanit, W.; Vattanaviboon, P.; Mongkolsuk, S. *Pseudomonas aeruginosa* Glutathione Biosynthesis Genes Play Multiple Roles in Stress Protection, Bacterial Virulence and Biofilm Formation. *PLoS One* **2018,** *13* (10), e0205815.

70. Romsang, A.; Duang-Nkern, J.; Khemsom, K.; Wongsaroj, L.; Saninjuk, K.; Fuangthong, M.; Vattanaviboon, P.; Mongkolsuk, S. *Pseudomonas aeruginosa* ttcA Encoding tRNA-Thiolating Protein Requires an Iron-Sulfur Cluster to Participate in Hydrogen Peroxide-Mediated Stress Protection and Pathogenicity. *Sci. Rep.* **2018,** *8* (1), 11882.

71. Seib, K. L.; Wu, H. J.; Kidd, S. P.; Apicella, M. A.; Jennings, M. P.; McEwan, A. G.; Defenses Against Oxidative Stress in *Neisseria gonorrhoeae*, A System Tailored for a Challenging Environment. *Microbiol. Mol. Biol. Rev.* **2006,** *70* (2), 344–361.

72. Lim, K. H.; Jones, C. E.; vanden Hoven, R. N.; Edwards, J. L.; Falsetta, M. L.; Apicella, M. A.; Jennings, M. P.; McEwan, A. G. Metal Binding Specificity of the MntABC Permease of *Neisseria gonorrhoeae* and its Influence on Bacterial Growth and Interaction with Cervical Epithelial Cells. *Infect. Immun.* **2008,** *76* (8), 3569–3576.

73. Wu, H. J.; Seib, K. L.; Srikhanta, Y. N.; Kidd, S. P.; Edwards, J. L.; Maguire, T. L.; Grimmond, S. M.; Apicella, M. A.; McEwan, A. G.; Jennings, M. P. PerR Controls Mn-Dependent Resistance to Oxidative Stress in *Neisseria gonorrhoeae*. *Mol. Microbiol.* **2006,** *60* (2), 401–416.

74. Skaar, E. P.; Tobiason, D. M.; Quick, J.; Judd, R. C.; Weissbach, H.; Etienne, F.; Brot, N.; Seifert, H. S. The Outer Membrane Localization of the *Neisseria gonorrhoeae* MsrA/B is Involved in Survival Against Reactive Oxygen Species. *Proc. Natl. Acad. Sci. U.S.A.* **2002,** *99* (15), 10108–10113.

75. Kidd, S. P.; Potter, A. J.; Apicella, M. A.; Jennings, M. P.; McEwan, A. G. NmlR of *Neisseria gonorrhoeae*, A Novel Redox Responsive Transcription Factor from the MerR Family. *Mol. Microbiol.* **2005,** *57* (6), 1676–1689.

76. Liu, G. Y.; Essex, A.; Buchanan, J. T.; Datta, V.; Hoffman, H. M.; Bastian, J. F.; Fierer, J.; Nizet, V. *Staphylococcus aureus* Golden Pigment Impairs Neutrophil Killing and

Promotes Virulence Through its Antioxidant Activity. *J. Exp. Med.* **2005,** *202* (2), 209–215.

77. Lalaouna, D.; Baude, J.; Wu, Z.; Tomasini, A.; Chicher, J.; Marzi, S.; Vandenesch, F.; Romby, P.; Caldelari, I.; Moreau, K. RsaC sRNA Modulates the Oxidative Stress Response of *Staphylococcus aureus* During Manganese Starvation. *Nucleic Acids Res.* **2019,** *47* (18), 9871–9887.

78. Cosgrove, K.; Coutts, G.; Jonsson, I. M.; Tarkowski, A.; Kokai-Kun, J. F.; Mond, J. J.; Foster, S. J. Catalase (KatA) and Alkyl Hydroperoxide Reductase (AhpC) Have Compensatory Roles in Peroxide Stress Resistance and are Required for Survival, Persistence, and Nasal Colonization in *Staphylococcus aureus*. *J. Bacteriol.* **2007,** *189* (3), 1025–1035.

79. Pang, Y. Y.; Schwartz, J.; Bloomberg, S.; Boyd, J. M.; Horswill, A. R.; Nauseef, W. M. Methionine Sulfoxide Reductases Protect Against Oxidative Stress in *Staphylococcus aureus* Encountering Exogenous Oxidants and Human Neutrophils. *J. Innate. Immun.* **2014,** *6* (3), 353–364.

80. Singh, V. K.; Vaish, M.; Johansson, T. R.; Baum, K. R.; Ring, R. P.; Singh, S.; Shukla, S. K.; Moskovitz, J. Significance of Four Methionine Sulfoxide Reductases in *Staphylococcus aureus*. *PLoS One* **2015,** *10* (2), e0117594.

81. Overton, T. W.; Justino, M. C.; Li, Y.; Baptista, J. M.; Melo, A. M.; Cole, J. A.; Saraiva, L. M. Widespread Distribution in Pathogenic Bacteria of Di-Iron Proteins that Repair Oxidative and Nitrosative Damage to Iron-Sulfur Centers. *J. Bacteriol.* **2008,** *190* (6), 2004–2013.

82. Ji, C. J.; Kim, J. H.; Won, Y. B.; Lee, Y. E.; Choi, T. W.; Ju, S. Y.; Youn, H.; Helmann, J. D.; Lee, J. W.; *Staphylococcus aureus* PerR Is a Hypersensitive Hydrogen Peroxide Sensor using Iron-mediated Histidine Oxidation. *J. Biol. Chem.* **2015,** *290* (33), 20374–20386.

83. Pineda, E.; Perdomo, D. *Entamoeba histolytica* under Oxidative Stress, What Countermeasure Mechanisms Are in Place? *Cells* **2017,** *6* (4), 44.

84. Fahey, R. C.; Newton, G. L.; Arrick, B.; Overdank-Bogart, T.; Aley, S. B. *Entamoeba histolytica*, A Eukaryote Without Glutathione Metabolism. *Science* **1984,** *224* (4644), 70–72.

85. Akbar, M. A.; Chatterjee, N. S.; Sen, P.; Debnath, A.; Pal, A.; Bera, T.; Das, P. Genes Induced by a High-Oxygen Environment in *Entamoeba histolytica*. *Mol. Biochem. Parasitol.* **2004,** *133* (2), 187–196.

86. Rastew, E.; Vicente, J. B.; Singh, U. Oxidative Stress Resistance Genes Contribute to the Pathogenic Potential of the Anaerobic Protozoan Parasite, *Entamoeba histolytica*. *Int. J. Parasitol.* **2012,** *42* (11), 1007–1015.

87. Sebbane, F.; Lemaitre, N.; Sturdevant, D. E.; Rebeil, R.; Virtaneva, K.; Porcella, S. F.; Hinnebusch, B. J. Adaptive Response of *Yersinia pestis* to Extracellular Effectors of Innate Immunity During Bubonic Plague. *Proc. Natl. Acad. Sci. U.S.A.* **2006,** *103* (31), 11766–11771.

88. Ni, B.; Zhang, Y.; Huang, X.; Yang, R.; Zhou, D. Transcriptional Regulation Mechanism of ter Operon by OxyR in *Yersinia pestis*. *Curr. Microbiol.* **2014,** *69* (1), 42–46.

89. Pha, K.; Navarro, L. Yersinia Type III Effectors Perturb Host Innate Immune Responses. *World J. Biol. Chem.* **2016,** *7* (1), 1–13.

90. Barnes, P. J.; Karin, M. Nuclear Factor-κB—A Pivotal Transcription Factor in Chronic Inflammatory Diseases. *N. Engl. J. Med.* **1997,** *336* (15), 1066–1071.
91. Good, R.; Yunis, E. Association of Autoimmunity, Immunodeficiency and Aging in Man, Rabbits, and Mice. *Immunol. Aging* **1974,** 33 (9), 2040–2050.
92. Änggård, E. Nitric Oxide, Mediator, Murderer, and Medicine. *Lancet* **1994,** *343* (8907), 1199–1206.
93. Zhu, L.; Gunn, C.; Beckman, J. S. Bactericidal Activity of Peroxynitrite. *Arch. Biochem. Biophys.* **1992,** *298* (2), 452–457.
94. Gregory, S. H.; Wing, E. J.; Hoffman, R. A.; Simmons, R. Reactive Nitrogen Intermediates Suppress the Primary Immunologic Response to Listeria. *J. Immunol.* **1993,** *150* (7), 2901–2909.
95. Moncada, S. Nitric Oxide, Physiology, Pathophysiology, and Pharmacology. *Pharmacol. Rev.* **1991,** *43,* 109–142.
96. Nathan, C. F.; Hibbs Jr, J. B. Role of Nitric Oxide Synthesis in Macrophage Antimicrobial Activity. *Curr. Opin. Immunol.* **1991,** *3* (1), 65–70.
97. Peterhans, E. Oxidants and Antioxidants in Viral Diseases, Disease Mechanisms and Metabolic Regulation. *J. Nutr.* **1997,** *127* (5), 962S–965S.
98. Knight, J. A. Free Radicals, Antioxidants, and the Immune System. *Ann. Clin. Lab. Sci.* **2000,** *30* (2), 145–158.
99. Semba, R. D. Vitamin A, Immunity, and Infection. *Clin. Infect. Dis.* **1994,** *19* (3), 489–499.
100. Baier-Bitterlich, G.; Fuchs, D.; Wachter, H. Chronic Immune Stimulation, Oxidative Stress, and Apoptosis in HIV Infection. *Biochem. Pharmacol.* **1997,** *53* (6), 755–763.
101. Allard, J. P.; Aghdassi, E.; Chau, J.; Salit, I.; Walmsley, S. Oxidative Stress and Plasma Antioxidant Micronutrients in Humans with HIV Infection. *Am. J. Clin. Nutr.* **1998,** *67* (1), 143–147.
102. Drain, P. K.; Kupka, R.; Mugusi, F.; Fawzi, W. W. Micronutrients in HIV-Positive Persons Receiving Highly Active Antiretroviral Therapy. *Am. J. Clin. Nutr.* **2007,** *85* (2), 333–345.
103. Puertollano, M. A.; Puertollano, E.; de Cienfuegos, G. A.; de Pablo, M. A. *Dietary Antioxidants, Immunity and Host Defense. Curr. Top. Med. Chem.* **2011,** *11* (14), 1752–1766.
104. Knight, J. A. Review, Free radicals, Antioxidants, and the Immune System. *Ann. Clin. Lab. Sci.* **2000,** *30* (2), 145–158.
105. Dinicola, S.; De Grazia, S.; Carlomagno, G.; Pintucci, J. P. *N*-Acetylcysteine as Powerful Molecule to Destroy Bacterial Biofilms. A Systematic Review. *Eur. Rev. Med. Pharmacol. Sci.* **2014,** *18* (19), 2942–2948.
106. Naguib, M. M.; Valvano, M. A. Vitamin E Increases Antimicrobial Sensitivity by Inhibiting Bacterial Lipocalin Antibiotic Binding. *mSphere* **2018,** *3* (6), e00564-18.
107. Prasad, A. S.; Zinc in Human Health, Effect of Zinc on Immune Cells. *Mol. Med.* **2008,** *14* (5–6), 353–357.
108. Wadhwa, N.; Basnet, S.; Natchu, U. C. M.; Shrestha, L. P.; Bhatnagar, S.; Sommerfelt, H.; Strand, T. A.; the zinc sepsis study group.; Ramji, S.; Aggarwal, K. C.; Chellani, H.; Govil, A.; Jajoo, M.; Mathur, N. B.; Bhatt, M.; Mohta, A.; Ansari, I.; Basnet, S.; Chapagain, R. H.; Shah, G. P.; Shrestha, B. M. Zinc as an Adjunct Treatment for

Reducing Case Fatality Due to Clinical Severe Infection in Young Infants, Study Protocol for a Randomized Controlled Trial. *BMC Pharmacol. Toxicol.* **2017,** *18* (1), 56.

109. Steinbrenner, H.; Al-Quraishy, S.; Dkhil, M. A.; Wunderlich, F.; Sies, H. Dietary Selenium in Adjuvant Therapy of Viral and Bacterial Infections. *Adv. Nutr.* **2015,** *6* (1), 73–82.

110. Palanisamy, G. S.; Kirk, N. M.; Ackart, D. F.; Shanley, C. A.; Orme, I. M.; Basaraba, R. J. Evidence for Oxidative Stress and Defective Antioxidant Response in Guinea Pigs with Tuberculosis. *PLoS One* **2011,** *6* (10), e26254.

CHAPTER 4

Role of Antioxidants in Diabetes

LALITA KUSHWAH[1*], RUPALI DUTT[1], GBKS PRASAD[1], and
D. K. SHARMA[2]

[1]*School of Studies in Biochemistry, Jiwaji University, Gwalior, India*

[2]*Department of Zoology, Government Model Science College, Gwalior*

Corresponding author. E-mail: lalitakuashwah@gmail.com

ABSTRACT

Diabetes is a chronic condition, produces little or no insulin, and usually develops in childhood or early childhood. Hyperglycemia triggers the generation of reactive oxygen species (ROS) and autoxidation of glucose leading to domination of the condition of oxidative stress. It also causes tissue damage through different mechanisms, including increased intracellular formation of advanced glycation end products (AGEs), increased expression of the receptor for AGEs, and activation of protein kinase C isoforms. Glucose can cause multiple secondary complications through a variety of pathways, which are appearing to lead to oxidative stress. Oxidative stress is an imbalance between radical engendering and scavenging systems. Overproduction of free radicals and a defect in antioxidant protection involved pathogenesis of diabetes. ROS level elevation in diabetes may be due to decrease in destruction or/and increase in the production by superoxide dismutase (SOD), glutathione peroxidase (GSHPx) antioxidants, and catalase (CAT—enzymatic/nonenzymatic). Oxidative stress causes cell damage both directly and indirectly through the activation of different pathways. Hyperglycemia promotes autoxidation of glucose to form free radicals. The generation of free radicals beyond the scavenging abilities of endogenous antioxidant defenses results in macro- and microvascular dysfunctions. Vitamin E is converted to tocopheroxyl radicals after acting as a free radical scavenger, which means the regeneration of vitamin E is required to prevent unwanted tocopheroxyl-mediated oxidative process. Vitamin E regeneration system is composed of ascorbic acid, reduced glutathione, and CoQ10.

4.1 INTRODUCTION

There are currently 425 million people suffering from diabetes worldwide, and this number is expected to reach 642 million by 2045, with type 2 diabetes mellitus (T2DM) (American Diabetes Association, 2018; International Diabetes Federation, 2017). Hence, efforts are to be taken to control the diabetes. Today, the synthetic drugs used for the treatment of hyperglycemia like acarbose, miglitol, biguanides, voglibose, and sulfonylureas are associated with various side effects and are effective at higher doses. Therefore, researchers focus on an alternative medicine system that reduces the major medical issues in the managements of diabetes, and traditional herbal and also antioxidant-based medicines are getting significant attention because of their effectiveness, fewer side effects, and relatively low cost (Samyal et al., 2017).

Diabetes mellitus (DM) is a disorder of blood sugar (glucose) metabolism whereby your body does not properly break down glucose in the bloodstream, a necessary function for cell nutrition. Diabetes caused either by inadequate insulin secretion from pancreatic beta cells or by the insufficient utilization of insulin or bath. Hyperglycemia triggers the generation of reactive oxygen species (ROS) and autoxidation of glucose leading to domination of the condition of oxidative stress, and it also causes tissue damage through different mechanisms, including increased intracellular formation of advanced glycation end products (AGEs), increased expression of the receptor for AGEs, and activation of protein kinase C is forms (Chen et al., 2017; Gurusamy and Mini, 2017).

Type 1 diabetes, also known as insulin-dependent diabetes, a chronic condition in which the beta cells of pancreas produce little or no insulin, usually develops in childhood or early childhood.

Type 2 diabetes comprises 90% of cases, wherein the body does not produce the insulin needed and/or cells do not respond to insulin, which is also called insulin resistance, making it ineffectual. Obesity is a major cause of type 2 diabetes.

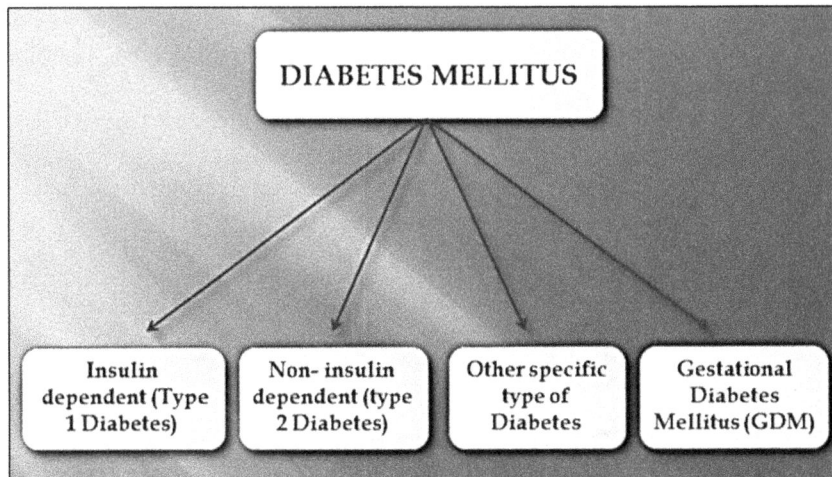

FIGURE 4.1   Classification of diabetes mellitus.

4.2   COMPLICATIONS OF DIABETES

Diabetes is a very serious condition, as it can lead to severe illness and even death. Variations in blood sugar level, too high and too low (hyperglycemia and hypoglycemia), can lead to atherosclerosis (fatty deposit buildup), neuropathy (loss of nerve function), nephropathy (kidney damage), and retinopathy (eye disease and leading cause of blindness) (Joseph et al., 2002). Glucose can cause multiple secondary complications through a variety of pathways, which are appearing to lead to oxidative stress.

4.3   OXIDATIVE STRESS AND DIABETES

Oxidative stress plays a key role in the development of wide range of diseases diabetes particularly *type 2 diabetes*. Oxidative stress is an imbalance between radical engendering and scavenging systems. Opara (2002) reported the overproduction of free radicals and a defect of antioxidant protection involved in the pathogenesis of diabetes. The mechanism of prooxidant–antioxidant imbalance in DM is autoxidation of glucose that increased the formation of glycation end products (AGEs), hexosamine pathway, polyol pathway, and mitochondrial respiratory chain. The enzymatic source of free radical generation includes nitric oxide synthase, nicotinamide adenine dinucleotide phosphate (NADPH), and xanthine oxidase (Singh et al., 2009).

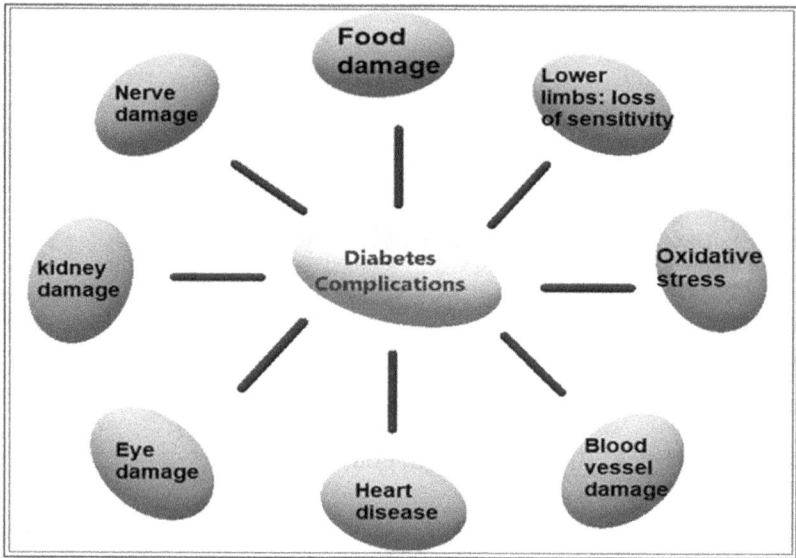

FIGURE 4.2   Complications of diabetes.

ROS level elevation in diabetes may be due to decrease in destruction or/and increase in the production by *superoxide dismutase* (SOD), *glutathione peroxidase* (GSHPx) antioxidants, and *catalase* (CAT— enzymatic/nonenzymatic). These enzymes make the tissues susceptible to oxidative stress leading to the development of *diabetic complications* (Lipinski, 2001). A number of previous experimental and clinical studies recommend that oxidative stress plays the main role in the pathogenesis of diabetes.

Oxidative stress-dependent activation of PKC in diabetic conditions. Diabetic causes high blood glucose that induces oxidative stress through the increase of mitochondrial ROS production. Oxidative stress causes cell damage both directly and indirectly through the activation of different pathways. One of these involves PKC that promotes insulin resistance and diabetic complication.

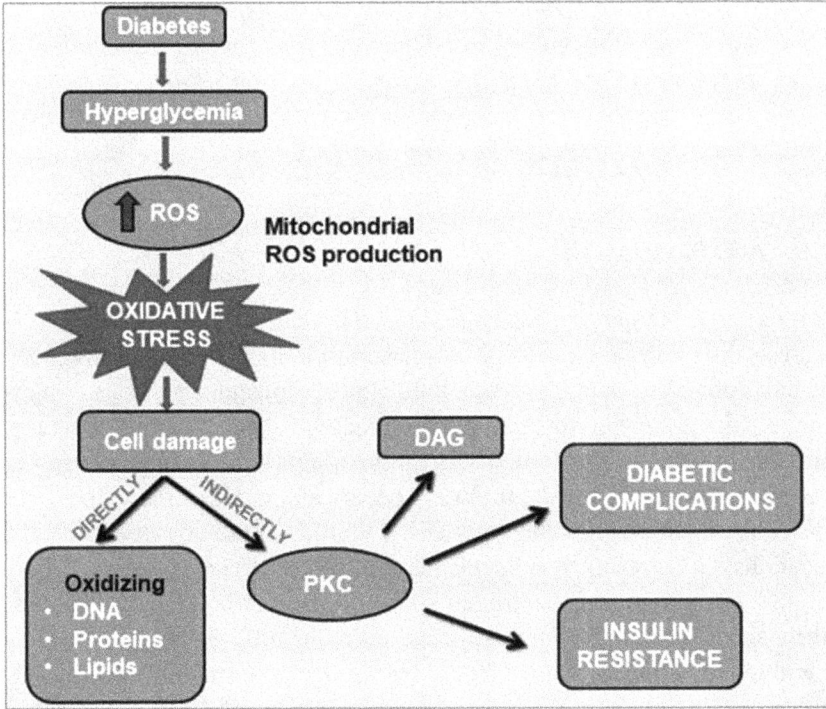

FIGURE 4.3 Effect of oxidative stress on diabetes.

4.4 THERAPY FOR DIABETES

Diabetic patients should receive healthy living advice, including physical activity, lifestyle modification, and particularly smoking cessation and healthy eating.

Therapies for diabetes are of the follo wing two types:

- *Non-pharmacotherapy*
  - Dietary therapy
  - Physical therapy

- *Pharmacotherapy*
  - Insulin therapy
  - Oral hypoglycemia agents

- *Stimulation of insulin by beta cells, for example, sulfonylureas*
- *Inhibitors of hepatic gluconeogenesis, for example, biguanides*
- *Inhibitors of intestinal alpha glucosidases, for example, acarbose*
- *Drugs are which reduce insulin resistance, for example, thiozoli-dinediones (Shan and Randeep, 2009)*

4.5 ANTIOXIDANTS

Antioxidants are natural substances that can *neutralize free radicals*. Free radicals are toxic chemicals that can do serious damage to cells and tissues, which is called oxidation process. Free radical molecules with one or more single pair of the electron can quickly react with the constituents such as proteins, nucleic acid, and lipids. So antioxidants remove these dangerous free radicals from the body. It always occurs along with a reduction—one substance is oxidized while another is reduced. These are termed "redox reactions." The reactive molecules comprise the derived oxygen species (ROS), whereas reactive nitrogen species was derived from oxygen and nitrogen, respectively. These reactive particles are generated in cellular membrane, mitochondria, nucleus, lysosome, peroxisome, endoplasmic reticulum, and cytoplasm. The enhanced generation of the reactive species is associated with hyperglycemia (Halliwe et al., 1999).

Hyperglycemia promotes autoxidation of glucose to form free radicals. The generation of free radicals beyond the scavenging abilities of endogenous antioxidant defenses results in macro- and microvascular dysfunction.

Antioxidants such as vitamin C, alpha-lipoic acid (ALA), and *N*-acetylcysteine are effective in reducing diabetic complications, indicating that it may be beneficial either by ingestion of natural antioxidants or through dietary supplementation.

The body has natural antioxidants (e.g., vitamin C, vitamin E, and glutathione) that normally sop up all these free radicals, reducing and often eliminating the damage caused. In chronic diseases, including diabetes, the levels of free radicals overcome the body's ability to soak or sop them up. The high level of antioxidants leads to a condition in the cells, tissues, and organs known as oxidative stress. Oxidative stress showed up as chronic inflammation and damage to nerves, blood vessels, tissues, and organs. In diabetes that the blood sugar glucose is heavily oxidized as are proteins and lipids (fats) leading to what is known as AGEs. In fact, A1c often followed to monitor how well someone is controlling their blood sugar levels is an AGE.

4.6 TYPES OF ANTIOXIDANTS

Antioxidants are classified into major two classes.

4.6.1 ENZYMATIC

There are three of the most important enzymes commonly present in most cells are SOD, catalase (CAT), and glutathione peroxidase (GSHPx). Superoxide catalyzes the dismutation of O_2^- to H_2O_2. Both catalase and glutathione peroxidase catalyze the reduction of H_2O to water, thereby preventing the formation of the potent OH^-.

4.6.2 NONENZYMATIC

Nonenzymatic antioxidants as vitamin C, vitamin E, and glutathione are most important. Vitamin E is an important micronutrient that also functions as an antioxidant; it acts to protect polyunsaturated fatty acids from oxidation by interrupting the chain of membrane lipid peroxidation and thus is also referred to as a chain-breaking antioxidant. The vitamin E radical is more stable and less reactive than the lipid radical which effectively terminates lipid peroxide–mediated chain reactions, and the resultant vitamin E radical is incapable of any further free radical scavenging activity. Thus, it must be regenerated back to a functional vitamin E molecule. The vitamin C is present in the water phase that regenerates vitamin E to the reduced form and therefore acts to spare the functional form of vitamin E.

The glutathione is present in the concentrations as reduced glutathione (GSH) with minor fractions being oxidized (GSSG) glutathione. Glutathione (GSH) as a co-substrate of glutathione peroxidase (GSHPx) plays an important role in the removal of H_2O_2 as well as other organic peroxide, thus preventing the peroxidation of membrane lipids. Glutathione status provides important information on cellular oxidative events and tissue accumulation or release of GSSG (Michael and Hill, 2008).

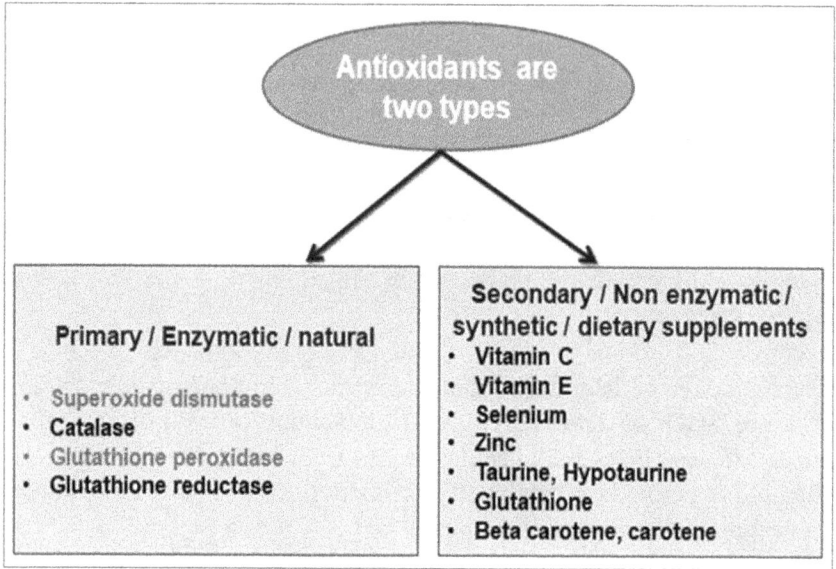

FIGURE 4.4   Types of antioxidants.

4.7   ROLE OF ANTIOXIDANTS IN DIABETES

Antioxidants are involved to reduce diabetic complications because they are involved to fight or destroy free radicals. The antioxidants that are scavengers are oxidants or free radicals that in hyperglycemia by glucose toxicity, glucose autoxidation, and oxidative phosphorylation produce ROS and release free radicals and are involved in oxidative stress and lead to destroy the pancreas. The beta cells are inhibited by their function and destroyed by free radicals.

The previous process will prone to diabetic complications so the antioxidants' role here is to inhibit the activity of free radicals and avoiding diabetic long-term complications.

Oxidative stress is strongly associated with diabetes and particularly with the complications of diabetes. Antioxidants may help one to prevent or potentially reverse damage from oxidative stress is by reducing damage to the endothelium; this is the layer of cells that line blood vessels. Antioxidants appear to act at the level of the endothelial cells, though it is not clear that adding antioxidants to the diet or as supplements directly acts on these cells (Christine, 2018).

The antioxidant therapy defends the beta cell against oxidative stress–induced apoptosis and preserves the function of the beta cell. Epidemiological studies revealed a strong association between the dietary antioxidants intake and protection against diabetes.

4.8 ANTIOXIDANT THERAPY

4.8.1 VITAMIN E

It is a naturally occurring antioxidant present as tocotrienol and tocopherol. It protects the cell against oxidative damage. It is believed that vitamin E plays an important role in controlling hyperglycemia. The studies in an animal model have shown that the administration of vitamin E decreases the hepatic lipid peroxide level in streptozotocin-induced diabetes (Seven et al., 2004).

Dietary vitamin and supplementation of vitamin E are positively associated with glucose concentration. The level of glucose decreased and the oral glucose tolerance test (OGTT) improved in diabetic condition by the administration of vitamin E (Shamsi et al., 2004). In diabetic condition, the antioxidant enzymes SOD, glutathione peroxidase (GPX), and CAT decreased. However, the oral administration of vitamin E (440 mg/kg of body weight) once in a week for 30 days significantly increased GSHPx and SOD activity and decreased the hydroperoxide level due to an improvement of glycaemia (Baragob et al., 2014).

During diabetic condition, the excess glucose gets attached to hemoglobin to produce glycosylated hemoglobin. Glycosylated hemoglobin is an important marker for diabetes which is prevented vitamin E–treated rat in diabetic condition (Je et al., 2001). Vitamin E has been shown to control hyperglycemia and also lowering the HbA1c by inhibiting the sequence of oxidative stress in diabetic rats (Ihara et al., 2000). The mechanism by which antioxidants reduced the glucose level is not clear, but the plasma glucose level is decreased by increasing the glucose metabolism in peripheral tissues (Roldi et al., 2009).

The administration of vitamin E (1800 IU/day) showed that the serum level of vitamin E increased in type 1 diabetes and control rats, whereas the retinal blood flow significantly increased and elevated baseline creatinine clearance to normal level, but the HbA1c level was not affected in the same experiment. It is achieved by unchanged glycemic control and normalization of DAG/PKC pathway through the activation of DAG kinase in diabetic patients (Bursell et al., 1999). In synergy with β-carotene and vitamin C, it reduced the risk of diabetes and cancer. The antioxidant property of vitamin E associated with the prevention of hyperglycemia minimizes the macrovascular and microvascular complications in individuals with diabetes (Milman et al., 2008).

4.8.2 VITAMIN C

It is powerful antioxidant scavenging free radicals in aqueous compartment. It is essential to convert vitamin E free radicals to vitamin E, as a cofactor required for hydroxylation reaction in human. The most important function of vitamin C is key chain-breaking antioxidants in the aqueous phase. It provides stability to the cell membrane.

It is reported that totally 84 diabetic patients received 500 or 1000 mg of ascorbic acid daily for 6 weeks; this research is conducted by Yazd Diabetes Research Center, Iran. Daily consumption of 1000 mg of vitamin C may be beneficial in reducing blood glucose level and lipids, whereas 500 mg not significantly made any change during the parameter studied (Afkham et al., 2007).

Eriksson and Kohvakka studied the effect of vitamin C supplementation (2 g/day for 90 days) in 56 diabetic patients; the result has shown that the high-dose supplementation reduced the level of fasting blood glucose, HbA1c and improved glycemic control (Eriksson et al., 1995). Frequent intake of vitamin C dietary source was found to decrease the risk of type 2 diabetes in a population-based study (Williams et al., 1999).

Administration of vitamin C and E (100 mg/kg of body weight of rat) significantly reduced the blood glucose level (Tanko et al., 2013). However, lowered level of ascorbic acid and SOD was observed in the diabetic subject when compared to the nondiabetic person (Will et al., 1999). In diabetes, the level of vitamin C is increased due to increased utilization in training the oxyradicals. Some of the studies have been reported that diabetes may result in decreased plasma vitamin C and E due to increased oxidative stress (Hisalkar et al., 2012).

4.8.3   ALPHA-LIPOIC ACID

A potent antioxidant, it is also known as 1, 2-dithiolane-3-pentanoic acid or thioctic acid. ALA fights cellular injuries triggered by free radicals, those unstable, highly reactive molecules that are derivatives of both normal and frazzled cell activity. It has a capability to restore endogenous antioxidants such as vitamin C, glutathione, and vitamin E. It is effective in many pathological conditions such as cardiovascular disease, DM, and liver disease (Wollin et al., 2003; Bustamante et al., 1998).

ALA has been reported to progress glucose metabolism in type 2 DM patient by directly activating lipid, tyrosine, and serine/threonine kinases in target cells, due to these mechanisms that stimulate glucose uptake and glycogenesis. In vitro studies have reported that the ALA increases the translocation of GLUT1 and GLUT4 to the plasmatic membrane of adipo-cytes and skeletal muscle. It is related to an improved activity of proteins of insulin signaling pathway (Lester et al., 2011).

The intake of ALA reduced the glucose level and total cholesterol in STZ-induced diabetes in rats (Budin et al., 2007). ALA also regenerates the other antioxidants such as vitamin C, vitamin E, and SOD in diabetic condition. The same results have been previously reported in experimental animals (Arambasic et al., 2013).

Jacob and his colleagues have been reported that the administration of 500 mg of ALA in type 2 diabetes patients for 10 days has shown a significant increase of insulin-stimulated glucose disposal (30%) and no changes were observed in fasting plasma glucose level or insulin. A clinical study shows that the administration of 500 mg ALA is capable to improve insulin resistance in non-insulin dependent diabetes mellitus (NIDDM) (Jacob et al., 1996). Same results were obtained by chronic administration (100 mg/kg) of antioxidant in type 2 DM (Bitar et al., 2004).

In another study, the oral supplementation of ALA (600 mg twice daily for 4 weeks) treatment increases the plasma insulin sensitivity (Kamenova et al., 2006). According to Packer, ALA is capable of scavenging ROS, produced during the lipid peroxidation, and guards the cell structure against damage. The continued supplementations of the ALA in diabetic rats were associated with diminution of both hyperglycemia and diabetic nephropathy (Packer et al., 2001).

4.8.4 SELENIUM

It is important trace element, naturally present in many foods. It exists in organic and inorganic forms. Selenomethionine and selenocysteine belong to organic form, whereas selenate and selenite are inorganic forms. Mostly the inorganic selenite presents in the soil. Selenium plays a major role in thyroid hormone metabolism and immune functions. Based on previous experimental and clinical studies, selenium focused on the prevention of many diseases due to their antioxidant activity (Sunde et al., 2006).

Previously, selenium was found as a toxic component due to Se poisoning in animals and humans; thereafter, it was recognized as essential element since selenium deficiency considered a major problem in animal and human (Whanger et al., 1996). The supplementation of selenium with low doses has a beneficial effect on glucose metabolism, which mimics insulin-like actions in the animal experimental model. While the mechanism behind the mimicking insulin is not clear, however, the previous report showed that Se activates the key protein responsible for insulin signal cascade (Stapleton, 2000).

The inorganic selenium compounds sodium selenate and sodium selenite are involved in insulin signaling cascade by the activation of kinases. In animal, experimental studies have shown selenate stimulate glucose uptake and involved phosphorylation of insulin receptor and insulin receptor substrate 1 (Steinbrenner et al., 2011; Wiernsperger et al., 2010) and the oral administration or intraperitoneal injection of daily doses of selenate for 3–8 weeks in streptozotocin-induced diabetic rat; the result has shown the raised glucose level to be reduced (McNeill et al., 1991; Battell et al., 1998).

In another study stated the above-mentioned insulin-like activity of selenium due to increased glucose tolerance and alteration in the activity of gluconeogenic and glycolytic maker enzyme. In the same way, selenomethionine also studied their antioxidant activity in a diabetic animal, supplementation of selenomethionine, vitamin E plus selenomethionine in type I diabetic rat for 24 weeks effectively decreased the glucose and glycosylated hemoglobin level (Douillet et al., 1999).

Numerous studies have reported that vitamin E, C, ALA, and selenium frequently used antioxidants in the management of diabetes. Nowadays, the antioxidant-based formulation has developed for the treatment of various diseases.

4.8.5   COENZYME Q10

Coenzyme Q10 is a fat-soluble, vitamin-like quinone, also known as ubiquinone, CoQ, or vitamin Q10, that was first isolated from beef mitochondria in 1957 (Tran et al., 2001; Greenberg et al., 1990). The most important biological feature of Q10 is its role in the mitochondrial electron transport chain that accepts electrons from several donors such as nicotinamide adenine dinucleotide (NADH), succinate, and glycerol-3-phosphate and then transfers them to the cytochrome system. This induces a proton gradient (chemiosmosis) that is essential for the production of ATP (Crane et al., 1997). Humans are able to synthesize CoQ10 endogenously or derive it from dietary sources. A recommended daily intake of CoQ has not been established, and since no deficiency symptoms have been reported, endogenous synthesis and dietary sources are likely be sufficient in healthy individuals (Overvad et al., 1999). However, there may be some benefit in increasing in intake in individuals with particular disease states where endogenous CoQ synthesis is either not sufficient or when requirements are increased. Impaired CoQ synthesis can result from a limited supply of phenylalanine and a decreased rate of cholesterol biosynthesis. An increased requirement can occur in disorders that uncouple oxidative phosphorylation or under conditions of increase cellular energy demand. For example, absolute and relative cellular deficiencies in CoQ can occur in patients with heart failure and diabetes and also in the elderly (Langsjoen et al., 1999). These findings suggest the possibility of improving glycemic control with CoQ in diabetic patients through various mechanisms, including a decrease in oxidative stress. Unfortunately, the evidence is too inconsistent to recommend the use of CoQ for improving glycemic control or even ameliorating diabetic complications.

4.8.6   L-CARNITINE

Carnitine, an L-β-hydroxy-γ-N-trimethylaminobutyric acid, is synthesized primarily in the liver and kidneys from lysine and methionine and has an important role in lipid metabolism by acting as an obligatory cofactor for β-oxidation of fatty acids through enabling the transport of long-chain fatty acids across the mitochondrial membrane as acylcarnitine esters. Furthermore, since carnitine shuttles acetyl groups from the inside to the outside of mitochondrial membranes, it also plays a key role in glucose metabolism and assists in fuel sensing. A reduction of mitochondrial fatty acid transport results in the cytosolic accumulation of triglycerides and this has been implicated in the pathogenesis of insulin resistance (Krajcovicová et al., 2000). Acute hypercarnitinemia increases non-oxidative glucose disposal by 50% in healthy volunteers treated with insulin (Ferrannini et al., 1988). Whole-body glucose utilization is also increased by L-carnitine in type 2 diabetic patients; an effect that may be related to increases in both glucose uptake and glucose oxidation (Capaldo et al., 1991; Mingrone et al., 1999). Treatment with propionyl-L-carnitine (PC, 2 g/day for 12 months) significantly increased the maximal walking distance and the distance walked prior to the onset of claudication (in patients whose initial maximal walking distance was less than 250 m) in a randomized placebo-controlled study of 495 patients with intermittent claudication (Brevetti et al., 1999). Acute intravenous administration of PC to type 2 diabetic patients with peripheral arterial disease (PAD) improved PAD-related symptoms as well as glycaemic control (Ragozzino et al., 2004). Acetyl-L-carnitine is effective and well tolerated in a 1-year treatment plan where pain reduction was targeted in diabetic patients with neuropathy (Grandis et al., 2002). Larger studies (both animal and human) are required to establish the precise role of supplementation with carnitine in diabetic patients, and it has not been recommended routinely by any evidence-based guidelines or treatment algorithms. In addition to this, its long-term effects and complications have not been adequately investigated.

4.8.7   *RUBOXISTAURIN (LY 333531)*

As stated earlier, PKC activation and increased diacylglycerol (DAG) levels initiated by hyperglycemia are associated with many vascular abnormalities in retinal, renal, and cardiovascular tissues during diabetes. The PKC βI and βII isoforms appear to be activated preferentially in the vasculatures of diabetics, although other PKC isoforms are also increased in the renal glomeruli and retina. It has been suggested that the mechanisms for the preferential activation of PKC βI and βII may be related to the subcellular localization, differential tissue expression, and differential phosphorylation of the various isoforms by other kinases of the β isoforms (Das et al., 2007; Mellor et al., 1998; Keranen et al., 1995). Glucose-induced activation of PKC increases the production of the extracellular matrix proteins and various cytokines while also enhancing vascular contractility, increasing vascular permeability and cell proliferation, activation of cytosolic phospholipase A2, and inhibition of Na+/K+- ATPase (Koya et al., 1998). Ruboxistaurin has shown promising effects in the treatment of diabetic retinopathy in both preclinical and human studies, while the efficacy of ruboxistaurin for the treatment of peripheral neuropathy has not been successfully demonstrated in Phase III trials. Although a pilot study reported a beneficial effect of ruboxistaurin in treating diabetic nephropathy, this has not been confirmed in a controlled large-scale trail (Danis et al., 2009). Likewise, the encouraging results obtained with the use of ruboxistaurin in treating diabetic retinopathy have yet to receive approval by the FDA.

4.9   CONCLUSION

Hyperglycemia is accompanied by increasing oxidative stress, which is considered a mechanism for inflammation and endothelial dysfunction. An antioxidant supplement in diabetes individuals to prevent long-term complications by prompted several clinical trials. Antioxidants have the capacity to transform into prooxidants after reacting with ROS; a chain reaction is required to regenerate such antioxidants de novo. As vitamin E is converted to tocopheroxyl radicals after acting as a free radical scavenger, it means the regeneration of vitamin E is required to prevent unwanted tocopheroxyl-mediated oxidative process. Vitamin E regeneration system is composed of ascorbic acid, reduced glutathione, and CoQ10. Vitamins and mineral intakes for people with DM are similar to those for healthy subjects. Patients should be encouraged to obtain such nutrients primarily from natural sources and foods rather than supplements.

Side Effects of Antioxidants

We take as food; there are no known side effects to antioxidants, though it is possible that there may be some interactions with other medications. If you take supplements according to your pharmacist's and physician's instructions, there are few side effects and even fewer serious side effects. Some people experience constipation, diarrhea, or an upset stomach. Vitamin C taken in high doses (in grams) can cause diarrhea. In some people and in higher doses (800–1000 mg/day), vitamin E can cause bleeding problems. Coenzyme Q10 (CoQ10) can also increase bleeding in high doses and may interact with blood pressure medications. Alpha-lipoic acid (ALA) appears to have few reported side effects. Carnitine can increase bleeding in high doses. Always tell your physician and pharmacist all the medications and supplements you are taking and always follow your physician's instructions on dosage (Christine, 2018).

KEYWORDS

- **diabetes mellitus**
- **oxidative stress**
- **antioxidant**

REFERENCES

Afkhami-Ardekani, M.; Shojaoddiny-Ardekani, A. Effect of Vitamin C on Blood Glucose, Serum Lipids and Serum Insulin in Type 2 Diabetes Patients. *Indian J. Med. Res.* **2007,** *126,* 471–474.

Al Shamsi, MS.; Amin, A.; Adeghate, E. Beneficial Effect of Vitamin E on the Metabolic Parameters of Diabetic Rats. *Mol. Cell. Biochem.* **2004,** *261,* 35–42.

American Diabetes Association. Standards of Medical Care in Diabetes. *Diabetes Care* **2018,** *41,* 1–2.

Arambasic, J.; Mihailovic, M.; Uskokovic, A.; Dinic, S.; Grdovic, N.; Markovic, J. Alpha-Lipoic Acid Up Regulates Antioxidant Enzyme Gene Expression and Enzymatic Activity in Diabetic Rat Kidneys through an *O*-Glcnac-Dependent Mechanism. *Eur. J. Nutr.* **2013,** *52,* 1461–1473.

Bajaj, S.; Khan, A. Antioxidants and Diabetes. *Endocrinol. Metab.* **2012,** *16,* S267–S271.

Baragob, A. E.; Al Malki, W. H.; Alla, W. H.; Ibrahim, A.; Muhammed, S. K.; Abdella, S. Investigate Evaluation of Oxidative Stress and Lipid Profile in STZ-Induced Rats Treated with Antioxidant Vitamin. *Pharmacol. Pharm.* **2014,** *5,* 272–279.

Battell, M. L.; Delgatty, H. L.; McNeill, J. H. Sodium Selenate Corrects Glucose Tolerance and Heart Function in STZ Diabetic Rats. *Mol. Cell. Biochem.* **1998,** *179,* 27–34.

Bitar, M. S.; Wahid, S.; Pilcher, C. W.; Al-Saleh, E.; Al-Mulla, F. Alpha-Lipoic Acid Mitigates Insulin Resistance in Goto-Kakizaki Rats. *Horm. Metab. Res.* **2004,** *36,* 542–549.

Brevetti, G.; Diehm, C.; Lambert, D. European Multicenter Study on Propionyl-L-Carnitine in Intermittent Claudication. *J. Am. Coll. Cardiol.* **1999,** *34,* 1618–1624.

Budin, S. B.; Kee, K. P.; Eng, M. Y.; Osman, K.; Bakar, M. A.; Mohamed, J. Alpha Lipoic Acid Prevents Pancreatic Islet Cells Damage and Dyslipidemia in Streptozotocin-Induced Diabetic Rats. *Malays J. Med. Sci.* **2007**, *14*, 47–53.

Bursell, S. E.; Clermont, A. C.; Aiello, L. P.; Aiello, L. M.; Schlossman, D. K.; Feener, E. P. High-Dose Vitamin E Supplementation Normalizes Retinal Blood Flow and Creatinine Clearance in Patients with Type 1 Diabetes. *Diabetes Care* **1999**, *22*, 1245–1251.

Bustamante, J.; Lodge, J. K.; Marcocci, L.; Tritschler, H. J.; Packer, L.; Rihn, B. H. Alpha-Lipoic Acid in Liver Metabolism and Disease. *Free Radic. Biol. Med.* **1998**, *24*, 1023–1039.

Capaldo, B.; Napoli, R.; Di Bonito, P.; Albano, G.; Saccà, L. Carnitine Improves Peripheral Glucose Disposal in Non-Insulin-Dependent Diabetic Patients. *Diabetes Res. Clin. Pract.* **1991**, *14*, 191–195.

Crane, F. L.; Navas, P. The Diversity of Coenzyme Q Function. *Mol. Aspects Med.* 1997, *18*, 51–56.

Danis, R. P.; Sheetz, M. J. Ruboxistaurin, PKC-Beta Inhibition for Complications of Diabetes. *Expert Opin. Pharmacother.* **2009**, *10*, 2913–2925.

Das Evcimen, N., King, G. L. The Role of Protein Kinase C Activation and the Vascular Complications of Diabetes. *Pharmacol. Res.* **2007**, *55*, 498–510.

De Grandis, D.; Minardi, C. Acetyl-L-Carnitine (Levacecarnine) in the Treatment of Diabetic Neuropathy. A Long-Term, Randomised, Doubleblind, Placebo-Controlled Study. *Drugs Res. Dev.* **2002**, *3*, 223–331.

Dipiro, J. T.; Talbert, R. L.; Yee, G. C.; Matzke, G. R.; Wells, B. G.; Posey, L. M., Eds. *Pharmacotherapy: A Pathophysiologic Approach*, 5th ed.; Mcgraw-Hill, 2002; pp 1335–1355.

Douillet, C.; Tabib, A.; Bost, M.; Accominotti, M.; Borson-Chazot, F.; Ciavatti, M. Selenium in Diabetes. Effects of Selenium on Nephropathy in Type I Streptozotocin-Induced Diabetic Rats. *Trace Elem. Exp. Med.* **1999**, *12*, 379–392.

Eriksson, J.; Kohvakka, A. Magnesium and Ascorbic Acid Supplementation in Diabetes Mellitus. *Nutr. Metab.* **1995**, *39*, 217–223.

Ferrannini, E.; Buzzigoli, G.; Bevilacqua, S. Interaction of Carnitine with Insulin Stimulated Glucose Metabolism in Humans. *Am. J. Physiol.* **1988**, *255*, E946–E952.

Greenberg, S.; Frishman, W. H. Co-Enzyme Q10, A New Drug for Cardiovascular Disease. *Clin. Pharmacol.* **1990**, *30*, 596–608.

Halliwell, B.; Guttreridge, J. M., Eds. *Free Radical in Biology and Medicine*; Clarendon Press: Oxford and New York, NY, 1999.

Hill, M. F. Emerging Role for Antioxidants Therapy in Protection against Diabetic Cardiac Complications, Experimental and Clinical Evidence for Utilization of Classic and New Antioxidants. *Curr. Cardiol. Rev.* **2008**, *4*, 259–268.

Hisalkar, P. J.; Patne, A. B.; Fawade, M. M. Assessment of Plasma Antioxidant Levels in Type 2 Diabetes Patients. *Biol. Med. Res.* **2012**, *3*, 1796–1800.

Ihara, Y.; Yamada, Y.; Toyokuni, S.; Miyawaki, K.; Ban, N.; Adachi, T. Antioxidant Alpha-Tocopherol Ameliorates Glycemic Control of GK Rats, A Model of Type 2 Diabetes. *FEBS Lett.* **2000**, *473*, 24–26.

International Diabetes Federation. *IDF Diabetes Atlas,* 8th ed.; IDF: Brussels, 2017.

Jacob, S.; Henriksen, E. J.; Tritschler, H. J.; Augustin, H. J.; Dietze, G. J. Improvement of Insulin-Stimulated Glucose-Disposal in Type 2 Diabetes After Repeated Parenteral Administration of Thioctic Acid. *Exp. Clin. Endocrinol. Diabetes* **1996**, *104*, 284–288.

Je, H. D.; Shin, C. Y.; Park, H. S.; Huh, I. H.; Sohn, U. D. The Comparison of Vitamin C and Vitamin E on the Protein Oxidation of Diabetic Rats. *Auton. Pharmacol.* **2001**, *21*, 231–236.

Kamenova, P. Improvement of Insulin Sensitivity in Patients with Type 2 Diabetes Mellitus after Oral Administration of Alpha-Lipoic Acid. *Hormones (Athens)* **2006**, *5*, 251–258.

Keranen, L. M.; Dutil, E. M.; Newton, A. C. Protein Kinase C is Regulated *In Vivo* By Three Functionally Distinct Phosphorylations. *Curr. Biol.* **1995**, *5*, 1394–1403.

Koya, D.; King, G. L. Protein Kinase C Activation and the Development of Diabetic Complications. *J. Diabetes* **1998**, *47*, 859–866.

Krajcovicová-Kudláčková, M.; Simoncic, R.; Béderová, A.; Babinská, K.; Béder, I. Correlation of Carnitine Levels to Methionine and Lysine Intake. *Physiol. Res.* **2000**, *49*, 399–402.

Langsjoen, P. H.; Langsjoen, A. M. Overview of the Use of CoQ10 in Cardiovascular Disease. *Biofactors* **1999**, *9*, 273–284.

Lipinski, B. Pathophysiology of Oxidative Stress in Diabetes Mellitus and Diabetes its Complications. *Res. Soc. Promot Health* **2001**, *15*, 203–210.

McNeill, J. H.; Delgatty, H. L.; Battell, M. L. Insulin-Like Effects of Sodium Selenate in Streptozotocin-Induced Diabetic Rats. *J. Diabetes* **1991**, *40*, 1675–1678.

Mellor, H.; Parker, P. J. The Extended Protein Kinase C Superfamily. *Biochem. J.* **1998**, *332*, 281–292.

Milman, U.; Blum, S.; Shapira, C.; Aronson, D.; Miller-Lotan, R.; Anbinder, Y. Vitamin E Supplementation Reduces Cardiovascular Events in a Subgroup of Middle-Aged Individuals with Both Type 2 Diabetes Mellitus and the Haptoglobin 2-2 Genotype, a Prospective Double-Blinded Clinical Trial. *Arterioscler. Thromb. Vasc. Biol.* **2008**, *28*, 341–347.

Mingrone, G.; Greco, A. V.; Capristo, E. L. Carnitine Improves Glucose Disposal in Type 2 Diabetic Patients. *Coll. Nutr.* **1999**, *18*, 77–82.

Opara, E. C. Oxidative Stress, Micronutrients, Diabetes Mellitus and its Complications. *Res. Soc. Promot Health* **2001**, *122*, 28–34.

Overvad, K.; Diamant, B.; Holm, L.; Holmer, G.; Mortensen, S. A.; Stender, S. Coenzyme Q10 in Health and Disease. *Eur. Clin. Nutr.* **1999**, *53*, 764–770.

Packer, L.; Kraemer, K.; Rimbach, G. Molecular Aspects of Lipoic Acid in the Prevention of Diabetes Complications. *Nutrition* **2001**, *17*, 888–895.

Packer, L.; Cadenas, E. Lipoic Acid, Energy Metabolism and Redox Regulation of Transcription and Cell Signaling. *Clin. Biochem. Nutr.* **2011**, *48*, 26–32.

Ragozzino, G.; Mattera, E.; Madrid, E. Effects of Propionyl-carnitine in Patients With Type 2 Diabetes and Peripheral Vascular Disease, Results of a Pilot Trial. *Drugs Res. Dev.* **2004**, *5*, 185–190.

Roldi, L. P.; Pereira, R. V.; Tronchini, E. A.; Rizo, G. V.; Scoaris, C. R.; Zanoni, J. N. Vitamin E (Alpha-Tocopherol) Supplementation in Diabetic Rats, Effects on the Proximal Colon. *BMC Gastroenterol.* **2009**, *9*, 88.

Seven, A.; Guzel, S.; Seymen, O.; Civelek, S.; Bolayirli, M.; Uncu, M. Effects of Vitamin E Supplementation on Oxidative Stress in Streptozotocin Induced Diabetic Rats, Investigation of Liver and Plasma. *Yonsei Med J.*. **2004**, *45*, 703–710.

Shan, H. H. M.; Rajendran, R. Effect of Antioxidant Therapy on Diabetes Mellitus. *B. Pharma Projects Rev. Articels,* **2009**, *1*, 1680–1721.

Singh, P. P.; Mahadi, F.; Roy, A.; Sharma, P. Reactive Nitrogen Species and Antioxidants in Etiopathogenesis of Diabetes Mellitus Type 2. *Clin. Biochem.* **2009,** *24*, 324–342.

Stapleton, S. R. Selenium, An Insulin-Mimetic. *Cell. Mol. Life Sci.* **2000,** *57*, 1874–1879.

Steinbrenner, H.; Speckmann, B.; Pinto, A.; Sies, H. High Selenium Intake and Increased Diabetes Risk, Experimental Evidence for Interplay between Selenium and Carbohydrate Metabolism. *Clin. Biochem. Nutr.* **2011,** *48*, 40–45.

Sunde, R. A.; Bowman, B.; Russell, R., Eds. Selenium. In *Present Knowledge in Nutrition*, 9th ed.; International Life Sciences Institute: Washington, DC, 2006; pp 480–497.

Tanko, Y.; Eze, E. D.; Chukwuemeka, U. E.; Jimoh, A.; Mohammed, A.; Abdulrazak, A. Modulatory Roles of Vitamin C and E on Blood Glucose and Serum Electrolytes Levels in Fructose-Induced Insulin Resistance (Type 2) Diabetes Mellitus in Wistar Rats. *Pharm. Lett.* **2013,** *5*, 259–263.

Tran, M. T.; Mitchell, T. M.; Kennedy, D. T.; Giles, J. T. Role of Coenzyme Q10 in Chronic Heart Failure, Angina, and Hypertension. *Pharmacotherapy* **2001,** *21*, 797–806.

Traxler, C. *Antioxidants for Diabetes. The Diabetes Council Article Reviewed. 14, 2018.*

Whanger, P.; Vendeland, S.; Park, Y. C.; Xia, Y. Metabolism of Subtoxic Levels of Selenium in Animals and Humans. *Ann. Clin. Lab. Sci.* **1996,** *26*, 99–113.

Wiernsperger, N.; Rapin, J. Trace Elements in Glucometabolic Disorders, an Update. *Diabetol. Metab. Syndr.* **2010,** *2*, 70.

Will, J. C.; Bowman, B. A. Serum Vitamin-C Concentrations and Diabetes, Finding from the Third National Health and Nutrition Examination Survey, 1988–1994. *Clin. Nutr.* **1999,** *70*, 49–52.

Williams, D. E.; Wareham, N. J.; Cox, B. D.; Bryne, C. D.; Hales, C. N.; Day, N. E. Frequent Salad Vegetable Consumption is Associated with a Reduction in the Risk of Diabetes Mellitus. *Clin. Epidemiol.* **1999,** *52*, 329–335.

Wollin, S. D.; Jones, P. J. Alpha Lipoic Acid and Cardiovascular Disease. *J. Nutr.* **2003,** *133*, 3327–3330.

CHAPTER 5

Extraction and Quantification of Antioxidants

NEHA CHAUHAN* and SURBHI ANTARKAR

Department of Life Sciences, ITM University, Gwalior, India

Corresponding author. E-mail: nehachauhan.sols@itmuniversity.ac.in

ABSTRACT

Members of the Food and Nutrition Board of the National Research Council in the United States have recently defined a dietary antioxidant as "a substance in foods that reduces the adverse effects of reactive oxygen species, reactive nitrogen species, or both on general physiology function in humans." The continuous consumption of used oil, unhealthy diet, and stress adversely affect the human body by generating free radicals. Free radical causes tissue damage, alters lipids, proteins, DNA, and trigger a number of human diseases. Antioxidants are free radical scavengers that neutralize these free radical autoxidation reactions. Antioxidants are secondary metabolites, and most of them are obtained by natural sources such as roots, leaves, fruits, seeds, and herbs. Natural plant pigments also contribute their antioxidant properties in human benefits. There are several techniques to extract, purify, and quantify antioxidants. Nowadays, there is a vast variety of oral supplements that can be procured from the market. Natural (functional foods) as well as synthetic antioxidants can serve their essential role in the management of human health.

5.1 INTRODUCTION

The importance of oxidation in the body and in foods has been widely recognized. Oxidative metabolism is essential for the survival of cells.

A side effect of this dependence is the production of free radicals and other reactive oxygen species (ROS), which causes oxidative changes. Incorporating such species into various types of in vivo regulatory systems has been reported in many researches. When more free radicals are formed, they overwhelm protective enzymes such as super oxyridismutase, caterase, and peroxidase and exert destructive and lethal cellular effects (e.g., apoptosis) by oxidation of membranous lipids, cellular proteins, DNA, and enzymes, resulting in cellular respiratory failure. These ROS affect cell signaling pathways in ways that are only now being unpublished. Oxidation due to chemical spoilage can also affect foods, resulting in hardness and/or deterioration in the quality, color, taste, texture, and safety of foods. It is estimated that half of the world's fruit and vegetable crops are lost due to postharvest damage.

Potential beneficial effects from antioxidants in protecting against the disease have been used as an argument for recommending increased intake of many nutrients derived from traditional methods. If it is possible to determine the amount of such claims, antioxidant properties should be considered in decisions related to the daily requirements of these nutrients. This section examines important aspects of the most important dietary antioxidants—vitamin C, vitamin E, carotenoids, and many minerals—and tries to define populations that should have antioxidant properties and may be at risk of insufficiency to determine what may be considered in establishing the requirement. In addition, the importance of pro-oxidant metabolism and iron is also considered.

Members of the Food and Nutrition Board of the National Research Council in the United States have recently defined a dietary antioxidant as a substance in foods that reduces the adverse effects of ROS, reactive nitrogen species, or both on general physiology function in humans.

Generally, antioxidants can be divided into two major categories, such as *synthetic* and *natural*. The main target site of these free radical damage and defensive approaches is at the cellular level. Based on this, these antioxidants can also be classified as *enzymatic* and *nonzymatic antioxidants* (as shown in Figure 5.1). Enzymatic antioxidants mainly include glutathione peroxidase, catalase, and superoxide dismutase. There are also many other enzymes in the body that contribute to the total antioxidant capacity, which is regenerated in the serum. Nonzymatic antioxidants have several subdivisions that primarily contain vitamins A, E, C, and to a lesser extent vitamin D, enzyme cofactors, peptides, and some minerals (zinc and selenium). The major elements from natural sources are polyphenolic compounds, which are reported to have significant antioxidant capacity.

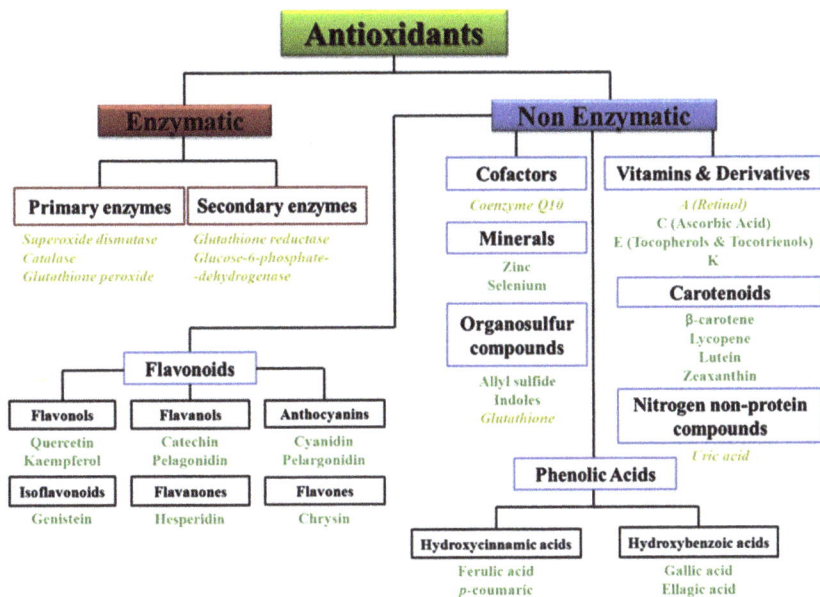

FIGURE 5.1 Antioxidants.

Source: Reprinted with permission from Carocho, et al. 2013. © Elsevier.

Natural antioxidants are mainly phenolics that can occur in all parts of plants, such as fruits, vegetables, nuts, seeds, leaves, roots, and bark. The literature regarding the use of synthetic antioxidants showed their unwanted or adverse effects. These reports have urged researchers to focus their studies on the discovery of natural sources with appropriate antioxidant potential and in the context of the use of these natural antioxidants. Antioxidants by nature can be classified into various subclassifications. However, the two major categories typically include antioxidants from consumed or regular natural diets (e.g., vegetables, fruits, grains, and beans) and antioxidants from a plant or herb sources that have reasonable antioxidant potential but are not regular dietary sources (e.g., medicinal plants and wild herbs). Among these, regular dietary sources are very important as they may be readily available and may have more needles.

5.2   METHODS OF EXTRACTION OF ANTIOXIDANTS

Extraction is a separation process that is used to separate solutes, that is, bioactive constituents from solutions using specific solvents by adoption of standard procedures. The main pure currency of this extraction method is to separate soluble solutes from plant by-products for efficient extraction performance process. Crude extracts obtained using these methods use a complex mixture of many plant metabolites: alkaloids, glycosides, phenolics, terpenoids, and flavonoids. These extracts are being used as a medicinal agents as a cool tincture and fluid extracts. There are several methods available to extract antioxidants from the plant by processing products.

5.2.1   TRADITIONAL EXTRACTION TECHNIQUES

Classical/traditional extraction techniques are being used at a small scale to extract bioactive components from many plants. These techniques are usually based on the extraction efficiency of different solvents, which are being used for this purpose.

There is a three-process approach, consisting of (1) Soxhlet extraction, (2) maceration, and (3) hydrodistillation (HD).

- Soxhlet extraction technique has been widely used extracting several bioactive compounds from various plant materials. Samples of dry plant material will have to be placed in the thimble. The thimble is then placed in a distillation flask containing the solvent selective solvent when the overflow level of the solvent is reached. Solution of the thimble-holder is aspirated by a siphon. Siphon removes the solution back to the distillation flask. This solvent solution carries the extracted solute in bulk liquid. The solute remains in distillation flask and solvent goes back to the bed of the plant. The extraction runs repeatedly until completion.
- Maceration stage was used at home level to prepare tonic since the old days. It is a popular and the cheapest way to get many essential oils and bioactive compounds from various plant materials. For small scales of extraction, the maceration process typically consists of several stages. First, materials are ground, that is, their size is being reduced, increase in surface area for uniform mixing with

the chosen solvent. As a second step, in the maceration process, the appropriate solvent, that is, menstruum, is added to a closed pot. Third, the liquid is strained closed, but marc, which is the solid residue of this extraction process, is pressed to fix a solution of a large amount of solution. The received strained and pressed out liquid are mixed and separated from impurities by filtration. The simultaneous shaking process will facilitate extraction in two ways: first, it will increase diffusion, and second, it will remove the concentrated solution from the sample surface to bring new solvent into the menstruum to achieve more extraction yield.

• HD is one of the traditional methods used to extract bioactive compounds and essential oils from many plant materials. In this process, organic solvents are not included, and this can be done before dehydration of any plant material. There are three types of HD: water distillation, water and steam distillation, and direct steam distillation. In HD, first, the plant material is still packed in a box; second, a sufficient amount of water is added and then brought to a boil. Alternatively, direct steam is also injected into the plant sample. Both hot water and steam can act as the main influencing factors. Release of bioactive compounds from many plant tissues takes place. Indirect when cooled by water, condensation of vapor mixture of water and oil occurs. Condensed current flows from the condenser to a separator, where the oil and bioactive compounds are spontaneously separated. HD consists of three main physiochemical processes: (1) hydrodiffusion, (2) hydrolysis, and (3) decomposition with heat. At high extraction temperatures, some volatile components will be lost. Therefore, this limitation limits its use for the extraction of various thermolabile compounds from different plant tissues. The extraction rate of any conventional method depends mainly on the option of using selective solvents. Solvent polarity is one of the most important factors for the target compound, and when choosing a solvent, the molecular affinity between the chosen, the solvent, and solute.

5.2.2 NONTRADITIONAL EXTRACTION TECHNIQUES

The major challenges of conventional extraction are now additional time and the need for expensive and high purity solvents, evaporation rations of large amounts of solvent, low extraction selectivity, and thermal decomposition of material. These techniques are generally based on the extraction effect of various solvents, which are being used for this purpose. These techniques are referred to nontraditional extraction techniques. Some of the most prominent techniques are,

1. Ultrasound-assisted extraction (UAE),
2. Pulsed electric field (PEF) extraction,
3. Enzyme-assisted extraction (EAE),
4. Microwave-assisted extraction (MAE),
5. Pressurized extraction (PLE), and
6. Supercritical fluid extraction (SFE).

Some of these techniques are considered "Green techniques" because they are compliant with standards set by the Environmental Protection Agency (2015).

5.2.2.1   ULTRASOUND-ASSISTED EXTRACTION

Ultrasound is a special type of sound wave that goes beyond human hearing and has a frequency ranging from 20 kHz to 100 MHz. Like other waves, it can pass through a medium creating compression and expansion. Therefore, this process produces known phenomena in the form of cavitation, which subsequently leads to the production, growth, and collapse of bubbles. Large amounts of energy can be produced during conversion of kinetic energy of motion, and thus, it helps heating the contents of the bubbles (Herrera and Luque-de-Castro, 2004). Intensification of extraction process by using ultrasound has been attributed to cavitation events. The effects caused by ultrasonic waves are compression and extend the expansion cycle during passage through the fluid, creating bubbles or cavities in a liquid. This happens when the negative pressure increased, which is higher than the local tensile strength of the streak, may vary depending on its nature and purity. Formation of growing bubbles, undergo implantation known as cavitation. The conditions within these trapping bubbles can be dramatic with temperatures up to 4500°C and pressures up to 100 MPa, which in turn produces very high shear energy waves and disturbance in cavity area (Patist and Bates, 2008). Combination of these factors (pressure, heat, and turbulence) is used to accelerate mass transfer.

The extraction mechanism by ultrasound process includes two main types of physical phenomena:

1. Cell dispersal rinsing the contents of the cell after breaking the wall
2. Rinsing the contents of after breaking the wall (Mason et al., 1996).

Moisture content of sample, milling degree, and particle size are very important factors for obtaining effective extraction. In addition, temperature, frequency, and time of sonication were the governing factors for the action of ultrasound. The UAE is also included along with various classical techniques they have reported to increase the efficiency of a traditional system. In a solvent extraction unit, an ultrasound device is placed in an appropriate position to increase extraction efficiency. The benefits of UAE include reduction in extraction time, energy, and the use of solvent. Ultrasound energy for extraction is also more effective mixing, faster energy transfer, thermal decreases gradient and extraction temperature, selective extraction, low tool size, rapid response extraction process, quick to process start-up, increased production, and it eliminates process steps. UAE appears to be an effective extraction technique for bioactive compound extraction from by-products of fruit and vegetable processing industries (Herrera and Luque-de-Castro, 2004).

UAE is interested in low cost due to the reduction in extraction time, a more effective and concentrated use of strength, a better yield, and comparatively more concentrated extracts S/L (solid–liquid) ratio. Traditional maceration process is quiet a time- and energy-consuming process but cannot be adopted at a professional level for efficient extraction of antioxidants. Extraction process takes a reasonable amount of time (30 min), so it is possible to convert batch system toward a constant system. Experimental pilot study was done in a continuous piston apparatus for the extraction of antioxidants from boldo leaves. It is found that 30 min is required to perform effective and relevant extraction of soluble material, which is similar to a traditional maceration process. Therefore, this time of extraction is more optimized for constant extraction (Petigny et al., 2013).

5.2.2.2 PULSED ELECTRIC FIELD EXTRACTION

The PEF extraction method was one of the well-known techniques to improve drying, extraction, and diffusion processes from the last decade

(Barsotti and Cheftel, 1998; Angersbach et al., 2000; Vorobiev et al., 2005; Vorobiev and Lebovka, 2006). The principle of PEF extraction is to decompose the cell structure. Membranes are used to increase the rate of extraction. The cell passes through the membrane when it is suspended in an electric field, and this electric potential separates membrane molecules depending on the nature of the dipole, that is, according to their charge in cell membrane. After exceeding the critical value of about 1 V for transmitter capacitance, there is a repulsion, which may occur between the molecules and charges that make holes in weak areas of membrane, and therefore, it causes a huge increase in permeability (Bryant and Wolfe, 1987). For PEF treatment of plant material, a simple circuit with exponential decay pulses is used. The plant materials are kept in a treatment room, which includes two electrode, depending on the treatment room design, PEF process can be operated in continuous or batch mode (Puertolas et al., 2010). The effectiveness of PEF treatment depends on the process parameters, including field strength, specific energy input, pulse number, treatment temperature, and properties of the occurring material treated (Heinz et al., 2003).

Membrane structure of plant material is beneficial to achieve enhanced extraction and thereby reducing extraction time. PEF applied to improve the release of intracellular compounds from plant tissues helps to increase the permeability of cell membrane (Toepfl et al., 2006). PEF treatment at moderate electric field is found to damage plant tissue's cell membrane with slight increase in temperature. PEF can reduce corrosion of heat sensitive compounds (Fincan and Dejmek, 2002; Lebovka et al., 2002). This is also applicable to plant material in a pretreatment process before the traditional extraction method to reduce the extraction effort. PEF treatment is (1 kV/cm with low energy consumption of 7 kJ/kg) a procedure for solid liquid extraction (Fincan et al., 2004; Corrales et al., 2008b).

Application of a PEF maceration may reduce the healing period on grape skin before step improvement in maceration and stability of bioactives (anthocyanin and polyphenols) during vinification (Lopez et al., 2008). Merlot results from skin permeation by PEF treatment in increased clearance of polyphenols and anthocyanin. For example, in the case of grape skins, it showed that both PEF and high voltage electrical discharge (HVED) treatments had a positive effect on the extraction of polyphenols and total solutes from the skin of chardonnay grapes. Quantity of polyphenol extracts was high (Boussetta et al., 2009, 2015).

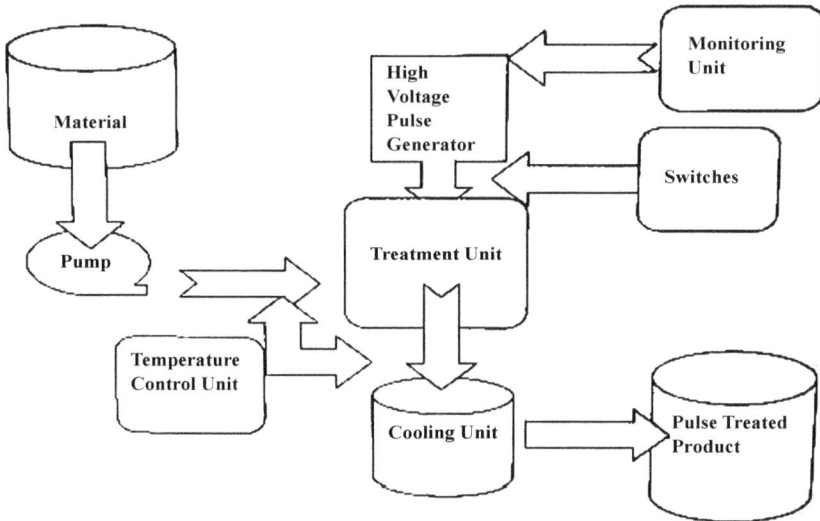

FIGURE 5.2   Components of pulsed electric field treatment and flow chart of process.
Source: Reprinted from Gamli, 2014. https://creativecommons.org/licenses/by/4.0/

The PEF technology is a mild food processing technology suitable for preserving liquid and semiliquid food products. This processing method uses short electric pulses to achieve microbial inactivation in food products while preserving the fresh characteristics.

5.2.2.3   ENZYME-ASSISTED EXTRACTION

In plant matrices, some phytochemicals are dispersed in the cell. Cytoplasm and some compounds are retained in polysaccharide lignin network by hydrogen bonding or hydrophobic interactions, which are not accessible with a solvent in a routine extraction process. Enzymatic pretreatment is considered a novel and an effective way to release and increase bonded compounds overall yield (Rosenthal et al., 1996). Apart from specific enzymes such as cellulase and α-amylase, pectinase during extraction increases recovery by breaking the cell wall and hydrolyzing structural polysaccharides and lipid bodies (Rosenthal et al., 1996; Singh et al., 1999).

There are two approaches for EAE process:

1.   Enzyme-assisted aqueous extraction (EAAE)
2.   Enzyme-assisted cold pressing (EACP) (Latif and Anwar, 2009).

EAAE methods have been developed primarily for extraction of oil from various seeds (Rosenthal et al., 1996, 2001; Hanmoungjai et al., 2001; Sharma et al., 2002). In EACP technology, enzymes are used to hydrolyze the seed cell wall because in it the polysaccharide-protein colloid is not available, which is obvious in EAEE (Concha et al., 2004). Various factors including enzymes composition and concentration, particle size of plant material, solids water ratios, and hydrolysis time are identified as major factors for extraction (Niranjan and Hanmoungjai, 2004). It is reported that the moisture of plant material is also an important factor for enzymatic hydrolysis. The process of EAE method from natural products was shown in Figure 5.3. Breakdown of cell walls is an important phase for the extraction of many bioactive compounds, which are extant inside the cell walls. EAE is based on the ability of enzymes to hydrolyze and inhibit the structural integrity of cell wall components under the mild process conditions, allowing efficient extraction and release of bioactive compounds (Pinelo et al., 2006; Gardossi et al., 2010). Direct proportionality by enzyme between rate and substrate concentration becomes limited (Sowbhagya and Chitra, 2010). Several parameters are needed to be considered to make this process efficient. The extraction process involves the time of reaction, temperature of extraction, system pH, enzyme concentration, the substrate's particle size. EACP is described as an ideal option because it is nontoxic to extract bioactive components from oilseeds as well as its nonflammable properties. Enzyme-extracted oils methods found high amounts of free fatty acid and phosphorus content compared to conventional hexane extracted oil (Dominguez et al., 1995). EAAE is recognized as eco-friendly technology for extraction of bioactive compounds from oil. It uses water as a solvent instead of organic chemicals (Puri et al., 2012). EAAE of phenolic antioxidants from grape pomace during wine production was tested (Meyer et al., 1998), which found a correlation between the yield of total phenols and the degree of plant cell wall breakdown by enzyme (Landbo and Meyer, 2001).

Industrial applications:

1. Enzymes are widely used on an industrial scale but mainly as catalysts, and the applications mainly concern the synthesis of pharmaceuticals, compounds for chemistry of specialty, polymers, etc.
2. At the industrial scale, one advantage of EAEP (enzyme assisted extraction process) is environmental benefit because it can avoid the risk of organic solvents and particularly hexane.

3. The quality of the products produced by the smooth process is usually higher.
4. EAEP technique is considered as an alternative method to produce valuable products without loss of quality at moderate conditions.
5. Compared with solvent extraction, EAEP is more eco-friendly. Besides that, one of the main advantages of EAEP is the specificity of enzymes

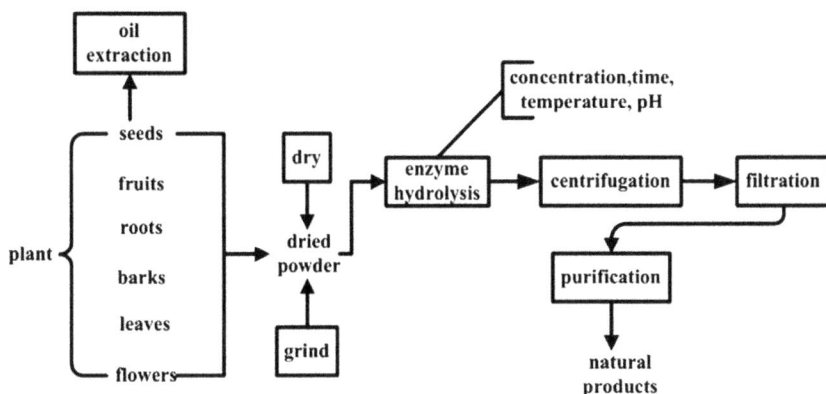

FIGURE 5.3 The process of enzyme-assisted extraction method from the natural products.

Source: Reprinted from Cheng et al., 2015.

5.2.2.4 *MICROWAVE-ASSISTED EXTRACTION*

MAE is also considered a novel method for soluble removal products in a fluid from a wide range of materials using microwave energy (Pare et al., 1994). Microwave has electromagnetic fields frequencies range from 300 MHz to 300 GHz. They are made of two oscillating fields that are perpendicular such as electric field and magnetic field (Letellier and Budzinski, 1999).

The principle of heating using microwave is based on its direct effect on polar material after ionic conduction (Jain, 2009). Electromagnetic energy is converted into heat and bipolar rotating mechanisms. During ionic conduction due to the resistance of the system, heat is generated in the medium. On the other hand, the ions carry their direction along field signs, which change frequently. This constant change of directions results in collisions between molecules and results in warmth (Kaufmann and

Christen, 2002). The larger the dielectric constant of the solvent, more optimal will be the heating. In the case of extraction, the advantage of microwave heating is dissolution. Weak hydrogen boundary promoted by dipole rotation molecules. The high viscosity of the medium reduces this mechanism affecting molecular rotation. Migration of dissolved ions increases solvent penetration into the matrix and thus facilitates solvent analysis of the extraction system (Kaufmann and Christen, 2002). The three sequential steps described in MAE are to be included by, first, separation of solutes from active sites of sample matrix under increased temperature and pressure, second, diffusion of solvent into the sample matrix, and third, the release of solutes from solvent matrix to solvent (Cravottoa et al., 2008). MAE has many advantages, such as early heating extraction of bioactive substances from plant materials, thermally reduced gradient, reduced equipment size, and extracts yield increased. MAE can remove bioactive compounds more quickly, and a better recovery is possible compared to traditional extraction processes. MAE is also referred to as green technology as it reduces its use organic solvent (Alupului et al., 2012) showed increased extraction efficiency MAE is a flavoliganin, removing silibinin from Silybum marianum compared with traditional extraction techniques as Soxhlet extraction and maceration (Asghari et al., 2011). Something removed bioactive compounds (E- and Z-guggolsterone, cinnamaldehyde, and tannins) from different plants under different conditions and shown is a faster and simpler method than MAE for traditional extraction processes. MAE process from Chinese quince (*Chaenomeles sinensis*) was optimized for solvent concentration, extraction time, and is designed using microwave power experiments to maximize the recovery of flavonoids and phenolics and also increase the electron donating capacity of extracts (Hui et al., 2009; Liazid et al., 2011).

MAE systems are classified into multimode system and focus-mode system (monomode); multimode system allows random dispersion of microwave radiation into the cavity by a mode stirrer, while focused system (monomode) allows focused microwave radiation over a restricted area in the cavity. Typically, multimode systems are associated with high pressure (HP), while the monomode system operating at atmospheric operating pressure. However, the monomode system can also run on HP. So that confusion can be avoided, MAE is generally classified as "closed system" and "open system" used to refer to a system that operates above atmospheric pressure and under atmospheric pressure, respectively.

Closed and open system are depicted in Figure 5.4 (Dean and Xiong, 2000; Garcia and Castro, 2003). In a closed MAE system, the extract is carried out in a sealed vessel with different modes of microwave radiation. High pressure and system temperature fast and efficient extraction. Pressure inside the extraction vessel is controlled in such a way that it is more than work vessel pressure while temperature can be regulated above the normal boiling point of the extraction solvent. In recent progress, it has been demonstrated that the hyper pressure has developed in closed system MAE (Wang et al., 2008). Increases in temperature and pressure are accelerated MAE due to the ability of the extraction solvent to absorb microwaves.

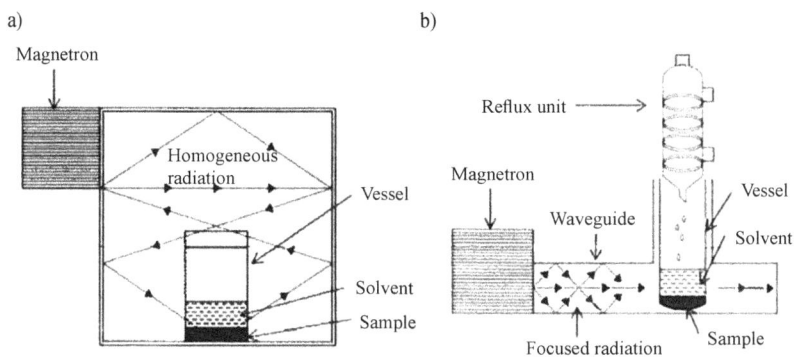

FIGURE 5.4 (a) Closed type microwave system and (b) open type microwave system.
Source: Reprinted from Mandal et al., 2007.

5.2.2.5 PRESSURIZED LIQUID EXTRACTION

PLE was first described by Richter et al. (1996). This is the way now known by many names, pressurized fluid extraction, accelerated fluid extraction, increased solvent extraction, subcritical water extraction (SWE), and HP solvent extraction (Nieto et al., 2010). The concept of PLE in HP's application is to keep the solvents liquid beyond their normal boiling point, in HP extraction facility process. Automation technology is the main reason for greater development of PLE-based technologies along with scarcity of extraction resolves time and requirement. PLE technology requires less amount of solvents a combination of HP and temperature, which provides faster extraction. Higher extraction temperatures may promote higher analyte solubility by increasing both solubility and mass transfer rate (Ibanez et al., 2012) and, thus also reducing the viscosity and surface tension of solvents improvement in extraction rate. Compared to traditional Soxhlet extraction (Richter et al., 1996), PLE was found to dramatically reduce time consumption and solvent. Therefore, for the extraction of polar compounds, PLE is considered one of the possible alternatives technique for the SFE process. Precedent is also useful for the extraction of organic pollutants from the environment matrices that are stable at high temperatures. PLE has also been used for the extraction of bioactive compounds from marine sponges. PLE technology has applications for obtaining natural products often available in literature Additionally, due to the low amount of organic solvent used, PLE becomes extensive recognition as a green extraction technique. PLE has been successfully applied to extract bioactive compounds from various plant materials in terms of yield, reproducibility, extraction time, and solvent consumption. For example, flavonoids extracted from spinach by PLE solvent at 50–150C using a mixture of ethanol and water (70:30) were more effective than water solvent at 50–130°C using the PLE method (Howard and Pandjaitan, 2008; Luthria, 2008).

The PLE setup is shown in Figure 5.5. Solvent the extraction was pumped into the cell, which was placed in an electric heating jacket at a desired temperature until the required pressure was obtained. Extraction samples were placed in 6.57 cm^3 extraction cell containing a sintered metal filter at the bottom and upper part. The cell containing the sample was heated, filled with extraction solvent, and then pressurized. Sample was kept in the heating system for 5 min to ensure that the extraction cell is at the desired temperature (313–393K) during filling and pressure process. After pressure, sample the pressurized solvent was statistically placed at the desired pressure (5–10 MPa) for the desired time (3–15 min). After PLE, extracts are rapidly cooled to 5°C in ice water using an amber flask to prevent anthocyanin degradation SWE process that removes antioxidant flavonoids from agriculture by-products such as *Citrus unshiu* Markovich. Operational impact parameters (extraction temperature, extraction time, material type, solute/solvent ratio and pressure on SWE of flavonoids) studied with satsuma mandarin peel. From a practical aspect, the optimal position of pilon to receive flavonoids he SWEs were as follows: extraction temperature of 130°C, extraction 15 min time, and a solute/solvent ratio of 1/34. Yields of the flavonoids obtained under laboratory and pilot conditions were similar, 11, 113, and 113.4 mg/g satsuma mandarin peel, respectively. The ratio of flavonoids recovered by SWE in the pilot plant was 96.3%, and large-scale experiments are demonstrated using this method. SWE is an excellent technique for selective flavonoid extract using dielectric constant properties dependent on the temperature of water.

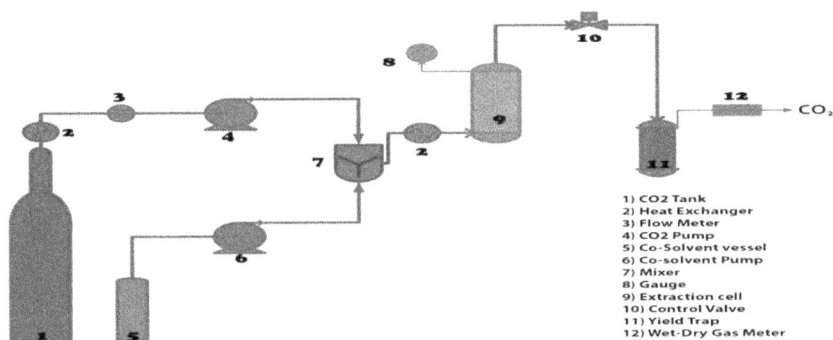

1) CO2 Tank
2) Heat Exchanger
3) Flow Meter
4) CO2 Pump
5) Co-Solvent vessel
6) Co-solvent Pump
7) Mixer
8) Gauge
9) Extraction cell
10) Control Valve
11) Yield Trap
12) Wet-Dry Gas Meter

FIGURE 5.5 Effects of supercritical fluid extraction parameters on lycopene yield and antioxidant activity.

5.2.2.6 SUPERCRITICAL FLUID EXTRACTION

The SFE technique has attracted widespread scientific interest, and it was successfully used in pharmaceutical, polymer, and food applications (Zougagh et al., 2004). Many industries are using this technology for several years, in particular, the preparation of decaffeinated coffee industry (Ndiomu and Simpson, 1988). The supercritical state is a typical state and can be attained only when subject to a substance temperature and pressure beyond its critical point. Important point is the above characteristic is defined as temperature (Tc) and pressure (Pc) in which specific gas and liquid phases are not present (Inczedy et al., 1998). Typical properties of gas and/or in the supercritical state fluid transformation are that supercritical fluid cannot be liquefied by modifying temperature and pressure. Near supercritical fluid properties like gas, viscosity, and surface tension, and liquid-like density and solvent power. These qualities make it suitable for extracting compound in a short period of time with high yields (Sihvonen et al., 1999). A basic SFE system includes the following parts, a tank of mobile phase, usually CO_2, a pump to suppress the pressure gas, co-solvent vessel and pump, an oven containing extraction vessel, a controller to maintain HP inside the system, and a trap vessel. Usually different types of meters like flow meter, dry/wet gas meters can be connected to the system. A symmetric diagram typical SFE instrumentation is given in Figure 5.5. CO_2 is considered an ideal solvent for SFE. Critical CO_2 (31°C) temperature is close to room temperature and provides possibility to operate at low critical pressure (74 bar) medium pressure, typically between 100 and 450 bar (Temelli and Guclu-Ustundag, 2005). The main drawback of CO_2 is its low polarity, which makes it ideal for lipids, fats, and nonpolar substances, but unsuitable for polar materials. Lower limit coating of CO_2 has been successfully overcome with the use of chemical modifiers. In general, a small amount of the modifier (Lang and Wai, 2001; Ghafoor et al., 2010) is considered to be significantly useful increases the polarity of CO_2. For example, 0.5 mol of dichloromethane (CH_2Cl_2) can enhance extraction, which is the same for 4-H HD (Hawthorne et al., 1994). Extraction of bioactive compounds from plant materials SFE depends on many parameters (Raverchon and Marco, 2006; Raynie, 2006, 2010), and most importantly, the major variables affecting extraction efficiency are temperature, pressure, particle size and feed moisture material, extraction time, CO_2 flow rate, and solvent-to-feed ratio (Temelli and Guclu-Ustundag, 2005; Ibanez et al., 2012). Advantages of using supercritical fluids for extraction of bioactive compounds can be understood by (Lang and Wai, 2001) considering the following points:

1. Supercritical fluid diffusion is high coefficient and lower viscosity and surface tension than a leading to liquid solvent, sample matrix, and greater penetration favorable mass transfer. Extraction time can be reduced to a great extent by SFE when compared to traditional methods.

2. The repeated reflux of supercritical fluid to the sample provides complete extraction.

3. Selectivity of supercritical fluid is greater than liquid the solvent as its solvent strength can be either tuned by changing temperature or pressure.

4. Separation of solutes from solvent in conventional the extraction process can be easily passed by sedimentation supercritical fluid, which will save time.

5. SFE is operated room temperature, hence an ideal method for thermolabile compound extraction.

6. In SFE, a smaller quantity of sample can be extracted with solvent extraction methods.
7. SFE does not use organic considered solvent and environmentally friendly.
8. Recycling and supercritical fluid reuse is possible and thus minimizing waste generation.
9. SFE scale can be organized with specific purpose some milligram samples in industries in the laboratory.
10. The SFE process provides information about the extraction process and mechanisms, which can be manipulated to optimize extraction process.

For example, modified supercritical carbon dioxide (SC-CO$_2$) with ethanol (15 wt.%) yielded high extraction of naringin (flavonoid) from citrus heaven compared to pure SC-CO$_2$ at 9.5 MPa and 58.6°C (Giannuzzo et al., 2003). Polyphenols and procyanidins were extracted from grape seeds (Khorassani and Taylor, 2004; Pascual-Marti et al. (2001) using SFE, where methanol was used modifiers and methanol released over modified CO$_2$ (40%) the 79% of catechin and epicatechin rated and adapted SFE conditions (pressure [80–110 bar], temperature [40°C], ethanol concentrations [5–15%], and extraction time [5–25 min]) recover resveratrol from the grape skin of *Vitis vinifera*. They found that optimal SFE extraction conditions were obtained at 110 bars, 40°C, 7.5% ethanol, and an extraction time of 15 min. Under these conditions, resveratrol content was fully recovered (100%). The impact of a combined process of liquid and supercritical solvent extraction to recover antioxidant compounds from winery by-products (Casas et al., 2010).

Comparing the two methods of purification, crude extract solid-phase extraction (SPE) and with SFE was intended to improve the quality of final extracts for potential use safe food additives, functional food ingredients, or nutraceuticals. They found that the major fraction generated by SPE was the highest active, and fraction separated with 30% (v/v) of methanol highest antioxidant activity (0.20 g/l). Most active ingredient the yield by SFE (EC50 of 0.23 g/l) was obtained under conditions, temperature 40°C, pressure 140 bars, extraction time 30 min, ethanol (6%) as a modifier, and modifier flow 0.2 ml/min. Finally, they concluded that the most appropriate procedure for SFE is purifying raw extracts. Therefore, natural extracts obtained can be used by SFE as residual stream and pure to natural antioxidant with potential applications in food, cosmetic, and pharmaceutical industry (Barbosa-Pereira et al., 2013). Pentacyclic triterpene α,β-amyrin is a promising bioactive natural product (Bensebia et al., 2016).

Process system. SC-CO$_2$ fluid extraction process is controlled by four major steps, extraction, expansion, dissociation, and solvent conditioning. Steps comprises of four primary components:

- Extractor (HP vessel)
- Pressure and temperature control system
- Separator
- Pressure intensifier.

Raw materials are usually ground and charged in making a temperature controlled extractor to form a fixed bed, usually for a batch and single-phase mode (Shi et al., 2007a, 2007c; Kassama et al., 2008). The processes described above are half-batch continuous processes where SC-CO$_2$ flows in a continuous mode while it is removable. The solid feed is charged in batches to the extraction vessel. In commercial-scale processing plant, there are several extraction vessels sequentially used to increase process performance and output. Though arrangement of the process is interrupted at the end of the extraction period, switch to another vessel designed for extraction, unloading, and/or extraction may be performed while loading spent vessels, in progress, reducing downtime and improving production efficiency. A semicontinuous approach at commercial scale uses a several phase extraction processes involving running the system synchronously using a series of extraction vessels in tandem. In this system, the process is not interrupted at the end of extraction duration for each vessel as the process switches to the next ready when unloading the ship through the control valve for landing and/or loading spent vessels. Thus, SC-CO$_2$ technology is available single-step batch form that can be upgraded to multistage semicontinuous batch operation coupled with a multiple dissociation process. The design really needs to be improved in continuous compounds for the extraction process. Other's presence components such as lipids can disrupt the process or increase the cost due to a longer withdrawal time. Although usually a higher temperature in the extraction process supercritical CO$_2$ increases solubility of components in liquids, conditions under which thermolabile-targeted compounds are negative must be considered affected. The intensity and length of heat processing affect the promotion of health properties of bioactive. Therefore, ideally, the extraction time and the temperature should be minimum. Minimize such situations leads to a more economically viable process. Extremely high flow rates may reduce contact and restrict the time and fluid flow between solute and solvent in the specimen if it becomes compressed. Optimal flow rate appears variation with target molecule, relatively high flow rate negative effects on some components. Increasing pressure increases extraction yields. The sample matrix is an important parameter that affects solubility and mass transfer process during SC-CO$_2$ extraction. Particle size and size distribution, orifice-like properties and pore size distribution, surface area, and moisture content effects solubility and mass transfer. Presence of water (moisture) material is also in the sample matrix during supercritical extraction an effect on the extraction result. To improve yield and the quality of the high value food components extracted from the raw material, a pretreatment of raw materials is an essential process. Cell dissolution is the most important pretreatment and is the process mechanical can be operated by many processes like ultrasonic, high electronic field pulse, and nonmechanical treatment. Together improved processing conditions and low cost, high value components extracted from natural materials by SC-CO$_2$ extraction process at higher throughput will become even more economical.

5.3   QUANTIFICATION OF ANTIOXIDANTS

Various analytical methods for evaluation of antioxidant capacity have three different categories: spectrometry, electrochemical assays, and chromatography. It is worth mentioning that many techniques are currently applied for antioxidant assays and show the most common assay in this regard. ABTS (2,2'-azino-bis(3-ethylbenzothiazoline-6-sulfonic acid), DH, ferric reducing ability of plasma (FRAP), and oxygen radial absorption capacity (ORAC) assays gave comparable results for antioxidant activity methanolic extracts are measured. FRAP technology high reproducibility was simple, performed rapidly, and showed the highest correlations with both ascorbic acid and total phenolics; therefore, it would be a suitable technique to determine antioxidants in fruit extracts. Antioxidant methanol extract may have measured activity can also be estimated indirectly. Since they are using ascorbic acid showed high correlation with all assays, the use of proposed screening methods online HPLC-DH (high-performance liquid chromatography with donepezil hydrochloride) is useful for detection antioxidants due to being highly sensitive and ease of handling. This method is beneficial for sensitive determinations of individual antioxidants in complex mixtures with sample operations.

5.3.1   DH ASSAY (DONEPEZIL HYDROCHLORIDE)

This method was developed by Blois (1958) with the viewpoint to determine the antioxidant activity in a like manner by using a stable free radical α,α-diphenyl-β-picrylhydrazyl (DH $C_{18}H_{12}N_5O_6$, M H HC18H12N5O6-picrylhydrazylical α the antioxidant activity in a /" \l "CR5" in complex mixtures w it. The odd electron of nitrogen atom in DH is reduced by receiving a hydrogen atom from antioxidants to the corresponding hydrazine.

DH is characterized as a stable free radical by virtue of the delocalization of the spare electron over the molecule as a whole, so that the molecules do not dimerize like most other free radicals. The delocalization also gives rise to the deep violet color, with an absorption in ethanol solution at around 520 nm. On mixing DH solution with a substance that can donate a hydrogen atom, it gives rise to the reduced form with the loss of violet color. Representing the DH radical by R• and the donor molecule by AH, the primary reaction is

$$R• + AH = RH + A•$$

where RH is the reduced form and A• is free radical produced in the first step. The latter radical will then undergo further reactions that control the overall stoichiometry. The reaction (1) is therefore intended to provide the link with the reactions taking place in an oxidizing system, such as the autoxidation of a lipid or other unsaturated substance; the DH molecule R• is thus intended to represent the free radicals formed in the system whose activity is to be suppressed by the substance AH.

The ferric antioxidant power (FRAP) mechanism is based on electron transfer rather than hydrogen atom transfer (East et al., 2005). The FRAP assay is based on PH's ability to reduce Fe^{3+} to PH^{2+}. The FRAP reaction is conducted at acidic pH 3.6 to maintain the solubility of iron, so the reaction at low pH decreases the ionization potential which drives hydrogen atom transfer and increases the redox potential, which is the major reaction mechanism. When the reduction of Fe^{3+} to Fe^{2+} occurs in the presence of 2,4,6-trypyridyl-*s*-triazine, the reaction is accompanied by the formation of a colored complex with Fe^{2+} (absorption at 593 nm). The reducing power appears to be related to the degree of hydroxylation at pH and the extent of conjugation. Because the reaction detects compounds with a redox potential of <700 mV, comparable with ABTS$^{\cdot+}$ (680 mV), similar compounds react in both TEAC and FRAP assays. FRAP cannot detect compounds that act by radical quenching (hydrogen transfer), particularly thiols (as glutathione) and proteins. However, FRAP can be simple, rapid (typically 4–6 min), inexpensive, and done using semiautomatic or automated protocols.

A variant of the FRAP assay using Cu instead of Fe is known as CUPRAC (copper reduction assay), which is based on the reduction of Cu^{2+} to Cu^+ by the combined action of reducing agents in the sample. Batho-cuproine (2,9-dimethyl-4,7-diphenyl-1,10-phenanthroline) or neocuproine (2,9-dimethyl-1,10-phenanthroline) is used for Cu+ absorbs at 490 nm or 450 nm, respectively. CUPRAC values for pH are generally comparable to TEAC values. The low redox potential of copper in both free and complex forms makes it more selective in reactions than iron and may also indicate a possible pro-oxidant activity of pH.

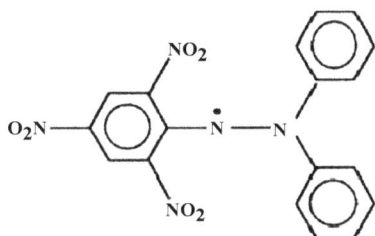

1: Diphenylpicrylhydrazyl (free radical)   2: Diphenylpicrylhydrazine (nonradical)

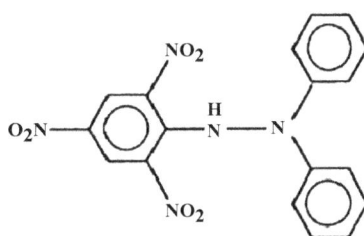

It is a fast, simple, inexpensive, and widely used method to measure the ability of compounds to act as free radical scavengers or hydrogen donors and to evaluate the antioxidant activity of foods. It can also be used to determine the amount of antioxidants in complex biological systems, for solid or liquid samples. This method is easy and applied to measure the overall antioxidant capacity and free radical scavenging activity of fruit and vegetable juices. This assay has been successfully used to investigate the antioxidant properties of wheat grains and bran, vegetables, conju-gated linoleic acids, herbs, edible seed oils, and many different, including ethanol, aqueous acetone, methanol, aqueous alcohols, and benzene (Kedare and Singh, 2011).

5.3.2 FRAP ASSAY (FERRIC REDUCING ABILITY OF PLASMA)

FRAP (conjointly metal particle–reducing inhibitor power) is associate inhibitor capability assay that uses Trolox as a customary (Benzie et al., 1996). The FRAP assay was initially performed by Iris Benzie and J. J. Strain of the human nutrition analysis cluster at the University of Ulster, Coleraine. The strategy relies on the formation of *o*-phenanthroline-Fe(2+) advanced and its disruption within the presence of chelating agents. This assay is usually accustomed to live foods, beverages, and nutritionary supplements containing polyphenols.

5.3.2.1 EXPERIMENTAL PROCEDURE

A reaction mixture containing one ml. of .05% *o*-phenanthroline in wood spirit, a pair of mil metal chloride (200 M) and a couple of mil of assorted concentrations starting from 10 to 1000 g was incubated at temperature for 10 min and also the absorbance of identical was measured at 510 nm. EDTA was used as a classical metal chelator. The experiment was performed in triplicates. The metal reducing activity of date seed extract calculably supported the strategy of Benzie and Strain (1999).

The FRAP reagent was prepared by mixing 50 ml of acetate buffer (0.3 M) at pH 3.6, 5 ml of tripyridyltriazine (TPTZ) solution 10 mM prepared in HCl (40 mM), and 5 ml of ferric chloride solution ($FeCl_3$) (20 mM). An amount of 2 ml of the freshly prepared FRAP reagent was added to 10 L of the extract. Then the absorbance was measured at 593 nm against the blank after 10 min at room temperature. The standard curve was constructed using Trolox. The result was expressed as Trolox equivalent in mg/100 g of dry weight date seed.

5.3.3 ORAC ASSAY

The ORAC assay is a method that measures the antioxidant capacity of a substance (Cao et al., 1993). The ORAC assay measures a fluorescent signal from a probe that is quenched in the presence of ROS. Addition of an antioxidant absorbs the generated ROS, allowing the fluorescent signal to be retained. Trolox (6-hydroxy-2,5,7,8-tetramethylchromane-2-carboxylic acid) is a vitamin E analog and a known antioxidant. It is used as a standard by which all unknown antioxidants are compared. Modifications of the ORAC assay include the use of fluorescein as a fluorescent probe (ORACFL - Oxygen Radical Absorbance Capacity fluorescent probe), the separation of hydrophilic and lipophilic antioxidants to achieve total antioxidant capacity, and an adaptation to a high-throughput platform.

The ORAC assay is unique in that its ROS generator, AAPH (2,2′-azobis (2-methylpropionamidine) dihydrochloride), produces a peroxyl-free radical upon thermal decomposition. This free radical is usually found in the body, making this reaction biologically relevant. In addition, AAPH is reactive with water and lipid soluble substances, so it can measure total antioxidant capacity (Huang et al., 2005).

The assay measures oxidative degradation of the fluorescent molecule (Kohri et al., 2005) (either beta-phycoarthrin or fluorescein) after being mixed with free radical generators such as azo-initiating compounds. Azo-initiators are believed to produce a peroxyl radical by heating, which damages the fluorescent molecule, resulting in loss of fluorescence. Antioxidants are believed to protect the fluorescent molecule from oxidative degeneration. The amount of protection is determined using a fluorometer. Fluorescence is currently used as a fluorescent probe.

The drawbacks of this method are

1. Only antioxidant activity against specifically (perhaps mainly peroxyl) radical is measured, However, peroxyl radical formation has never been proven.
2. The nature of the harmful reaction is not characterized.
3. There is no evidence that free radicals are involved in this reaction.
4. There is no evidence that ORAC values have any biological significance after consumption of any food. Furthermore, a relationship between ORAC values and convalescence has not been established.

5.4   IMPORTANCE OF PHYTONUTRIENTS

The idea of growing crops for health instead of food or fiber is gradually changing plant biotechnology and medicine. The connection between plants and health is reconnected. Responsible for launching new generation of vegetation therapeutics that include plant-derived pharmaceuticals are multipurpose botanical medicines, dietary supplements, functional foods, and plant-produced recombinant proteins. Among polyphenols, flavonoids are most commonly formed important single groups with more than 5000 compounds. Thus far it has been identified. In addition to nutrient components such as carotene, vitamins C and E, and selenium, compounds such as phenol, flavonoids, isoflavones, isothiocyanates, detraps, methylxanthine, dithiol, and coumarin appear to be through its role on important role in cancer prevention and inhibition of tumor production.

5.5 FUNCTIONAL FOODS

The very concept of food is changing from a previous emphasis on health maintenance for the promising use of foods promoting better health to prevent chronic diseases. Functional foods are those that provide more than ordinary nutrition; they provide additional physical benefits to the consumer. Because dietary habits are specific to the population and variations broadly, it is necessary to study the preventive efficiency of functional micronutrients in regional diets. Indian food components such as spices as well as medicinal plants with increased levels of essential vitamins and nutrients (e.g., vitamin E, lycopene, vitamin C, bioflavonoids, thioredoxin, etc.) provide a rich source of compounds such as antioxidants. That can be used in functional foods.

5.6 CONCLUSION

Antioxidants are chemicals and secondary metabolites that bind with free radicals and eliminate their effects from causing damage to biological molecules. Endogenous antioxidants are produced by our body, which are used to combat various free radical generated reactions. However, most of them are obtained from external sources, primarily through diet known as exogenous or dietary antioxidants. Major sources of this class of antioxidants are colored vegetables, fruits, and grains. Other very effective sources are berries (blue berries, straw berries, raspberries), beans, green tea, beat roots, spinach, and dark chocolate. Nowadays, many oral supplements are available in the market sold as dietary antioxidants.

Antioxidants bind with free radical by giving up their own free electrons. These results in the termination of autoxidation reactions, and the free radicals are no longer able to attack the cell. Antioxidant attains free radical state after donating its electron. Antioxidants prevent free radical induced tissue damage by preventing the formation of radicals, chelating them, or by promoting their decomposition. Synthetic antioxidants are recently marked to be dangerous to human health. Thus, the search for effective, nontoxic natural compounds with antioxidative activity has been boomed in recent years. In addition to endogenous antioxidant defense systems, consumption of dietary and plant-derived antioxidants appears to be a suitable alternative of synthetic sources. The traditional Indian diet, spices, and medicinal plants are rich sources of natural antioxidants, higher intake of foods with functional properties includes high level of antioxidants. New approaches utilizing collaborative research and modern technology in combination with established traditional health principles will reap dividends in the near future in improving health, especially among those who are not up to the use of expensive Western systems of medicine.

KEYWORDS

- **antioxidants**
- **traditional and nontraditional antioxidants**
- **extraction and quantification**

REFERENCES

Alupului, A.; Calinescu, I.; Lavric, V. Microwave Extraction of Active Principles from Medicinal Plants. *UPB Sci. Bull. Ser. B* **2012**, *74*, 129–142.

Asghari, J.; Ondruschka, B.; Mazaheritehrani, M. Extraction of Bioactive Chemical Compounds from the Medicinal Asian Plants by Microwave Irradiation. *J. Med. Plants Res.* **2011**, *5*, 495–506.

Angersbach, A.; Heinz, V.; Knorr, D. Effects of Pulsed Electric Fields on Cell Membranes in Real Food Systems. *Innovative Food Sci. Emerg. Technol.* **2000**, *2*, 135–149.

Barsotti, L.; Cheftel, J. C. Treatment of Food by Electric Fields Pulses. *Sci. Aliments* **1998**, *18*, 584–601.

Bryant, G.; Wolfe, J. Electromechanical Stress Produced in the Plasma Membranes of Suspended Cells by Applied Electrical Fields. *J. Membr. Biol.* **1987**, *96*, 129–139.

Bensebia, O.; Bensebia, B.; Allia, K. H.; Barth, D. Supercritical CO_2 Extraction of Triterpenes from Rosemary Leaves, Kinetics and Modeling. *Sep. Sci. Technol.* **2016**, *51*, 2174–2182.

Barbosa-Pereira, L.; Pocheville, A.; Angulo, I.; Paseiro-Losada, P.; Cruz, J. M. Fractionation and Purification of Bioactive Compounds Obtained from a Brewery Waste Stream. *BioMed Res. Int.* **2013**, *40*, 84–91.

Boussetta, N.; Grimi, N.; Vorobiev, E. Pulsed Electrical Technologies Assisted Polyphenols Extraction from Agricultural Plants and Bioresources, A Review. *Int. Food Process. Technol.* **2015**, *2*, 1–10.

Boussetta, N.; Lebovka, N.; Vorobiev, E.; Adenier, H.; Bedel-Cloutour, C.; Lanoiselle, J. L. Electrically Assisted Extraction of Soluble Matter from Chardonnay Grape Skins for Polyphenol Recovery. *J. Agric. Food Chem.* **2009**, *57*, 1491–1497.

Benzie, I. F.; Strain, J. J. The Ferric Reducing Ability of Plasma (FRAP) as a Measure of "Antioxidant Power: The FRAP Assay. *Anal. Biochem.* **1996**, *239* (1), 70–76.

Carocho, M., Ferreira, I. C.F.R. A review on antioxidants, prooxidants and related controversy: Natural and synthetic compounds, screening and analysis methodologies and future perspectives. Food and Chemical Toxicology, Volume 51, 2013, 15–25.

Cheng, X., Bi, L., Zhao, Z., Chen, Y. (2015). Advances in enzyme assisted extraction of natural products. 3rd International Conference on Material,Mechanical and Manufacturing Engineering (IC3ME 2015). Atlantis Press, Guangzhou, China, pp. 371–375.

Concha, J.; Soto, C.; Chamy, R.; Zuniga, M. E. Enzymatic Pretreatment on Rose-Hip Oil Extraction, Hydrolysis and Pressing Conditions. *J. Am. Oil Chem. Soc.* **2004**, *81*, 549–552.

Cravottoa, G.; Boffaa, L.; Mantegnaa, S.; Peregob, P.; Avogadrob, M.; Cintasc, P. Improved Extraction of Vegetable Oils Under High-Intensity Ultrasound and/or Microwaves. *Ultrason. Sonochem.* **2008**, *15*, 898–902.

Corrales, M.; Butza, P. Tauschera, B. Anthocyanin Condensation Reactions under High Hydrostatic Pressure. *Food Chem.* **2008**, *110*, 627–635.

Casas, L.; Mantell, C.; Rodríguez, M.; De-la-Oss, E. J. M.; Roldan, A.; De Ory, I.; Caro, I.; Blandino, A. Extraction of Resveratrol from the Pomace of Palomino Fino Grapes by Supercritical Carbon Dioxide. *J. Food Eng.* **2010**, *96*, 304–308.

Cao, G.; Alessio, H. M.; Cutler, R. G. Oxygen-Radical Absorbance Capacity Assay for Antioxidants. *Free Radic. Biol. Med.* **1993**, *14* (3), 303–311.

Carocho, M.; Ferreira, I. C. A Review on Antioxidants, Prooxidants and Related Controversy, Natural and Synthetic Compounds, Screening and Analysis Methodologies and Future Perspectives. *Food Chem. Toxicol.* **2013**, *51*, 15–25.

Dean, J. R.; Xiong, G. Extraction of Organic Pollutants from Environmental Matrices, Selection of Extraction Technique. *Trends Anal. Chem.* **2000**, *19*, 553–564.

Dominguez, H.; Ntiiiez, M. J.; Lema, J. M. Enzyme-Assisted Hexane Extraction of Soybean Oil. *Food Chem.* **1995**, *54*, 223–231.

Fincan, M.; Dejmek, P. In Situ Visualization of the Effect of a Pulsed Electric Field on Plant Tissue. *J. Food Eng.* **2002**, *55*, 223–230.

Fincan, M.; De-Vito, F.; Dejmek, P. Pulsed Electric Field Treatment for Solid–Liquid Extraction of Red Beetroot Pigment. *J. Food Eng.* **2004**, *64*, 381–388.

Garcia, J. L.; Castro, M. D. Where is Microwave-Based Analytical Equipment for Solid Sample Pre-Treatment Going? *Trends Anal. Chem.* **2003**, *22*, 90–98.

Gardossi, L.; Poulsen, P. B.; Ballesteros, A.; Hult, K.; Svedas, V. K.; Vasic-Racki, D.; Carrea, G.; Magnusson, A.; Schmid, A.; Wohlgemuth, R.; Halling, P. J. Guidelines for Reporting of Biocatalytic Reactions. *Trends Biotechnol.* **2010**, *28*, 171–180.

Giannuzzo, A. N.; Boggetti, H. J.; Nazareno, M. A.; Mishima, H. T. Supercritical Fluid Extraction of Naringin from the Peel of *Citrus paradise. Phytochem. Anal.* **2003**, *14*, 221–223.

Gamli, F. A Review of Application of Pulsed Electric Field in the Production of Liquid/ Semi-Liquid Food Materials. *Adv. Res. Agric. Vet. Sci.* **2014**, *1*, 54–61.

Ghafoor, K.; Park, J.; Choi, Y. H. Optimization of Supercritical Carbon Dioxide Extraction of Bioactive Compounds from Grape Peel (*Vitis labrusca* B.) by using Response Surface Methodology. *Innovative Food Sci. Emerg. Technol.* **2010**, *11*, 485–490.

Heinz, V.; Toepfl, S.; Knorr, D. Impact of Temperature on Lethality and Energy Efficiency of Apple Juice Pasteurization by Pulsed Electric Fields Treatment. *Innovative Food Sci. Emerg. Technol.* **2003**, *4*, 167–175.

Hanmoungjai, P.; Pyle, D. L.; Niranjan, K. Enzymatic Process for Extracting Oil and Protein from Rice Bran. *J. Am. Oil Chem. Soc.* **2001**, *78*, 817–821.

Howard, L.; Pandjaitan, N. Pressurized Liquid Extraction of Flavonoids from Spinach. *J. Food Sci.* **2008**, *73*, C151–C157.

Herrera, M. C.; Luque-de-Castro, M. D. Ultrasound-Assisted Extraction for the Analysis of Phenolic Compounds in Strawberries. *Anal. Bioanal. Chem.* **2004**, *379*, 1106–1112.

Huang, D.; Ou, B.; Prior, R. L. The Chemistry Behind Antioxidant Capacity Assays. *J. Agric. Food Chem.* **2005**, *53* (6), 1841–1856.

Ibanez, E.; Herrero, M.; Mendiola, J. A.; Castro-Puyana. M. Extraction and Characterization of Bioactive Compounds with Health Benefits from Marine Resources, Macro and Micro Algae, Cyanobacteria, and Invertebrates. In *Marine Bioactive Compounds, Sources, Characterization and Applications*; Hayes, M., Ed.; Springer: New York, NY, 2012; pp 55–98.

Inczedy, J.; Lengyel, T.; Ure, A. M. *Supercritical Fluid Chromatography and Extraction. Compendium of Analytical Nomenclature (Definitive Rules 1997)*; Blackwell Science, Oxford, UK, 1998.

Landbo, A. K.; Meyer, A. S. Enzyme-Assisted Extraction of Antioxidative Phenols from Black Currant Juice Press Residues (*Ribes nigrum*). *J. Agric. Food Chem.* **2001**, *49*, 3169–3177.

Letellier, M.; Budzinski, H. Microwave Assisted Extraction of Organic Compounds. *Analusis* **1999**, *27*, 259–270.

Latif, S.; Anwar, F. Physicochemical Studies of Hemp (*Cannabis sativa*) Seed Oil Using Enzyme-Assisted Cold-Pressing. *Eur. J. Lipid Sci. Technol.* **2009**, *111*, 1042–1048.

Lebovka, N. I.; Bazhal, M. I.; Vorobiev, E. Estimation of Characteristic Damage Time of Food Materials in Pulsed-Electric Fields. *J. Food Eng.* **2002**, *54*, 337–346.

Lopez, N.; Puertolas, E.; Condon, S.; Alvarez, I.; Raso, J. Effects of Pulsed Electric Fields on the Extraction of Phenolic Compounds during the Fermentation of Must of Tempranillo grapes. *Innovative Food Sci. Emerg. Technol.* **2008**, *9*, 477–482.

Kaufmann, B., Christen, P. Recent Extraction Techniques for Natural Products, Microwave-Assisted Extraction and Pressurized Solvent Extraction. *Phytochem. Anal.* **2002**, *13*, 105–113.

Khorassani, M. A.; Taylor, L. T. Sequential Fractionation of Grape Seeds into Oils, Polyphenols, and Procyanidins via a Single System Employing CO_2-Based Fluids. *J. Agric. Food Chem.* **2004,** *52,* 2440–2444.

Kohri, S.; Fujii, H.; Oowada, S.; Endoh, N.; Sueishi, Y.; Kusakabe, M.; Shimmei, M.; Kotake, Y. An Oxygen Radical Absorbance Capacity-Like Assay that Directly Quantifies the Antioxidant's Scavenging Capacity Against AAPH-Derived Free Radicals. *Anal. Biochem.* **2009,** *386* (2), 167–171.

Liazid, A.; Guerrero, R. F.; Cantos, E.; Palma, M.; Barroso, C. G. Microwave Assisted Extraction of Anthocyanins from Grape Skins. *Food Chem.* **2011,** *124,* 1238–1243.

Luthria, D. L. Influence of Experimental Conditions on the Extraction of Phenolic Compounds from Parsley (*Petroselinum crispum*) Flakes Using a Pressurized Liquid Extractor. *Food Chem.* **2008,** *107,* 745–752.

Lang, Q.; Wai, C. M.. Supercritical Fluid Extraction in Herbal and Natural Product Studies—a Practical Review. *Talanta* **2001,** *53,* 771–782.

Mandal, V.; Mohan, Y.; Hemalatha, S. Microwave Assisted Extraction – An innovative and Promising Extraction Tool for Medicinal Plant Research. *Pharmacogn. Rev.* **2007,** *1,* 7–18.

Mason, T. J.; Paniwnyk, L.; Lorimer, J. P. The Uses of Ultrasound in Food Technology. *Ultrason. Sonochem.* **1996,** *3,* 253–260.

Meyer, A. S.; Jepsen, S. M.; Sorensen, N. S. Enzymatic Release of Antioxidants for Human Low-Density Lipoprotein from Grape Pomace. *J. Agric. Food Chem.* **1998,** *46,* 2439–2446.

Niranjan, K.; Hanmoungjai, P. Enzyme-Aided Aqueous Extraction. In *Nutritionally Enhanced Edible Oil Processing*; Dunford, N. T., Dunford, H. B., Eds.; AOCS Publishing: IL, 2004.

Ndiomu, D. P.; Simpson, C. F. Some Applications of Supercritical Fluid Extraction. *Anal. Chim. Acta* **1988,** *213,* 237–243.

Nieto, A.; Borrull, F.; Pocurull, E.; Marce, R. M. Pressurized Liquid Extraction, A Useful Technique to Extract Pharmaceuticals and Personal Care Products from Sewage Sludge. *Trends Anal. Chem.* **2010,** *29,* 752–764.

Pascual-Marti, M. C.; Salvador, A.; Chafer, A.; Berna, A. Supercritical Fluid Extraction of Resveratrol from Grape Skin of *Vitis vinifera* and Determination by HPLC. *Talanta* **2001,** *54,* 735–740.

Pare, J. J. R.; Belanger, J. M. R.; Stafford, S. S. Microwave-Assisted Process (MAP™), A New Tool for the Analytical Laboratory. *Trends Anal. Chem.* **1994,** *13,* 176–184.

Puri, M.; Sharma, D.; Barrow, C. J. Enzyme-Assisted Extraction of Bioactives from Plants. *Trends Biotechnol.* **2012,** *30,* 37–44.

Pinelo, M.; Arnous, A.; Meyer, A. S. Upgrading of Grape Skins, Significance of Plant Cell Wall Structural Components and Extraction Techniques for Phenol Release. *Trends Food Sci. Technol.* **2006,** *17,* 579–590.

Patist, A.; Bates, D. Ultrasonic Innovations in the Food Industry, From the Laboratory to Commercial Production. *Innovative Food Sci. Emerg. Technol.* **2008,** *9,* 147–154.

Petigny, L.; Perino, S.; Minuti, M.; Visinoni, F.; Wajsman, J.; Chemat, F. Molecular Sciences Simultaneous Microwave Extraction and Separation of Volatile and Non-Volatile Organic Compounds of Boldo Leaves from Lab to Industrial Scale. *Int. J. Mol. Sci.* **2014,** *15,* 7183–7198.

Puertolas, E.; Lopez, N.; Saldana, G.; Alvarez, I.; Raso, J. Evaluation of Phenolic Extraction during Fermentation of Red Grapes Treated by a Continuous Pulsed Electric Fields Process At Pilot-Plant Scale. *J. Food Eng.* **2010,** *119,* 1063–1070.

Rosenthal, A.; Pyle, D. L.; Niranjan, K. Aqueous and Enzymatic Processes for Edible Oil Extraction. *Enzyme Microb. Technol.* **1996,** *19,* 402–420.

Rosenthal, A.; Pyle, D. L.; Niranjan, K.; Gilmour. S.; Trinca, L. Combined Effect of Operational Variables and Enzyme Activity on Aqueous Enzymatic Extraction of Oil and Protein from Soybean. *Enzyme Microb. Technol.* **2006,** *28,* 499–509.

Raverchon, E.; Marco, I. D.; Review, Supercritical Fluid Extraction and Fractionation of Natural Matter. *J. Supercrit. Fluids* **2006,** *38,* 146–166.

Richter, B. E.; Jones, B. A.; Ezzell, J. L.; Porter, N. L.; Avdalovic, N.; Pohl, C. Accelerated Solvent Extraction, A Technology for Sample Preparation. *Anal. Chem.* **1996,** *68,* 1033–1039.

Sharma, A.; Khare, S. K.; Gupta, M. N. Enzyme-Assisted Aqueous Extraction of Peanut Oil. *J. Am. Oil Chem. Soc.* **2010,** *79,* 215–218.

Sowbhagya, H.; Chitra, V. Enzyme-Assisted Extraction of Flavorings and Colorants from Plant Materials. *Crit. Rev. Food Sci. Nutr.* **2010,** *50,* 146–161.

Sihvonen, M.; Jarvenpaa, E.; Hietaniemi, V.; Huopalahti, R. Advances in Supercritical Carbon Dioxide Technologies. *Trends Food Sci. Technol.* **1999,** *10,* 217–222.

Shi, J.; Yi, C.; Ye, X.; Xue, S.; Jiang, Y.; Maa, Y.; Liu, D. Effects of Supercritical CO_2 Fluid Parameters on Chemical Composition and Yield of Carotenoids Extracted from Pumpkin. *LWT – Food Sci. Technol.* **2010,** *43,* 39–44.

Temelli, F.; Guclu-Ustundag, O. *Supercritical Technologies for Further Processing of Edible Oils. Bailey's Industrial Oil and Fat Products*; John Wiley & Sons Inc.: TX, 2005.

Toepfl, S.; Heinz, V.; Knorr, D. High Intensity Pulsed Electric Fields Applied for Food Preservation. *Chem. Eng. Process.* **2007,** *46,* 537–546.

Vorobiev, E.; Jemai, A. B.; Bouzrara, H.; Lebovka, N. I.; Bazhal, M. I. Pulsed Electric Field Assisted Extraction of Juice from Food Plants. In *Novel Food Processing Technologies*; Barbosa-Canovas, G., Tapia, M. S., Cano, M. P., Eds.; CRC Press: New York, NY, 2005; pp 105–130.

Vorobiev, E.; Lebovka, N. I. Extraction of Intercellular Components by Pulsed Electric Fields. In *Pulsed Electric Field Technology for the Food Industry, Fundamentals and Applications*; Raso, J., Heinz, V., Eds.; Springer: New York, NY, 2006; pp 153–194.

Wang, Y., You, J.; Yu, Y.; Qu, C.; Zhang, H.; Ding, L.; Zhang, H. Li, X. Analysis of Ginsenosides in *Panax ginseng* in High Pressure Microwave Assisted Extraction. *Food Chem.* **2008,** *110,* 161–167.

CHAPTER 6

Comparative Estimation of Antioxidant and Antimicrobial Activity of Bioactive Components with Special Reference to Urinary Tract Infection

PALLAVI SINGH CHAUHAN[1*], ANUJ DUBEY[2], and SONIA JOHRI[1]

[1]*Department of Life Sciences, ITM University, Gwalior, Madhya Pradesh, India*

[2]*Department of Chemistry, ITM University, Gwalior, Madhya Pradesh, India*

[3]*Department of Life Sciences, ITM University, Gwalior, Madhya Pradesh, India*

Corresponding author. E-mail: anujdubey.mail@gmail.com

ABSTRACT

In view of uncertainties regarding role of phytochemicals in treatment of urinary tract infection (UTI), the study aims at the evaluation of antimicrobial as well as antioxidant activity of chosen plant extracts. In the present study, *Cascabela thevetia, Tridax procumbens,* and *Arctium tomentosum* leaf extracts were prepared using various organic solvents. Both the qualitative and quantitative estimations of the plant extract have been done. The plant extract with best phytoconstituents was chosen for antioxidant analysis, that is, Dehydrogenase (DH) activity, as well as estimation of antimicrobial activity and MIC determination against UTI-associated pathogens, that is, *Klebsiella pneumonia* and *Enterococcus faecalis*. The results obtained showed that the *T. procumbens* leaf extract has a wide range of phytochemicals. Various leaf extracts of *T. procumbens*, that is, ethanolic, methanolic, toluenoic, benzenoic, and acetone showed maximum *antioxidant activity* with 46.3 ± 0.23, 51.4 ± 0.32, 49 ± 0.76, 55.6 ± 0.24, and 56.54 ± 1.12% inhibition, respectively. The antimicrobial activity of *T. procumbens* leaf extract showed that maximum zone of inhibition was found in case of benzene extract of *T. procumbens* leaf extract. MIC results thus obtained showed that the MIC value for benzene extract of *T. procumbens* leaf extract is 5 mg/ml. To understand the mode of action, it is a prerequisite condition to first understand the availability as well as composition of phytoconstituents within plants. Thus, this study may provide a new insight to develop an eco-friendly and economically viable strategy-based research in order to treat UTI infection.

6.1   INTRODUCTION

Bioactive compounds in plant play an active role in treatment of various diseases. Organic compounds present in medicinal plants are known to provide various useful effects on human body.[2] Bioactive components reported in plant extracts are polyphenols, tannins, terpenoids, alkaloids, steroids, carbohydrates, and flavonoids.[3] To develop novel and efficient therapies, preliminary phytochemical estimation is needed.[4] Mode of action of bioactive components in treatment of cancer and other degenerative diseases is still unclear.[5] At industrial level, extraction of phytoconstituent and drug development are being done regularly these days.[6] Traditional medicines always paved a path to develop advanced form of the existing drugs. Previous studies have showed that few urinary tract infection (UTI)-associated pathogens have developed resistance toward preexisting drug.[7] Although some cases are reported where few phytoconstituents are known to have potential antimicrobial, it was reported that chemical-based therapies have some disadvantages related to the toxicity level. So, it was thought worthwhile to explore bio-assisted pathway to reduce their toxicity effect and then to provide better therapy to avoid the resistance related problem.[8] Thus, in view of uncertainties regarding the role of phytoconstituents against allergic or infectious diseases, this study may provide a new insight into the development of effective antiallergic and anti-infective agents.[9,10]

Cascabela thevetia belongs to genus, *Cascabela*; family, Apocynaceae; kingdom, Plantae. The medicinal uses of oleander leaves and the flowers are cardiotonic, diaphoretic, diuretic, emetic, expectorant, and sternutatory.

A decoction of the leaves has been applied externally in the treatment of scabies and to reduce swellings. This is a very poisonous plant, containing a powerful cardiac toxin, and should only be used with extreme caution. The root is a powerful resolvent. Because of its poisonous nature, it is only used externally. It is beaten into a paste with water and applied to chancres and ulcers on the penis. An oil prepared from the root bark is used in the treatment of leprosy and skin diseases of a scaly nature.[11,12] *Tridax procumbens* belongs to genus, *Tridax*; family, Asteraceae; order, Asterales; kingdom, Plantae. Medicinal uses of *T. procumbens* are for wound healing and as an anticoagulant, antifungal, and insect repellent. The juice extracted from the leaves is directly applied on wounds. Its leaf extracts were used for infectious skin diseases in folk medicines. It is used in Ayurvedic medicine for liver disorders, hepatoprotection, gastritis, and heartburn. *T. procumbens* is also used as treatment for boils, blisters, and cuts by local healers in parts of India.[13,14] *Arctium tomentosum* belongs to genus, *Ancitum*; family, Asteraceae; clade, Angiosperms; kingdom, Plantae. Medicinal benefits of *A. tomentosum* root are that it is a power-house of antioxidant, removes toxins from the blood, may inhibit some types of cancer, may be an aphrodisiac, and can help treat skin issues.[15] Solvent plays a very significant role in the isolation of plant metabolites because the quality and quantity of phytochemicals extracted depend on nature of extracting organic solvent.[16] In view of uncertainties regarding the role of phytochemicals in the treatment of UTI, the study aims at the evaluation of antimicrobial as well as antioxidant activity of chosen plant extracts.

6.2 MATERIALS AND METHODS

6.2.1 COLLECTION OF LEAVES AND EXTRACT PREPARATION

Fresh leaves of *C. thevetia, T. procumbens,* and *A. tomentosum* were collected from Botanical Garden, Jiwaji University, Gwalior, Madhya Pradesh, in the month of March having voucher specimen numbers 090124, 090325b, and 090516, respectively. Fresh leaves of chosen plant were washed thoroughly and chopped into fine pieces. About 20 g of the chopped and crushed leaves were taken into 100 ml (20%) of five different organic solvents, that is, ethanol, methanol, toluene, benzene, and acetone, in a conical flask. It was then allowed to mix well and then kept on rotary shaker. The sample is then filtered and dried by using a Soxhlet extractor. The dried samples were stored in 4°C for further use.[17]

6.2.2 PHYTOCHEMICAL ANALYSIS OF PLANT EXTRACT

Qualitative and quantitative estimations of phytochemicals present in *C. thevetia, T. procumbens,* and *A. tomentosum* plant leaf extract were done using standard methods. The details are as follows:

6.2.2.1 QUALITATIVE ESTIMATION OF PHYTOCHEMICALS

The qualitative estimation of the phytochemicals present within plant leaf extract was done using flavonoids test (lead acetate test), alkaloids test (Hager's test and Wagner's test), glycosides test (Borntrager's test), steroids test (Liebermann–Burchard test and Salkowski's test), phenols test (ferric chloride test), terpenoid test (Salkowski's test), saponins test (foam test), resins test (ferric chloride test), tannins test (gelatin test), cardiac glycosides (legal test and Keller–Kiliani test), phytosterols and triterpenoids test (Libermann–Burchard test), carbohydrates test (Molisch's test, Benedict's test, Fehling's test, Barfoed's test), and fixed oils and fats test (iodine value).[18]

6.2.2.2 QUANTITATIVE ESTIMATION OF PHYTOCHEMICALS

The quantitative estimation was done by estimating total phenolics (mg/g) and total flavonoids (mg/g) content in solvent extracts of plant leaves, with best phytochemical composition. Quantitative estimation of total phenol content and total flavanoid content was done by comparing with the absorbance against standards, that is, gallic acid and quercetin solution respectively.[19–21]

6.2.2.2.1 Total Flavanoid Content

Aluminum chloride colorimetric assay was used for determining the total content of flavanoids in per gram of dried powder. For estimation, extraction

(2 mg/ml) and make-up were done with 1 ml of methanol and then finally make-up with 4 ml of double distilled water. Amounts of 0.15 ml $NaNO_2$ (0.5 M), 3.4 ml methanol (30%), and 0.15 ml of aluminum chloride (0.3 M) were mixed in a test tube and kept for 5 min for stabilization. An amount of 1 ml sodium hydroxide (1 mol/l) was then added. The final make-up was done up to 10 ml and kept for 15 min. The solution absorbance was then taken at 506 nm against blank. A standard curve was made with reference to the standard quercetin solution (prepared at different concentration in methanol). The total content of flavonoid was expressed as milligram quercetin equivalent (QUE) per gram of dry weight.[22]

6.2.2.2.2 *Total Phenol Content*

Total phenol content was determined by Folin–Ciocalteu method, in per gram dried powder, where the gallic acid was kept as standard. An amount of 200 μl of extract (2 mg/ml) was added to 3 ml in distilled water; to this, 0.1 ml Folin–Ciocalteu (FC) reagent and 2.5 ml Na_2CO_3 (0.2 N) were added. For standardization of the sample, incubation (in dark for 60 min) at optimum room temperature was done. Distilled water was kept as blank. Absorbance measurement at 650 nm was done keeping distilled water as blank and gallic acid as standard (by preparing standard curve of gallic acid using different concentration). The results thus obtained were expressed as milligrams of gallic acid, which is equivalents to per gram of dried extract (DE) (μg gallic acid equivalents (GAE)/g DE).[23]

6.2.3 *ANTIOXIDANT ACTIVITY*

DH (2,2-diphenyl-1-picrylhydrazyl) was used to determine free radical scavenging activity of different solvent extracts of the plant leaves (with best phytochemical composition). Methanol was used to make 0.2 mM DH. The standard used was ascorbic acid. To design a standard curve, different concentrations were used ranging from 0.2 to 1 ml. To prepare test samples, each extract (10 μg) was dissolved in parent solvent (2 ml). DH (1 ml) was then added to each tube. Tubes were kept in dark condition of 60 min and absorbance was measured (515 nm).[24] Inhibition percentage was calculated using the following formula:

$$\% \text{ Inhibition} = \text{Absorbance of control} - \text{Absorbance of extract} / \text{Absorbance of control} \times 100$$

6.2.3.1 ANTIMICROBIAL ACTIVITY OF PLANT EXTRACT AGAINST UTI-ASSOCIATED PATHOGENS

Kirby–Bauer well diffusion method was used to evaluate antimicrobial activity of plant extract[25–27] against UTI-associated bacterial strains (*Klebsiella pneumonia* and *Enterococcus faecalis*) collected from MTCC, Chandigarh. An amount of 5 mg/ml concentration of the plant extract was kept to evaluate the antimicrobial activity. The 0.5 McFarland standard was kept.[28]

6.2.3.2 MINIMUM INHIBITORY CONCENTRATION OF PLANT EXTRACT AGAINST UTI-ASSOCIATED PATHOGENS

Different concentrations of plant extract ranging as 1, 3, 5, 7, and 9 mg/ml were used to evaluate MIC value of plant extracts against *K. pneumonia* and *E. faecalis*. Broth dilution method in nutrient broth was used to carry out the analysis. Control was used as standard. Turbidity of the tubes was analyzed to detect MIC value.[29] A small aliquot from the tubes was poured in agar plate for analyzing bacterial growth. The experiment was performed in triplicates.

6.3 RESULTS

6.3.1 PHYTOCHEMICAL EVALUATION OF PLANT EXTRACT

Among the three different plant leaf extracts of *C. thevetia, T. procumbens,* and *A. tomentosum, T. procumbens* leaf extract has shown the best phytochemicals composition. The results obtained from the quantitative estimation of leaf extract support the previous studies, whereas few studies have shown slight variation from the result obtained. Few studies have also shown the solvent-based variation in the phytoconstituents of the plant leaf extract. The results obtained from both qualitative and quantitative estimation of plant extract are as follows:

6.3.2 QUALITATIVE PHYTOCHEMICAL ANALYSIS

The result obtained from phytochemical estimation of solvent extracts of *C. thevetia, T. procumbens,* and *A. tomentosum* leaf extract showed the availability of various phytochemicals as shown in Table 6.1. Several qualitative tests were performed to check the availability of various phyto-chemicals. The tests showed that the *T. procumbens* leaf extract has a wide range of phytochemical compounds as compared to other extracts.

6.3.3 QUANTITATIVE PHYTOCHEMICAL ANALYSIS

Plant extract with best phytochemical constituent, that is, *T. procumbens* leaf extract, was chosen for quantitative estimation of different phytochemicals. The quantitative estimation revealed the phenols and flavonoids contents in the leaf extract, and the results are shown in Figure 6.1. Phenols content in benzene extract of plant leaf was 56.3 ± 1.6 mg GA/g, 38.4 ± 1.4 mg GA/g in ethanolic extract, 51.2 ± 3.6 mg GA/g in methanol extract, 35.9 ± 4.2 mg GA/g in toluene extract, and 52.7 ± 5.4 mg GA/g in acetone extract. Flavonoids content in benzene extract of plant leaf was 34.3 ± 1.8 mg GA/g, 18.5 ± 1.8 mg GA/g in ethanolic extract, 24.6 ± 2.9 mg GA/g in methanol extract, 22.1 ± 5.8 mg GA/g in toluene extract, and 31.7 ± 6.4 mg GA/g in acetone extract.

6.3.4 ANTIOXIDANT ACTIVITY

In the results obtained from DH assay, it was observed that plant leaf extracts obtained from different solvents, that is, ethanol, methanol, toluene, benzene, and acetone show maximum antioxidant activity with 46.3 ± 0.23, 51.4 ± 0.32, 49 ± 0.76, 55.6 ± 0.24, and $56.54 \pm 1.12\%$ inhibition, respectively (Graph 6.1).

6.3.5 ANTIMICROBIAL ACTIVITY OF PLANT EXTRACT

Figure 6.2 clearly shows the result obtained from evaluation of antimicrobial activity of plant extracts against UTI-associated pathogens, that is, *K. pneumonia* and *E. faecalis*.

TABLE 6.1 Qualitative Screening of Phytochemicals in Three Different Plant Leaf Extract.

Sr. no.	Phytoconstituents	Plant leaf extracts														
		Cascabela thevetia					Tridax procumbens					Arctium tomentosum				
		E	M	T	B	A	E	M	T	B	A	E	M	T	B	A
1.	Flavonoids (lead acetate test)	+	+	+	+	+	+	+	+	+	+	−	+	−	+	−
2.	Alkaloids															
	A. Hager's test	−	−	+	+	−	−	+	+	+	+	−	−	−	+	+
	B. Wagner's test	−	+	+	+	+	−	+	−	−	+	−	+	−	−	+
3.	Glycosides (Borntrager's test)	−	−	−	+	+	+	+	+	+	+	+	+	+	+	+
4.	Steroids															
	A. Liebermann–Burchard test	+	−	+	+	−	+	+	−	+	+	+	−	−	+	+
	B. Salkowski's test	+	+	+	+	+	+	+	+	+	+	−	−	+	+	+
5.	Phenols (ferric chloride test)	+	+	+	+	+	+	+	+	+	+	−	+	+	−	+
6.	Terpenoid (Salkowski's test)	−	+	−	+	+	−	+	−	+	+	+	−	+	+	+
7.	Saponins (foam test)	+	+	+	+	+	+	+	+	+	+	−	+	+	+	+
8.	Resins (ferric chloride test)	−	−	+	+	−	−	+	+	+	+	+	+	−	+	+
9.	Tannins (gelatin test)	−	−	−	+	+	+	+	+	+	+	+	+	+	+	+
10.	Cardiac glycosides															
	A. Legal test	+	−	+	+	−	+	+	−	+	+	−	−	−	+	−
	B. Keller–Kiliani test	+	+	+	+	+	+	+	+	+	+	+	−	+	+	−

TABLE 6.1 *(Continued)*

Sr. no.	Phytoconstituents	Plant leaf extracts														
		Cascabela thevetia					Tridax procumbens					Arctium tomentosum				
		E	M	T	B	A	E	M	T	B	A	E	M	T	B	A
11.	Phytosterols and triterpenoids (Liebermann–Burchard test)	+	+	+	+	+	+	+	+	+	+	-	-	+	-	-
12.	Carbohydrates															
	A. Molisch's test	-	++	-	+	+	-	++	-	+	+	+	+	-	+	+
	B. Fehling's test	-	-	-	+	-	+	-	+	+	-	+	+	+	+	+
	C. Benedict's test	-	-	-	-	+	-	+	-	-	-	+	+	-	+	+
	D. Barfoed's test	+	+					+					+			+
13.	Fixed oils and fats (iodine value)	-	-	+	+	-	+	+	+	+	+	+	+	-	+	+

Data is represented as +, present; -, absent; E, ethanol; M, methanol; T, toluene; B, benzene; A, acetone

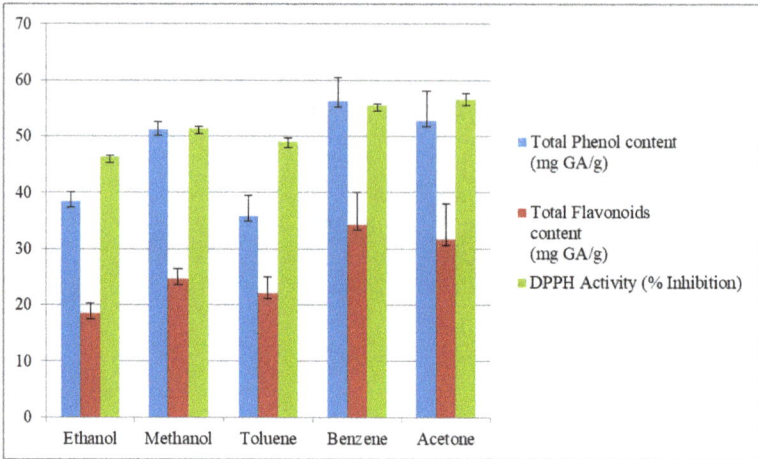

FIGURE 6.1 Quantitative estimation of different phytochemicals in various organic solvents of *Tridax procumbens* leaves and its antioxidant activity. (Results are expressed as Mean ± S.E.)

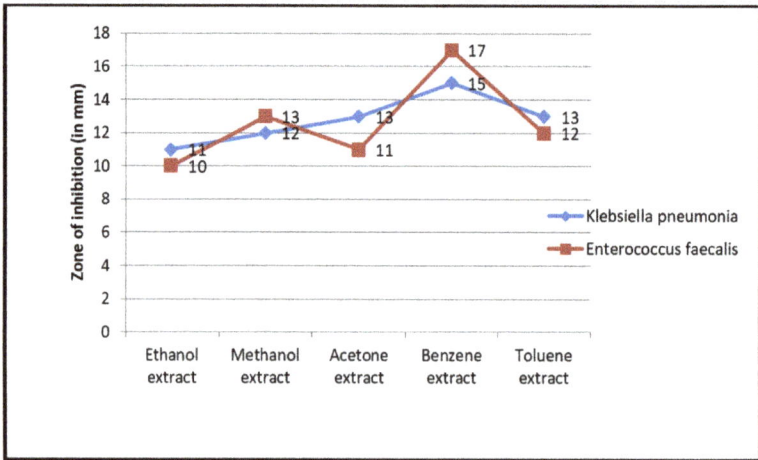

FIGURE 6.2 Antimicrobial activity of various plant extracts against UTI-associated microbial flora.

6.3.6 *MINIMUM INHIBITORY CONCENTRATION OF PLANT EXTRACT*

Table 6.2 clearly shows the result obtained from evaluation of minimum inhibitory concentration of plant extracts against UTI-associated pathogens.

TABLE 6.2 Minimum Inhibitory Concentration of Various Plant Extracts Against UTI-associated Microbial Flora.

Dilution for same bacterial concentration	Sets	Bacterial growth at different concentrations of *Tridax procumbens* plant extracts																							
		Toluene extract (mg/ml)					Benzene extract (mg/ml)					Acetone extract (mg/ml)					Methanol extract (mg/ml)					Ethanol extract (mg/ml)				
		9	7	5	3	1	9	7	5	3	1	9	7	5	3	1	9	7	5	3	1	9	7	5	3	1
Klebsiella pneumonia	1	–	–	–	+	+	–	–	–	+	+	–	–	+	+	+	–	–	–	+	+	–	–	–	+	+
	2	–	+	+	+	+	–	–	–	–	+	–	–	+	+	+	–	–	–	+	+	–	+	+	+	+
	3	–	+	+	+	+	–	–	–	+	+	–	+	+	+	+	–	–	+	+	+	–	+	+	+	+
Enterococcus faecalis	1	–	+	+	+	+	–	–	–	+	+	–	+	+	+	+	–	–	–	+	+	–	–	+	+	+
	2	–	–	–	+	+	–	–	–	+	+	–	–	+	+	+	–	+	+	+	+	–	–	–	+	+
	3	–	–	+	+	+	–	–	–	+	+	–	–	+	+	+	–	–	–	+	+	–	–	–	+	+

Data is presented as +, present; -, absent.

6.4 DISCUSSION

Traditional medicine nowadays is considered as a potent and safe alternate therapy.[30] In several urban and rural areas, including some countries like Thailand, plants-based medicinal therapies are in regular practice.[31] But for fulfilling standard drug criteria, very few reports are available on qualitative as well as quantitative data on plants, which makes them officially unrecognized. Because of various pharmacological activities, bioactive components such as secondary metabolites are considered as suitable markers for effective drug therapy.[32] Few reports are available, which have shown plants as an effective traditional medicine with potent antioxidant activity.[33,34]

The present study provides a new insight into the investigation of the availability of potent phytochemicals, within the natural resources, that is, green plants. The findings of our study showed that among the three different plant extracts chosen, the *T. procumbens* leaf extract was found to be the best with respect to availability of various phytochemical constituents. The composition of phytochemicals within the plant extract can be correlated with its antioxidant activity as mentioned in Figure 6.1. The antibacterial activity of various organic solvents of *T. procumbens* leaf extract has been investigated.

Oxidative stress markers include several parameters, and generation of ROS is one of the well-known oxidative stress markers.[35] Oxidative stress may lead to decrease in the kinetics of antioxidative defense mechanism, which ultimately leads to generation of several chronic diseases.[36] For example, phytoconstituents like phenolic compounds have redox potential that has been potent in antioxidant activity. This property makes them an important source to donate H^+ to reactive oxygen species and ultimately neutralizing free radicals.[37]

The reason for choosing the two microbial strains, that is, *K. pneumonia* and *E. faecalis* is that they are common microbial strains associated with UTI. Among these two microbial strains, maximum activity was found against *E. faecalis*. Possible reason for this may be that Gram-positive bacteria are more susceptible for antimicrobial therapy[38] as compared to Gram-negative strains, that is, *K. pneumonia*, because it is easier for an antibiotic to penetrate the cell wall. Gram-negative bacteria are known to contain lipopolysacharide in the outer membrane, which makes it a difficult task for an antibiotic to penetrate within the cell wall. The results from the earlier study may provide a new insight into the development of a new and potential antibiotic source.

Differences at the solvent level were made because of the variability they show in phytochemical extraction. The benzene extract of *T. procumbens* showed potent antimicrobial activity against chosen microbial flora, followed by toluene and methanol. The MIC of plant leaf extract was evaluated by analyzing the turbidity of culture tubes. Culture tubes containing plant extract ranging from 0.1 to 0.3 mg/ml showed bacterial growth, whereas no growth was seen in culture tubes containing plant extract ranging from 0.5 to 0.9 mg/ml in benzene extract. Small aliquots of the sample from culture tubes containing plant extract ranging from 0.5 to 0.9 mg/ml were collected and poured in agar plates, which were allowed to grow for 24 h at optimum temperature condition. No bacterial growth was seen, thus indicating bactericidal property of benzene extract at this particular concentration. Thus, it can be concluded that both MIC and MBC (minimum bactericidal concentration) of benzene extract are effective at concentration of 0.5 mg/ml, whereas for methanol and acetone extract it is 0.7 mg/ml and for toluene and ethanol extract it is 0.9 mg/ml.

There are a few oxidation parameters that provide a clear evidence of local and systemic oxidative stress.[39] UTI infection is known as a causative agent for oxidative stress, along with depletion of antioxidant enzymes.[40] As compared to the control urine sample collected from a patient with renal disease, it was reported that there is a decreased ratio of antioxidant enzyme activity, that is, Catalase (CAT) and Superoxide Dismutase (SOD) activities.[41] Thus, due to the lack of antioxidant enzymes, UTI is considered as a causative marker for oxidative stress. Antioxidant along with antibiotic therapy may provide a newer approach that gives protection against UTI.

6.5 CONCLUSIONS

The present study provides the insight to synthesize new, economically viable potential bio-therapy using plant as a therapeutic agent with high efficacy, less toxicity, feasibility, eco-friendliness, more stability, along with providing the approach to develop the medication with ease. This may provide a wide range of antimicrobial spectrum with greater efficacy. Likewise, this study may also indicate about the development of bio-based formulation with accelerated efficacy against UTI infection. This approach may be helpful to reduce health-care expenses in various forms, which may also be helpful for patients to apply it with all comfortably and easily continue. To understand the mode of action, it is a prerequisite condition to first understand the availability as well as composition of phytoconstituents within plants. Thus, this study may provide a new insight to develop an eco-friendly and economically viable strategy-based research in order to treat UTI infection.

ACKNOWLEDGMENT

We would like to acknowledge ITM University, Gwalior, India, Vice chancellor of ITM University, Gwalior, India, for providing necessary facility and their valuable support and encouragement throughout the work.

KEYWORDS

- plant extract
- organic solvents
- antioxidant activity
- antibacterial activity
- urinary tract infection

REFERENCES

1. Tungmunnithum, D.; Thongboonyou, A.; Pholboon, A.; Yangsabai, A. Flavonoids and Other Phenolic Compounds from Medicinal Plants for Pharmaceutical and Medical Aspects, An Overview. *Medicines (Basel)* **2018,** *5*, 93.
2. Panche, A. N.; Diwan, A. D.; Chandra, S. R. Flavonoids, An Overview. *J. Nutr. Sci.* **2016,** *5*, e47.
3. Ali, S.; Khan, M. R.; Irfanullah, S. M.; Zahra Z. Phytochemical Investigation and Antimicrobial Appraisal of *Parrotiopsis jacquemontiana* (Decne) Rehder. *BMC Complement Altern. Med.* **2018,** *18*, 43.
4. Hosseini, A.; Ghorbani, A. Cancer Therapy with Phytochemicals, Evidence from Clinical Studies. *Avicenna J. Phytomed.* **2015,** *5* (2), 84–97.

5. Rao, S.; Chinkwo, K. A.; Santhakumar, A. B.; Blanchard, C. L. Inhibitory Effects of Pulse Bioactive Compounds on Cancer Development Pathways. *Diseases* **2018**, *3*, 6.
6. Katiyar, C.; Gupta, A.; Kanjilal, S.; Katiyar, S. Drug Discovery from Plant Sources, An Integrated Approach. *Ayu* **2012**, *33*, 10–19.
7. Akgül, T.; Karakan, T. The Role of Probiotics in Women with Recurrent Urinary Tract Infections. *Turk. J. Urol.* **2018**, *44*, 377–383.
8. Abdul, W. M.; Hajrah, N. H.; Sabir, J. S.; Al-Garni, S. M.; Sabir, M. J.; Kabli, S. A.; Saini, K. S.; Bora, R. S. Therapeutic Role of *Ricinus communis* L. and Its Bioactive Compounds in Disease Prevention and Treatment. *Asian Pac. J. Trop. Med.* **2018**, *11*, 177–185.
9. Chauhan, P. S.; Shrivastava, V.; Prasad, G. B. K. S.; Tomar, R. S. Effect of Silver Nanoparticle-Mediated Wound Therapy on Biochemical, Hematological, and Histological Parameters. *APCR* **2018**, *11*, 251–258.
10. Shrivastava, V.; Chauhan, P. S.; Tomar, R. S. Bio-Fabrication of Metal Nanoparticles, A Review. *Int. J. Curr. Res. Life Sci.* **2018**, *7*, 1927–1932.
11. Morales-Luna, E.; Pérez-Ramírez, I. F.; Salgado, L. M.; Castaño-Tostado, E.; Gómez-Aldapa, C. A.; Reynoso-Camacho, R. The Main Beneficial Effect of Roselle (*Hibiscus sabdariffa*) on Obesity is Not Only Related to Its Anthocyanin Content. *J. Sci. Food. Agric.* **2019**, *99*, 596–605.
12. Anandhi, D.; Pandit, V. R.; Kadhiravan, T.; Soundaravally, R.; Raju, K. N. J. Cardiac Arrhythmias, Electrolyte Abnormalities and Serum Cardiac Glycoside Concentrations in Yellow Oleander (*Cascabela thevetia*) Poisoning – A Prospective Study. *Clin. Toxicol. (Phila.)* **2019**, *57*, 104–111.
13. Hickman, S.; Izzy, S.; Sen, P.; Morsett, L.; El Khoury J. Microglia in Neurodegeneration. *Nat. Neurosci.* **2018**, *21*, 1359–1369.
14. Andriana, Y.; Xuan, T. D.; Quy, T. N.; Minh, T. N.; Van, T. M.; Viet, T. D. Antihyperuricemia, Antioxidant, and Antibacterial Activities of *Tridax procumbens* L. *Foods* **2019**, *8*, 21.
15. Yen, C. H.; Chiu, H. F.; Huang, S. Y.; Lu, Y. Y.; Han, Y. C.; Shen, Y. C.; Venkatakrishnan, K.; Wang, C. K. Beneficial Effect of *Arctium tomentosum* Complex on Asymptomatic Helicobacter Pylori-infected Subjects, A Randomized, Double-Blind Placebo-Controlled Clinical Trial. *Helicobacter* **2018**, *23*, e12469.
16. Maroyi, A. A Review of Botany, Medicinal Uses, and Biological Activities of *Pentanisia prunelloides* (Rubiaceae). *Asian J. Pharm. Clin. Res.* **2019**, *12*, 4–9.
17. Saikia, T.; Das, B.; Das, P. Comparative In Vitro Anticancer Activity of Methanolic Extract of Traditionally Used Medicinal Plant of Mizoram. *Int. J. Curr. Pharm. Res.* **2019**, *11*, 84–87.
18. Verma, R.; Balaji, B. S.; Dixit, A. Phytochemical Analysis and Broad Spectrum Antimicrobial Activity of Ethanolic Extract of *Jasminum mesnyi* Hance Leaves and its Solventpartitioned Fractions. *Bioinformation* **2018**, *14*, 430–439.
19. Ohikhena, F. U.; Wintola, O. A.; Afolayan, A. J. Quantitative Phytochemical Constituents and Antioxidant Activities of the Mistletoe, *Phragmanthera capitata* (Sprengel) Balle Extracted with Different Solvents. *Pharmacogn. Res.* **2018**, *10*, 16–23.
20. Chauhan, P. S.; Shrivastava, V.; Tomar, R. S. Phytomediated Synthesis of Silver Nanoparticles and Evaluation of Its Antibacterial Activity Against *Bacillus subtilis* and *Staphylococcus aureus*. *Int. J. Pharma Bio Sci.* **2016**, 184–195.

21. Shrivastava, V.; Chauhan, P. S.; Tomar, R. S. A Biomimetic Approach for Synthesis of Silver Nanoparticles using *Murraya paniculata* Leaf Extract with Reference to Antimicrobial Activity. *J. Pharm. Sci. Res.* **2016**, *8*, 247–250.

22. Shi, P.; Du, W.; Wang, Y.; Teng, X.; Chen, X.; Ye, L. Total Phenolic, Flavonoid Content, and Antioxidant Activity of Bulbs, Leaves, and Flowers Made from *Eleutherine bulbosa* (Mill.) Urb. *Food Sci. Nutr.* **2019**, *7*, 148–154.

23. Derakhshan, Z.; Ferrante, M.; Tadi, M.; Ansari, F.; Heydari, A.; Hosseini, M. S.; Conti, G. O.; Sadrabad, E. K. Antioxidant Activity and Total Phenolic Content of Ethanolic Extract of Pomegranate Peels, Juice and Seeds. *Food Chem. Toxicol.* **2018**, *114*, 108–111.

24. Faraone, I.; Rai, D. K.; Chiummiento, L.; Fernandez, E.; Choudhary, A.; Prinzo, F.; Milella, L. Antioxidant Activity and Phytochemical Characterization of *Senecio clivicolus* Wedd. *Molecules* **2018**, *23*, 2497.

25. Gonelimali, F. D.; Lin, J.; Miao, W.; Xuan, J.; Charles, F.; Chen, M.; Hatab, S. R. Antimicrobial Properties and Mechanism of Action of Some Plant Extracts Against Food Pathogens and Spoilage Microorganisms. *Front. Microbiol.* **2018**, *9*, 1639.

26. Shrivastava, V.; Chauhan, P. S.; Tomar, R. S. Nanobiotechnology, A Potential Tool for Biomedics. *World J. Pharm. Pharm. Sci.* **2015**, *4*, 1929–1943.

27. Tomar, R. S.; Chauhan, P. S.; Shrivastava, V. A Critical Review on Nanoparticles Synthesis, Physicochemical v/s Biological Approach. *World J. Pharm. Res.* **2014**, *4*, 595–620.

28. Chauhan, P. S.; Tomar, R. S.; Shrivastava, V. Biofabrication of Copper Nanoparticles, A Next Generation Antibacterial Agent against Wound Associated Pathogens. *Turk. J. Pharm. Sci.* **2018**, 15.

29. Etame, R. E.; Mouokeu, R. S.; Pouaha, C. L. C.; Kenfack, I. V.; Tchientcheu, R. et al. Effect of Fractioning on Antibacterial Activity of *Enantia chlorantha* Oliver (Annonaceae) Methanol Extract and Mode of Action. *Evid. Based Complement. Alternat. Med.* **2018**, *2018*, 4831593.

30. Yuan, H.; Ma, Q.; Ye, L.; Piao, G. The Traditional Medicine and Modern Medicine from Natural Products. *Molecules* **2016**, *21*, 559.

31. Thorsen, R. S.; Pouliot, M. Traditional Medicine for the Rich and Knowledgeable, Challenging Assumptions about Treatment-Seeking Behaviour in Rural and Peri-Urban Nepal. *Health Policy Plan.* **2016**, *31*, 314–324.

32. Mushtaq, S.; Abbasi, B. H.; Uzair, B.; Abbasi, R. Natural Products as Reservoirs of Novel Therapeutic Agents. *Exp. Clin. Sci. J.* **2018**, *17*, 420–451.

33. Nguyen, V. B.; Wang, S. L.; Nguyen, A. D.; Lin, Z. H.; Doan, C. T.; Tran, T. N.; Huang, H. T.; Kuo, Y. H. Bioactivity-Guided Purification of Novel Herbal Antioxidant and Anti-NO Compounds from *Euonymus laxiflorus* Champ. *Molecules* **2019**, *24*, 120.

34. Belatrix, B.; Puspitawati, R.; Djais, A. A. Effect of Javanese Turmeric Ethanol Extract on the Eradication of *Candida albicans* Biofilms in Early, Intermediate, and Maturation Phases. *Int. J. Appl. Pharm.* **2019**, *11*, 1–4.

35. Alahmar, A. T. Role of Oxidative Stress in Male Infertility, An Updated Review. *J. Hum. Reprod. Sci.* **2019**, *12*, 4–18.

36. Kurutas, E. B. The Importance of Antioxidants Which Play the Role in Cellular Response Against Oxidative/Nitrosative Stress, Current State. *Nutr. J.* **2016**, *15*, 71.

37. Phaniendra, A.; Jestadi, D. B.; Periyasamy, L. Free Radicals, Properties, Sources, Targets, and Their Implication in Various Diseases. *Indian J. Clin. Biochem.* **2015,** *30,* 11–26.

38. Li, B.; Webster, T. J. Bacteria Antibiotic Resistance, New Challenges and Opportunities for Implant-Associated Orthopaedic Infections. *J. Orthop. Res.* **2018,** *36,* 22–32.

39. Nair, A.; Nair, B. J. Comparative Analysis of the Oxidative Stress and Antioxidant Status in Type II Diabetics and Nondiabetics, A Biochemical Study. *J. Oral Maxillofac. Pathol.* 2017, *21,* 394–401.

40. Flores-Mireles, A. L.; Walker, J. N.; Caparon, M.; Hultgren, S. Urinary Tract Infections, Epidemiology, Mechanisms of Infection and Treatment Options. *Nat. Rev. Microbiol.* **2015,** *13,* 269–284.

41. Dennis, J. M.; Witting, P. K. Protective Role for Antioxidants in Acute Kidney Disease. *Nutrients* **2017,** *9,* 718.

CHAPTER 7

Citrus Fruits and Their By-Products, Power House of Remedial Antioxidants

HRADESH RAJPUT[1*], PRATISTHA SRIVASTAVA[1], and RITA SHARMA[2]

[1]Department of Food Technology, ITM University, Gwalior, India

[2]Department of Life Sciences, ITM University, Gwalior, India

*Corresponding author. E-mail: hrdesh802@gmail.com

ABSTRACT

Citrus fruit is popular due to its characteristic flavor, taste, aroma, and multiple health benefits. The desert environment is conducive for citrus production provided that appropriate agronomic practices are followed for obtaining high-quality citrus fruit. By-products can also be maximizing the utilization of natural foods and at the same time, and it can also protect the environment. Citrus fruits are financially significant with a large-scale generation of both the new foods grown and processed products. Citriculture as a garden industry existed for quite a long time in India. It includes the third largest fruit industry. Citrus organic products are perceived as a significant part of the human eating routine, giving an assortment of constituents critical to human sustenance, including vitamin C, folic acid, potassium, flavonoids, coumarins, pectin, and dietary fibers. Citrus flavonoids have a wide range of natural exercises, including antibacterial, antioxidant, antidiabetic, anticancer cardiovascular, analgesic, anti-inflammatory, and antianxiety. This chapter details the health benefits of citrus and by-products of citrus especially in cancer and the active components that are thought to produce these health benefits, their mechanisms of action, and the level at which they are found in citrus fruits.

7.1 INTRODUCTION

In the context of India, agriculture and agriculture-based allied sectors continue to be of crucial importance not only to meet the food and nutrition demand of ever-growing 1.3 billion population of India but also for employment generation and thereby sustainable socioeconomic development of the country. In light of the changing dietary example, cultivation area is assuming a critical job with yearly development of about 7% against 3% development in grains. As zone under the cultivation crops is developing at the pace of 2.7% per annum with increment in efficiency by 37% somewhere in the year of 2004 and 2015, India has kept up the second most noteworthy position for the creation of agricultural harvests, after China. With 6.3 million ha territory under development (27% of all-out cultivation region), and all-out result of 88.8 million t, natural product crops record to 31% of all out agricultural yields (Anonymous, 2018). Despite that, India tops in the UN's World Hunger List 2015, with 194.6 million undernourished people exceeding China by 15% (Anonymous, 2018).

Citrus, the genus Citrus L. of the family Rutaceae, is one of the most significant organic product crops on the planet. This family has rich phytochemicals wellsprings of numerous bioactive mixes that are responsible for cell reinforcement and numerous other organic exercises (Fejzić and Ćavar, 2014). It is widely grown in the tropical and subtropical areas of the world, and many other areas, the significant amount of fruits produced globally include 124.73 MMT of citrus; 74.49 MMT of grapes; 45.22 MMT of mangoes, mangosteens, and guavas; and 25.43 MMT of pineapples (FAO, 2017). Horticultural by-products are excellent sources of pigments, phenolic compounds, dietary fibers, sugar derivatives, organic acids, and minerals, among other components. A few of these bioactive mixes have useful well-being traits, antibacterial, antitumor, antiviral, antimutagenic, and cardioprotective exercises (Yahia, 2010, 2017). Citrus natural products are well acknowledged by purchasers of everywhere throughout the world in light of their appealing hues, wonderful, flavors, and smell. Fruits yield about 25–30% of nonedible products such as peels and seeds (Ajila et al., 2010). As a rule, these loss side effects contain high substance of cell reinforcement and antimicrobial intensifies that can be effectively used as a wellspring of phytochemicals and cancer prevention agent operators.

Orange is created by an outside layer (peel) framed by flavedo (epicarp or exocarp) and albedo (mesocarp), and an inward material considered endocarp that contains vesicles with juice, flavedo, and albedo represent around 50, 10, and 25% (w/w) individually of the entire organic product. Lemon strip comprises two layers, the furthest layer called zest, and contains basic oils (6%) that are made for the most part out of limonene (90%) and citral (5%) and a modest quantity of cintronelene, alphaterpincol, linayl, and gernanyl acetic acid derivation alongside B-complex nutrients. Citrus fruits are rich sources of useful phytochemicals, such as vitamins A, C, and E; mineral elements; flavonoids; coumarins; limonoids; carotenoids; pectins; and other compounds (Zhou, 2012).

Citrus natural products are rich wellsprings of helpful phytochemicals, for example, nutrients A, C, and E, mineral components, flavonoids, coumarins, limonoids, carotenoids, gelatins, and different mixes (Zhou, 2012). Citrus foods grown from the ground containing citrus are known for various medical advantages and aversion of infections in human. The presence of important bioactive mixtures in citrus fruits is the significant purpose behind various natural properties (Al-Juhaimi and Ghafoor, 2013) that produce resistance against different diseases. The nearness of phenolic mixes in Citrus citrus fruits is likewise revealed and that they additionally add to the cell reinforcement properties like nutrient C and carotenoids type mixes (AL-Juhaimi and Ghafoor, 2013). Flavonoids and phenolic acids decide a significant piece of bioactive mixes for citrus natural products (Astell et al., 2013). Cancer preventive agent action indicates the capacity of a bioactive compound to keep up cell structure and capacity by adequately clearing free radicals, repressing lipid peroxidation responses, and forestalling other oxidative harm. It is also a foundation of many other biological functions, such as anticancers, anti-inflammation, and antiaging.

Risk of chronic diseases can be reduced by frequent consumption of fruits and vegetables. A typical part of nourishment items is a dietary fiber that comprises assortment of nonstarch polysaccharides, for example, cellulose, hemicelluloses, gelatin, b-glucans, gums, and lignin (Elleuch et al., 2011) because their helpful consequences for nourishment wholesome properties are devoured as food sources. To this respect, a few models about the utilization of citrus natural products as helpful cures can be referred to, oranges to fix scurvy (Magiorkinis et al., 2011); orange, lime, and lemon squeezes as solutions for the aversion of kidney stones development; grapefruits as operators ready to bring down pulse and to meddle with calcium channel blockers; citrus flavonoids as successful in vivo specialists ready to regulate hepatic lipid digestion; squeezed orange to forestall and balance incendiary procedures (Assis et al., 2013); kumquat strip polyphenolics as viable cell reinforcement operators; grapefruit juice that is hostile to genotoxic impacts (Alvarez-Gonzales et al., 2010); and a few others.

Due to increasing production and processing of fruits, disposal represents a growing problem since the plant material is usually prone to microbial spoilage, thus limiting further exploitation. On the other hand, expenses of drying, stockpiling, and shipment of side effects are financially restricting variables. Consequently, agro-mechanical waste is regularly used as feed or as compost (Varzakas et al., 2016). There is a pattern to discover new wellsprings of practical fixings, for example, plant nourishment side effects that have customarily been underestimated (Rodríguez et al., 2006). These results may stretch around 60% of collected plants. These deposits are truly transitory items that are hard to oversee on account of ecological issues in the enterprises (Arvanitoyannis and Varzakas, 2008).

The preparing of plant nourishments brings about the creation of results that are rich wellsprings of bioactive mixes, including phenolic mixes. The cell reinforcement mixes from squander result of nourishment industry could be utilized for expanding the soundness of nourishments by forestalling lipid peroxidation and furthermore for ensuring oxidative harm in living frameworks by searching oxygen free radicals (Makris et al., 2007). Although these buildups are typically disposed of, they could be utilized as an elective wellspring of supplements to expand the nutritive estimation of destitute individuals' weight control plans and to help diminish dietary inadequacies (da Silva et al., 2013) as useful nourishment showcase is one of the top patterns in the nourishment business (Helkar et al., 2016).

Therefore, overhauling frameworks for nourishment squander decrease, explicitly reusing, have been rehearsed for generation of numerous helpful items, for example, usage of products of the soil squanders as a wellspring of bioactive mixes. These mixes have high-esteem items, and their recuperation might be financially appealing (Hernandez-Carranze et al., 2016). The medical advantages of citrus natural products have been credited for the most part to the nearness of cell reinforcements, for example, phenolics and ascorbic corrosive (Kumar et al., 2015). The Jordan condition is rich and there is assorted variety in the Jordanian harvest creation (Qura'n, 2010). There is a developing acknowledgment that phenols, amino acids, fundamental oils, gelatin, carotenoids, flavonoids, and nutrient C present in citrus natural products apply valuable impacts in the counteractive action of degenerative maladies.

Routinely, the utilization of manufactured cancer preventive agents as butylated hydroxytoluene and butylated hydroxyanisole in nourishments is crippled because of their elevated levels of poisonous quality and cancer-causing nature (Noor et al., 2014). So, regular cell reinforcements from foods grown from the ground squander have concerned noteworthy consideration because of their well-being. In recent years, there is a global trend toward the use of phytochemicals from natural resources such as vegetables, fruits, oilseeds, and herbs, as antioxidants and functional ingredients. In addition, this research will give new information about bioactive compounds of fruit/vegetables and its waste. The extraction of bioactive compounds is present in pomegranate, mango, grapes, citrus peel, pineapple waste, tomato, potato, sweet potato, beetroot, processing waste, which are of economic importance in the national and international market. Accordingly, the interest for such significant nourishment wares has expanded fundamentally because of the developing total populace and the changing dietary propensity (Vilari ˜no et al., 2017).

7.2 STRUCTURE AND COMPOSITION OF CITRUS FRUIT

The plainly visible structure of the organic product comprises skin or strip made up of fingernail skin on outside, meagerly covering an epidermal layer (flavedo) containing various oil sacks loaded up with fragrant fundamental oil having high business esteem. Flavedo is followed by light layer parenchymatous cells. The albedo contains roughly 20% of citrus gelatin. The inward mash or substance (palatable part) of the organic product is framed of portions (locules), isolated by a film of meager epidermal tissue and containing various juice sacs (vesicles) and seeds. The focal white supple tissue like that of albedo is called hub (center) of the natural product. The center and section layers are on the whole called the (cloth) of the removed juice (Fig. 7.1).

The existence of important organic acids, sugars, and amino acids is the major reason for the popularity of the citrus fruits. Diet-rich organic product contains apparent measure of nutrients (C, An, and B), minerals, fiber, phenolic mixes, and phytochemicals, for example, carotenoids and limonoids, which have high medical advantages.

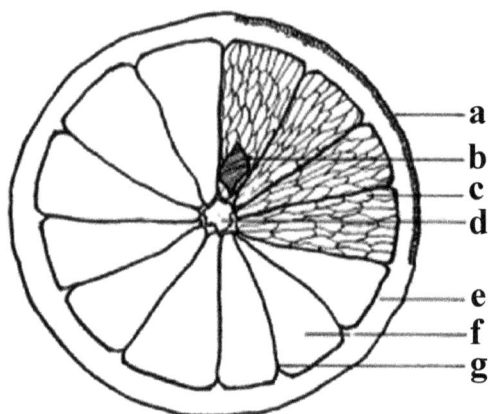

FIGURE 7.1   Schematic view of the cross section of an orange.

7.3 BIOACTIVE COMPOUNDS IN DIFFERENT CITRUS FRUITS

The antioxidant components of citrus fruits and their antioxidant activities are discussed in the following subsections.

7.3.1 VITAMINS IN CITRUS FRUITS

There are more than 170 cancer preventive agents from citrus natural products, including nutrients, mineral components, phenolic mixes, and terpenoids, and gelatin abridges their delegate types, synthetic structures, and cell reinforcement properties. Vitamins are found in citrus natural products, including vitamins A, B1, B2, C, E, and B3, of which, vitamins A, C, and E were assessed for their cell reinforcement exercises (Amitava and Kimberly, 2014). Vitamin A will be a class of fat-dissolvable natural mixes, which incorporates retinol, retinal, retinoic corrosive, and a few professional b-carotenes. Citrus fruits are wealthy in carotenes and cryptoxanthin. Vitamin C, L-ascorbic corrosive or essentially ascorbate, is a water solubility substance. It is a significant vitamin found in Citrus and wealthy in the fragile living creature and strip of natural products. Vitamin C is a characteristic free extreme scrounger, which can adequately rummage an assortment types of responsive oxygen species (ROS) and emit semidehydroascorbic corrosive and lessening sulfur radicals (Amitava and

Kimberly, 2014). Vitamin E, another fat-dissolvable nutrient, is a gathering of exacerbates that incorporate the two compounds, tocopherols and tocotrienols. Vitamin E is predominantly found in the strips and seeds of citrus natural products, and its substance in sugar-coated orange, tangerine, and lemon can arrive at 5.60, 4.50, and 11.40 mg/kg, individually.

7.3.2 MINERAL ELEMENTS IN CITRUS FRUITS

Mineral components are the chemical exacerbates that plants take from the dirt for their development and advancement except for carbon, hydrogen, and oxygen. Among the 81 chemical elements found in mammalian bodies, at least 19 are found in Citrus plants (Table 7.1), including calcium (Ca), phosphorus (P), magnesium (Mg), potassium (K), sulfur (S), sodium (Na), iron (Fe), manganese (Mn), nickel (Ni), boron (B), silicon (Si), copper (Cu), zinc (Zn), molybdenum (Mo), selenium (Se), cobalt (Co), chromium (Cr), germanium (Ge), and arsenic (As) (Zhou, 2012). These components, Mn, Fe, Cu, Zn, and Se, have been accounted for to be identified with the cancer preventive agent action of life forms (Amitava and Kimberly, 2014).

TABLE 7.1 Chemical Compositions of Citrus Fruits (per 100 g of Edible Portion).

	C. aurantifolia	*C. aurantium*	*C. Limon*	*C. paradisi*	*C. reticulate*	*C. Sinensis*
Moisture, g	84.6	87.6	85.0	88.5	87.8	88.4
Protein, g	1.5	0.7	1.0	1.0	0.9	0.8
Fat, g	1.0	0.2	0.9	0.1	0.3	0.3
Fiber, g	1.3	0.3	1.7	-	-	0.5
Carbohydrates, g	10.9	10.9	11.1	10.0	10.6	9.3
Minerals, g	0.7	0.3	0.3	0.4	0.4	0.7
Calcium, mg	90	26	70	30	50	40
Phosphorous, mg	20	20	10	30	20	30
Iron, mg	0.3	0.3	2.3	0.2	0.1	0.7
Thiamine, mg	0.02	-	0.02, Juice	0.12	40[*]	-
Riboflavin, mg	0.03	-	0.01, Juice	0.02	-	-
Niacin, mg	0.1	-	0.01, Juice	0.3	-	0
Vitamin C, mg	63	30	39, Juice	-	68	50
Carotene, μg	15	1104	0	-	350[*]	0
Energy, K cal	59	48	57	45	-	43

7.3.3   PHENOLIC COMPOUNDS IN CITRUS FRUITS

Polyphenols comprise a variety of bioactive compounds that are commonly divided into several classes, hydroxybenzoic acids, hydroxy-cinnamic acids, anthocyanins, proanthocyanidins, flavonoids, stilbenes, and lignans. Among the citrus fruits, phenolic compounds, the antioxidant activity of flavonoids, phenolic acid, and coumarins are the most studied in existing literature.

7.3.3.1   FLAVONOIDS

Flavonoids have an immediate job in rummaging receptive oxygen species, which can neutralize lipid oxidation in vitro and improve the body's cell reinforcement catalyst action, and diminishing peroxide arrangement in vivo (Nakao et al., 2011). Among the Citrus flavonoids, the antioxidants of naringin, hesperidin, and naringenin are regularly contemplated. Naringin can altogether upgrade the insusceptible framework's adequacy to dodge interior organs and tissue damage or malady brought about by oxidation by expanding the action of catalase (CAT), superoxide dismutase (SOD), glutathione peroxidase (GPx), paraoxonase (PON), and other cell reinforcement chemicals. Naringenin can hinder the b-oxidation of unsaturated fats in the liver by directing the chemicals of the unsaturated fat oxidation forms, for example, carnitine palmitoyl transferase (CPT, the rate-restricting protein of unsaturated fat oxidation), 3-hydroxy-3-methyl-glutaryl-CoA reductase, PON, and plasma cell reinforcement catalysts (Jung et al., 2006). Naringenins are more successful than hesperidin.

7.3.3.2   PHENOLIC ACIDS

The phenolic acids are wealthy in citrus foods grown from the ground various degrees of free radical rummaging. Citrus phenolic acids show solid cancer preventive agent properties through the dehydrogenation of hydroxyl gatherings and the impact of ortho-substitution on a benzene ring (Dai and Mumper, 2010).

7.3.3.3 COUMARINS

Coumarins are another class of phenolic compound wealthy in Citrus organic products. They are acquired from a part of the phenylalanine digestion pathway, which drives at last to furanocoumarin (psoralen) amalgamation. Coumarins have appeared to have solid cancer preventive agent exercises as a result of their phenolic hydroxyl gatherings.

7.3.4 TERPENOIDS IN CITRUS FRUITS

Among the citrus terpenoids, the antioxidant activities of limonoids and carotenoids are reported in the following subsections.

7.3.4.1 LIMONOIDS

Limonoids are a gathering of profoundly oxygenated, tetracyclic triterpene optional metabolite subsidiaries. A total of 36 limonoid aglycones and 17 limonoid glycosides have been accounted for in citrus natural products. Distinctive limonoids have variable cancer preventive agent limits and some are surprisingly better than nutrient C. For example, the free radical scavenging activity of four limonin glycosides, limonin 17-b-D-glucopyranoside (LG), obacunone 17-b-D-glucoside body (OG), millington acid 17-b-D-glucoside (NAG), and deacetylation millington acid 17-b-D-glucoside (DNAG), was evaluated, and it was discovered that each of them has cancer preventive agent exercises, among which NAG is the most grounded and LG is the weakest.

7.3.4.2 CAROTENOIDS

Carotenoids are a sort of tetraterpenoids. They have been accounted for to show cell reinforcement exercises through extinguishing and dispensing with unsafe free radicals. They may likewise shield insusceptible cell film lipids from oxidative harm, along these lines guaranteeing correspondence flag among cells and receptors on the cell layer to keep up ordinary cell capacity and upgrade human invulnerability.

7.3.5   PECTIN IN CITRUS FRUITS

Pectin is the significant segment of the cell divider in plants. It is synthetically a polysaccharide, comprising a direct chain of connected galacturonic corrosive. It has been accounted for that pectin diminished blood lipid level and peroxidative status and indicated cell reinforcement exercises in kidney danger incited by octylphenol (Koriem et al., 2014). The suppressive impact of pectin has all the earmarks of being through upgrade of endogenous cancer preventive agent catalysts and transfer of free radicals, where pectin at a higher portion was progressively intense (Koriem et al., 2014). In Citrus citrus fruits as a rule have higher pectin content, and their complete pectin substance runs from 36.0 ± 1.46 to 86.4 ± 3.36 mg/g db in the strips of Citrus natural products (Wang et al., 2008).

7.3.6   CONTRIBUTION OF DIFFERENT ANTIOXIDANT COMPONENTS OF CITRUS FRUITS

The absolute cancer preventive agent limit of plant separates is impacted by their compound pieces and substance of cell reinforcements. Various segments in plant separates contribute inconsistent to their complete cell reinforcement capacity. In a lipid peroxidation framework, the cell reinforcement limit of various Citrus natural product separates is emphatically connected with their complete polyphenol content, while no undeniable relationship was found with their nutrient C content. This outcome may propose that Citrus polyphenols might be the prevailing cancer preventive agent part. Nonetheless, the cancer preventive agent limit of Citrus products of various species and cultivars was unmistakably connected with the ascorbic corrosive substance as opposed to with the nearness of flavanone glycosides. In addition, Rekha et al. (2012) found that the cancer preventive agent limit of organic product juices was straightforwardly identified with the substance of absolute phenolics and nutrient C in some Citrus species.

7.3.6.1   METHODS FOR THE ANTIOXIDANT ACTIVITY EVALUATION OF CITRUS FRUITS

These days, the cell reinforcement limit of plant nourishments has been taken as a marker of their helpful consequences for human well-being

(Prior and Wu, 2013). Along these lines, a great strategy for the cell reinforcement movement assessment of Citrus natural products is vital. As a general perspective on the potential techniques that can be utilized for the cancer prevention agent movement assessment of Citrus organic products, we present the in vitro and in vivo examinations, HPLC-dependent online strategies, and nanoparticle-based as well as myoglobin-based strategies.

The application of these methods to Citrus fruits is presented in the following subsections.

7.3.6.2   CHEMICAL METHODS

Chemical methods are the most part worried about the free radical or oxide rummaging limit of the cancer preventive agents. In the current literature, the major in vitro methods used for plant samples are 1,1-diphenyl-2-pierylhydrazy (DH) (Alam et al., 2013), 2,20-azino-bis(3-ethylbenzthiazoline-6-sulfonic acid) (ABTS) (López-Alarcón and Denicola, 2013), oxygen radical absorbance capacity (ORAC) (López-Alarcón and Denicola, 2013), total radical-trapping antioxidant parameter (TRAP) (Alam et al., 2013), Trolox equivalent antioxidant capacity (TEAC) (Netzel et al., 2007), ferric reducing antioxidant power (FRAP) (Alam et al., 2013), cupric ion reducing antioxidant capacity (CUPRAC) (Alam et al., 2013), and photochemiluminescence (PCL) (Netzel et al., 2007). The main preferred positions of these techniques are speed and straightforwardness, yet the weakness is that their outcomes are affected by numerous elements, for example, cell reinforcements and cooperations, impedance materials, pH, activity time, creating framework with the expectation of complimentary radicals, etc. With respect to Citrus fruits, the DH, FRAP, ABTS, ORAC methods are often used to evaluate antioxidant activity (Zhang et al., 2014).

7.3.6.3   ONLINE METHODS BASED ON HPLC SYSTEM

Customary disconnected techniques for the cell reinforcement action assessment of plant tests have a few issues, chiefly tedious and high work power (Zhang et al., 2015). Then again, the online strategies dependent on HPLC, remembering for line HPLC-chemiluminescence (CL) discovery, HPLC-DH technique, online HPLC-ABTS strategy (He et al., 2010), and online HPLC-CUPRAC strategy, and online HPLC-CUPRAC method

(Çelik et al., 2010), can detect the antioxidant activity of a single constituent and its contribution to the overall activity of complex mixtures simultaneously. Along these lines, the filtration of each and every compound for disconnected tests is never again expected, prompting a huge decrease of time and cost to get results. To assess the cancer preventive agent action of Citrus natural products, our team built up an online elite fluid chromatography free radical rummaging identification (HPLC-FRSD) framework for the all-out cell reinforcement limit assessment of Citrus citrus fruits (Zhang et al., 2015).

7.3.6.4 MYOGLOBIN-BASED METHOD

Myoglobin is a novel fluorescence test. Terashima et al., (2012) proposed a myoglobin-based cell reinforcement action assessment technique, which estimated the cancer preventive agent action of tests by inspecting the adjustment in the fluorescence absorbance, which came about because of the response of myoglobin. The myoglobin defensive proportion (MPR) was characterized to express the cell reinforcement levels of the examples that are tried (Terashima et al., 2012). The technique was proposed to be quick, straightforward, and solid. At present, it is utilized to assess the cancer preventive agent movement of cooked Gomchwi (*Ligularia fischeri*) (An et al., 2014).

7.3.6.5 NANOPARTICLE-BASED METHOD

Novel chemical tests dependent on nanotechnology, especially utilizing nanoparticles, have been proposed to assess cancer preventive agent exercises (Scampicchio et al., 2006). This methodology is commonly founded on the decrease of metal buildings by normal cancer preventive agents to produce NPs. In a spearheading study, Özyürek et al. (2012) built up a silver nanoparticle cancer preventive agent limit (SNPAC) strategy for the cell reinforcement movement assessment of regular nourishment. Their technique utilizes Trolox as a standard cancer preventive agent to mirror the absolute cell reinforcement limit (TAC). Polyphenols going about as auxiliary lessening operators gave a more vigorous and reproducible technique than those utilizing metal particles by direct decrease by cell reinforcements. The upside of this technique is the great linearity with polyphenol focus, which is not influenced by the nearness of citrus fruits acids, lessening sugars, or amino acids in the concentrates. Although nanoparticle-based strategies open a promising field for the cell reinforcement movement assessment of characteristic items, as of recently, the commonsense use of these techniques is uncommon.

7.3.6.6   *FACTORS INFLUENCING THE ANTIOXIDANT CAPACITY OF CITRUS FRUITS*

The cancer preventive agent arrangement of a natural example is convoluted and may be affected by a wide exhibit of variables. The phytochemicals of Citrus plants are various and change with its species, starting point, and various tissues. In this way, their cell reinforcement abilities are likewise unique. For effortlessness of depiction, the inner and outside components that impact the cell reinforcement limit of Citrus leafy foods determined items are isolated into the accompanying classes, the substance structure of the cancer preventive agents, pre- and postharvest factors, and handling factors.

7.3.6.7   *THE CHEMICAL STRUCTURE*

The movement of cancer preventive agents is firmly identified with their substance structure. Among the cell reinforcements revealed in Citrus natural products, flavonoids, coumarins, limonoids, and phenolic acids are accounted for to have structure–action connections. The structure of flavonoids and their relationship to cancer preventive agent movement has been explained in numerous investigations. The glycosylation of flavonoid mixes normally diminished their cancer preventive agent limit. The hydroxyl structure on the B ring normally impacts the radical searching effectiveness of flavonoids or its subsidiaries, and the hydroxyl number expands such exercises. Also, a lower cancer preventive agent action of limonoids than different flavonoids was viewed as because of the absence of pigmented rings in limonoids. Despite the way that bound phenolic acids had higher cell reinforcement exercises, examination of cancer preventive agent possibilities and their association with phenolic corrosive substance indicated that free phenolics were progressively viable (Dai and Mumper, 2010).

7.3.6.8   PREHARVEST FACTORS

The preharvest factors that impact the cell reinforcement movement of Citrus citrus fruits incorporate natural conditions and agronomic conditions, which act by influencing the degree of phytochemicals (Tiwari and Cummins, 2013). The ecological conditions, for example, soil dampness, temperature variety, daylight radiation, and climatic conditions inside a topographical area, impact the degree of cancer preventive agents in Citrus organic products. Research has demonstrated that the sort and substance of Citrus phytochemicals differ with soil type and profundity. Temperature difference between day and night affects the substance of flavonoids, phenolic corrosive, and anthocyanin, along these lines influencing the cell reinforcement limit of Citrus organic products. In the development time frame, the substance of supplements and bioactive mixes goes together with the sun-based radiation and long stretches of sun. The agronomic conditions, including manure, planting date, water system, development stages, and ensuing collecting, impact the degree of cancer preventive agents in Citrus natural products. Gathering Citrus natural products at an overripened arrange causes higher phenolic and anthocyanins contents than those collected at unmatured stages (Pantelidis et al., 2007).

7.3.6.9   POSTHARVEST FACTORS

Fruit harvesting reaping and postharvest treatment are the primary factors that influence cell reinforcement movement. The postharvest factors that impact the cancer preventive agent limit of Citrus natural products basically incorporate capacity conditions, for example, time, temperature, mugginess, light force, and agro-synthetic substances. Citrus fruits have an expanded capacity to prompt flavonoid amassing (particularly anthocyanins) during cold stockpiling (Chaudhary et al., 2014). For instance, in blood oranges under low-temperature stockpiling, there is an expansion in flavanones, anthocyanins, and hydroxycinnamic acids and a gently decline in nutrient C (Rapisarda et al., 2008). Gas arrangement affects the cell reinforcement action of natural products, which implies the groupings of carbon dioxide, and oxygen should be controlled properly (Moretti et al., 2010). Under a high O_2 climate, the higher stockpiling quality conveys higher absolute phenolic substance and DH searching limit (Yang et al., 2008). Ethylene, a significant characteristic plant hormone utilized in farming to advance the maturing of natural products, assumes a significant job in animate movement of phenylalanine smelling salts lyase (PAL), a key catalyst in the biosynthesis of phenolic mixes and aggregation of phenolic constituents after Citrus citrus fruits were gathered. Citrus strips (CP) treated with methyl jasmonate and ethanol had more significant levels of absolute phenolics, flavonoids, anthocyanins just as higher radical searching exercises against DH, superoxide, and hydroxyl radicals than those in the control.

7.4 SOME HEALTH-RELATED PROPERTIES OF CITRUS FRUITS

7.4.1 ANTICARCINOGENIC PROPERTIES

Plant flavonoids have stood out as a significant dietary malignant growth chemo-defensive operator. Citrus flavonoids have anticarcinogenic and hostile to tumor exercises. Citrus flavonoids can hinder the intrusion of chick heart pieces and syngeneic mice liver. The polymethoxylated flavones have appeared in various in vitro investigations to apply solid antiproliferative activity against malignancy cells antigen–initiated T lymphocytes gastric disease cells, prostate malignancy cells squamous cell carcinoma and antimetastatic activities against human bosom malignant growth cells have additionally been seen with tangeretin. Naringin, hesperidin, nobiletin, and tangeretin restrain the bacterial mutagenesis. Quercetin in test consumes less calories brought down the occurrence of colon tumors in azoxymethanol-treated rodents and fibrosarcoma in mice. Naringenin lessens lung metastasis in a bosom disease resection model.

7.4.2 CARDIOVASCULAR PROPERTIES

Several studies indicate that certain flavonoids may have a protective and therapeutic effect on coronary heart disease.

1. Effect on capillary fragility: The effect of flavonoids on bleeding and capillary fragility is that capillary damage can be treated with flavonoids. Diosmin produces a significant decrease in venous capacitance, venous distensibility, and venous emptying time.

2. Effect of platelet aggregation: *Citrus* flavonoids show an antiadhesive and antiaggregation action against red cell clumping. Quercetin, fisetin, kaempferol, and myricetin inhibit platelet aggregation.
3. Effect on coronary heart disease: Flavonoids inhibit the oxidation of low-density lipoprotein (LDL) and reduces thrombotic tendencies. Flavonoids reduce the rate of oxidized compound formation, thus inhibiting the growth of atherosclerotic complications.
4. Hypercholesterolemia: Dietary intake of orange or grapefruit juices reduces hypercholesterolemia. Tangeretin, nobiletin, or polymethoxylated flavones significantly reduced serum triacylglycerols without altering HDL cholesterol level and causing toxic effect.

7.4.3   HYPERGLYCEMIA

Citrus flavonoids play important roles in preventing the progression of hyperglycemia, partly by binding to starch, increasing hepatic glycolysis and the glycogen concentration, and lowering hepatic gluconeogenesis (Shen et al., 2012). Hesperidin and naringin both significantly lowered the blood glucose level.

7.4.4   ANTI-INFLAMMATORY, ANTIALLERGIC, AND ANALGESIC ACTIVITY

Citrus flavonoids like hesperidin, diosmin, quercetin, and other flavonoids have shown dose-dependent anti-inflammatory activities by influencing metabolism of arachidonic acid and histamine. Hesperidin is an effective component with antiallergic action. Hesperidin inhibits bone loss and decreases serum and hepatic lipids in ovariectomized mice. Naringenin may provide neuroprotection through suppression of proinflammatory pathways in activated BV-2 microglial cells (Park et al., 2012).

7.4.5   ANTIMICROBIAL ACTIVITY

One of the properties of flavonoids with their physiological action in the plants is their antifungal and antiviral activities. Quercetin and hesperetin actively inhibit the infectivity and/or replication of herpes simplex virus, polioviruses, parainfluenza, and syncytial viruses. Bergamot peel is a potential source of natural antimicrobials that are active against Gram-negative bacteria (Mandalari et al., 2007).

7.5   BY-PRODUCTS OF CITRUS FRUITS

The measure of buildup acquired from the natural products represents half of the entire organic product mass. Subsequently, the nourishment business creates huge volumes of strong and fluid squanders. As indicated by Mamma et al. (2008), citrus squander has generally been dried and utilized as crude materials for gelatin extraction or utilized without treatment for making creature feed or composts. As of late, be that as it may, the expanding costs related to the capacity and transportation of citrus squander and the lower costs got from feed markets have brought about the declining enthusiasm with respect to industry for these employments. Simultaneously, the need to avert ecological contamination and to save vitality and crude materials has developed, and new strategies and arrangements for squander recuperation and bioconversion for increasingly helpful, high-esteem items are being presented. Various multifunctional fixings are being created from citrus side effects and citrus squander, strikingly, strip oil, oil and water-stage characters, mash sacs, and limonene. A few research bunches have been chipping away at the advancement of multifunctional fixings from citrus side effects and citrus squander. Besides, citrus waste could be utilized through enzymatic, cellulolytic, or pectinolytic hydrolysis or microbial change to acquire fluid biofuel. Consequently, the side effects and conventions coming about because of the undertaking were investigated through a natural and monetary appraisal, giving an assessment of the mechanical importance (Fava et al., 2013).

7.6   CHARACTERIZATION OF CITRUS WASTE

Citrus juice plentiful in nutrient C is the significant result of citrus preparing enterprises and is broadly utilized for creation of supplement rich drinks. Be that as it may, it has just half unadulterated juice yield of its weight and the rest is considered as a buildup (strip, mash, seeds, and entire orange citrus fruits that do not arrive at the quality prerequisites), which has dampness content up to 80% (Rezzadori et al., 2012). The yearly citrus squander produced in India is 7.8 million t while world normal is about 119.7 million t (Anonymous, 2017). Enormous measure of this waste is dumped on the neighboring landfill/streams or consumed causing natural contamination and consumption of broke down oxygen level in polluted water (Wadhwa and Bakshi, 2013). This strategy for squander the executives delivers exceptionally dirtied wastewater, causes extraordinary corruption of soil characteristics, and furthermore drives harm to the shallow water in the territory (Martín et al., 2010). A few research bunches have been taking a shot at the advancement of multifunctional fixings from citrus results and citrus squander. One option for the best administration of these buildups is the as far as strengthened supplement-rich creature feed, usage of fiber rich, gelatin generation, fundamental oil, and so on.

7.7 CITRUS WASTE VALORIZATION

Squander valorization is the way toward changing over waste and biomass into vitality, fuel, and other progressively helpful items, including synthetic chemicals, materials, and fills with specific spotlight on natural markers and maintainability objectives (Arancon et al., 2013). The buildup of citrus juice generation, for example, strip and seeds is extraordinary wellspring of a few mixes, as dissolvable sugars, amino acids, fiber, natural acids and oils and lipids, and nutrients. Deductively valorization of these items offers financial pick up just as natural projection. The present survey is predominantly centered around the advancements in squander valorization of citrus organic product modern buildup. Late advanced techniques for squander valorization, for example, fundamental oil extraction, creation of biofuels, nourishment grade kraft paper and bundling materials, adsorbents, and enacted carbons have been examined in subtleties (Fig. 7.2).

7.7.1 ANIMAL FEED

Solid waste generated from the citrus processing can be used as the ingredients for the animal feed. As the cheapest and easiest way of disposal, most of the industries worldwide are ending their waste in the fresh or dried form for the development of animal feed. For the generation of dried silage, the mash is squeezed twice to lessen the dampness content up to 65–70%, dried and pelletized for showcasing. Citrus buildup contains high measure of gelatin that ties the water in buildup. Lime and calcium hydroxide or calcium oxide are added during drying. Lime and calcium hydroxide or calcium oxide establishes pH in the range of 5.5–6.5 and destroys the hydrophilic nature of pectin that is added to the pulp and thus facilitates the separation of water and carbohydrate present in the pulp. Therefore, supplementation rich in pectin citrus by-product feed that is degradable neutral detergent fiber has no negative effect on rumen ecosystem and can be used as high energy feed in ration that supports growth as well as lactation in ruminants.

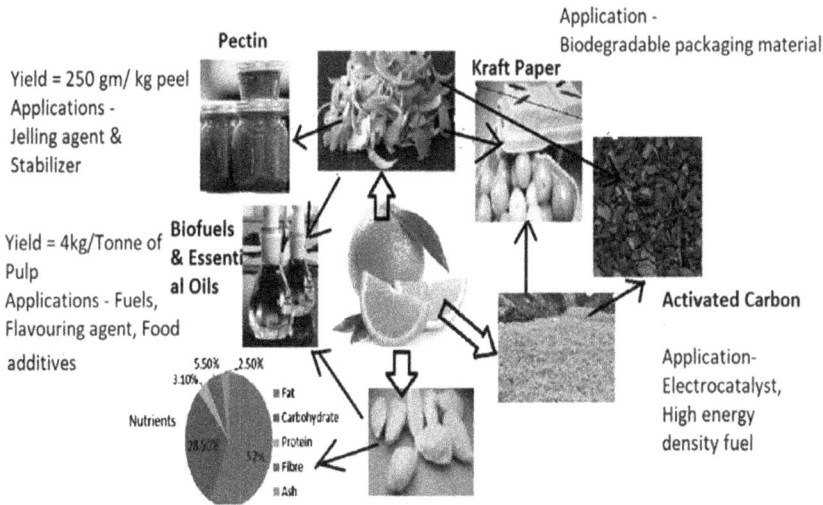

FIGURE 7.2 By-product of citrus industry and their utilization.

7.7.2 ESSENTIAL OIL EXTRACTION

Extraction of fundamental oil from the citrus buildup is prevalent field of research among numerous researchers nowadays (Fig. 7.3). Economy of the extraction of fundamental oil can be legitimized by its high incentive in more extensive pharmaceutical industry, as enhancing specialist in nourishment and drink industry and cleaning items (Anagnostopoulou et al., 2006). Bizzo (2009) has reported that a maximum of 4.0 g essential oil can be extracted per 100 kg of citrus waste. The primary constituent of this oil is a blend of unstable mixes like terpenes and oxygenated subsidiaries, for example, aldehydes (citral), alcohols, and esters. Endeavors were additionally made toward mixing lemon basic oils acquired by steam refining process with diesel oil in the proportion of 20, 80 (Nanthagopal et al., 2017). These essential oils are made up of compounds like D-limonene, α-terpinolene, α-pinene, citronellol, β-citronellol, etc. (Sahraoui et al., 2011). These oils have wider applications in food and pharmaceutical industry as a flavoring agent in beverages and other food additives and also have been used for preparation of perfumes, soaps, and other cosmetic products (Raeissi et al., 2008). The terpenes, which form a major part of citrus essential oil, have a strong antifungal activity.

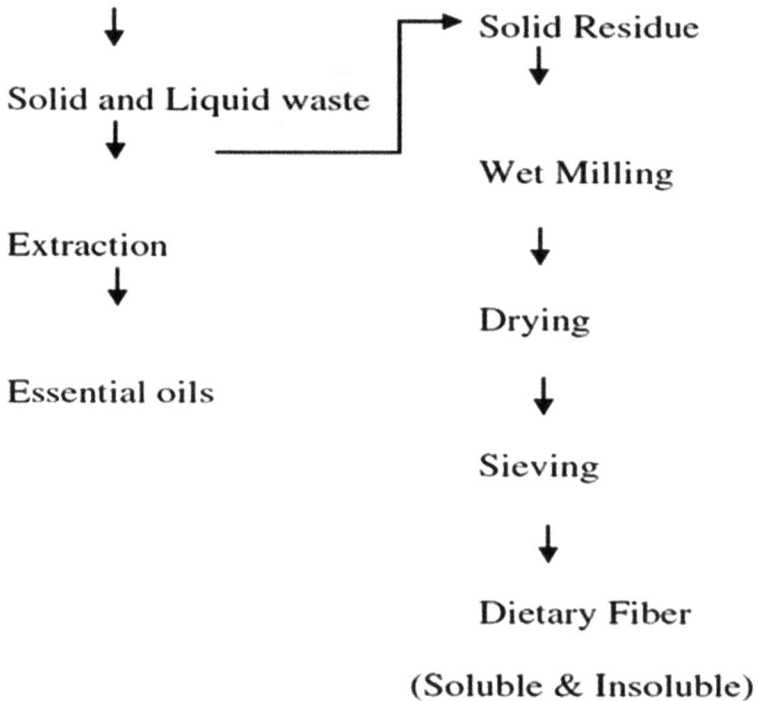

FIGURE 7.3 Flowchart for extraction of essential oils.

- Different extraction methods are used for essential oil production:
- Steam distillation method
- Ultrasound extraction

- Supercritical fluid extraction
- Subcritical water
- Microwave-assisted extraction
- Microwave-assisted hydrodistillation (MAHD) technique

7.7.3 PECTIN PRODUCTION

Citrus peel is a great source of pectin, which is soluble fiber and used in food industry as gelling agent particularly jam and jelly, medicines, sweets, and as stabilizer in fruit juices (Sulieman et al., 2013). About 25 g pectin yield is obtained from 100 g of citrus peel. Detailed process for extraction of pectin from the waste is described in Figure 7.4. Exceptionally, high measure of flavonoids present in citrus strip just as incredibly harsh compound naringin present in albedo grants harshness to the strip, which should be evacuated before gelatin extraction (Puril et al., 2008).

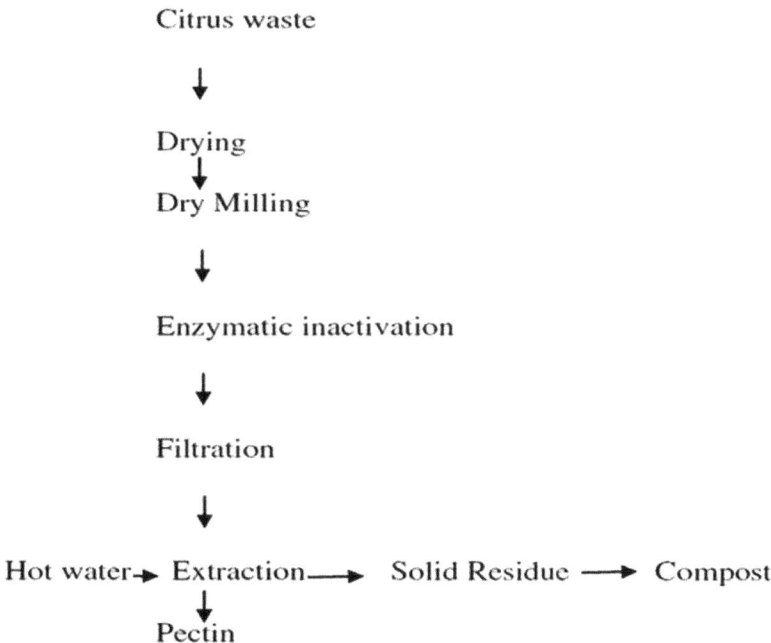

Citrus waste
↓
Drying
↓
Dry Milling
↓
Enzymatic inactivation
↓
Filtration
↓
Hot water→ Extraction──→ Solid Residue ──→ Compost
↓
Pectin

FIGURE 7.4 Flowchart for the extraction of pectin.

Pectin extraction techniques are as follows:

- Supercritical water extraction
- Enzymatic extraction
- Microwave extraction
- Ultrahigh pressure
- Ultrasound extraction
- High-intensity pulsed electric field
- Moderate electric field
- Attempted extraction of pectin using
- Electromagnetic
- Ohmic heating technique

7.7.4   PRODUCTION OF BIO-FUEL

Since the yearly citrus squander creation all-inclusive is 119.7 million t, there is an incredible potential for generation of bio-oil through thermochemical and biosynthetic procedures. Biochemical generations of fermentable sugars by hydrolysate of citrus strip and methane creation utilizing bioconversion strategies are the elective ways for the usage of the citrus squander. Different polymers of solvent and insoluble starches present in Citrus citrus fruits are exceptionally perfect material for transformation of waste into bioenergizes, for example, ethanol and biogas (Wikandari et al., 2015). Because of the quality of cellulose, hemicellulose, and lignin in the citrus squander that are significant vitality source in biomass, citrus squander is considered as a great hotspot for generation of biomass. Physico-warm procedure includes pulverizing, warming, and compelling, and biochemical procedure utilizes catalysts and microorganisms. Gasification process is used for the production of biofuels such as gasoline and electricity, whereas pyrolysis process produces bio-oils, chemicals, and charcoals (Alisaraei et al., 2017). Biochar produced from the process can be used as a fertilizer and other applications include decontamination of water bodies and soil affected by metals.

7.7.5   FOOD GRADE KRAFT PAPER

There is global demand for use of renewable sources instead of synthetic material for the food coating and food packaging. On the other hand, however, paper and paperboard materials are biodegradable and possess high mechanical strength, and they are not suitable for packaging of high moisture food due to their porous nature that makes it permeable to moisture and some gases. Increased accumulation of plastic waste yielded the attention for the development of moisture barrier biodegradable material. The combination of wax and lipid–hydroxypropyl methylcellulose-based composite films significantly reduces the water permeability of the composite film (Sothornvit, 2009). Research was conducted by Kasaai and Moosavi (2017) for the incorporation of citrus peel and leaf hydrophobic extracts (terpene hydrocarbons and limonene) into the paper and paperboard to enhance the water barrier properties without losing mechanical strength. The dissolvable was then completely vanished at 25°C utilizing a mechanical shaker (60 rpm, 24 h) and the paper was dried. The segments of the concentrates in the arrangement were mostly presented in the free volume and were put among cellulose strands of the papers. Another part of the concentrates framed a flimsy layer on the paper surface.

7.7.6 PREPARATION OF CITRUS PEEL PACKAGING FILMS

With the developing worry about nondegradable properties of oil-based polyester and their unfriendly impact on nature, advancement of biodegradable plastic has picked up prevalence among specialists. In such manner, analysts from the New York-based Cornell College have created plastic produced using citrus strip. The orange strip oil was oxidized to get limonene oxide, which can be utilized as building square. Limonene oxide structure, the citrus strip, was joined with another structure square carbon dioxide (which is turning out to be earth hurtful ozone harming substance generally) to make a novel polymer. Arrieta et al. (2013) who created nourishment bundling film having greater adaptability by researchers guarantee that created polymer is not just of comparative trademark to that of polystyrene yet, in addition, biodegradable and securing the carbon dioxide in the air.

7.7.7 ENCAPSULATING AGENT

Unsaturated securities in the subatomic structure of the polyphenols are helpless against light, warmth, and oxidants. Also, inferable from the low water and fluid dissolvability, the use of phenolic extricates in the nourishment is troublesome (Spigno et al., 2013). Along these lines, so as to expand the steadiness during capacity, improvement of their shading, and appropriateness for use as an added substance, phenolic mixes are exemplified for the most part with shower drying as the most basic strategy (Kaderides et al., 2015). The divider material chose for the exemplification ought to of properties, for example, low thickness even at exceptionally focused arrangement, successful emulsification, productive drying properties, film framing attributes, and ease. Variable materials utilized as embodying operators incorporate emulsifying starches, gums, and hydrolyzed starches (maltodextrins, corn syrup solids). It was accounted for that dissolvable fiber diminishes blood cholesterol and is related to intestinal retention of glucose, while insoluble fiber adds to appropriate working of the intestinal tract (Fang and Bhandari, 2010). The prescribed utilization of dietary strands is 30–45 g/day. Higher nearness of insoluble fiber can be utilized as perfect was material to seal the dynamic material inside its structure during embodiment.

### 7.7.8	DEVELOPMENT OF ACTIVATED CARBON

Polymer electrolyte membrane fuel cell is considered as next-generation potential power due to its characteristics like high energy density and low emission (Avgouropoulos et al., 2016). For electrocatalyst support, it is noted that carbon is more advantageous than metal oxide due to its more specific surface area, higher stability in acidic and basic medium, and easy recovery of metal catalyst by burning off carbon support. Numerous specialists have created high surface region initiated carbon from rural waste, for example, groundnut shell, coconut shell, mango nut, and banana fiber. In such manner, exertion was made by Dhelipan et al. (2017) to synthesize activated carbon from orange peel by chemical activation using orthophosphoric acid (H_3PO_4) using pyrolysis method at 600°C, and its stability as electrolyte support was examined. The procedure for development of activated carbon from citrus waste is described in Figure 7.5. Because of their good electrochemical stability and electrochemical properties, activated carbon can be used in commercial supercapacitor as an electrode material. As fossil fuels are nonrenewable, biowaste as precursor for production of activated carbon can meet the increasing demand for activated carbons.

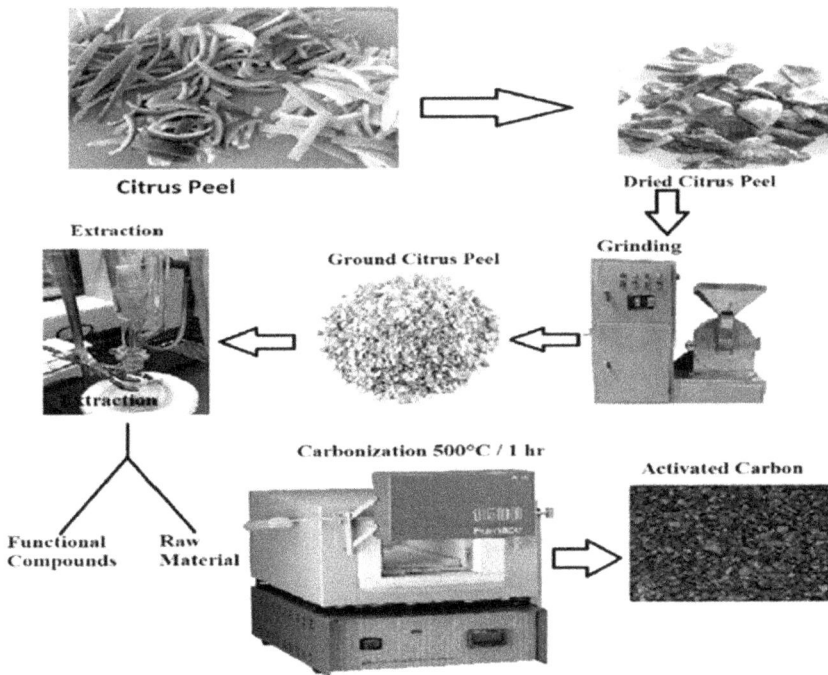

FIGURE 7.5   Orange peels based activated carbon.

7.7.9   UTILIZATION OF CITRUS SEED

Citrus seeds are commonly considered pointless and are arranged as a waste. The normal seed contained in dried citrus mash is 4.8%. As high in protein, these disposed seeds can be used monetarily as protein supplement for animals. Additionally, citrus seeds have roughly 30% oil (by weight) and have incredible potential in use as biodiesel. Proximate investigation of flour arranged from unhulled and dehulled citrus seeds contains fat 52%, starches 28.5%, rough fiber 5.5%, unrefined protein 3.1%, and debris 2.5% (dry premise). Rashid et al. (2013) have created citrus seed–based biodiesel oil by sodium methoxide–catalyzed transesterification with methanol and announced that delivered methyl esters fulfilled both ASTM D6751 and EN 14214 biodiesel benchmarks

7.8 BIOACTIVE COMPOUNDS FROM CITRUS FRUITS WASTE

Citrus natural product squanders are rich wellsprings of phytochemicals and have been read for the extraction of phenolic mixes, dietary filaments, and other bioactive mixes (Galanakis, 2012). In many foods grown from the ground, just the substance or mash is expended; however, ponders have uncovered that critical measures of phytochemicals and basic supplements are available in the seeds, strips, and different segments of natural products not regularly devoured (Rudra et al., 2015). For instance, the strips of lemons, grapes, and oranges and the seeds of avocados, jackfruits, longans, and mangoes contain over 15% higher phenolic fixations than that found in the natural product mash. All in all, squanders ought to be prepared utilizing warm (warming, microwave, radiofrequency, infrared warming, and disinfection) or nonthermal (high hydrostatic weight, ultrasound, beat electric fields [PEFs], illumination, and beat light) advancements, which may influence phytochemicals.

TABLE 7.2 Nature of Potential Fruits and Vegetable Losses and Waste.

Sr. No.	Commodity	Nature of waste	Typical losses and waste (%)
1.	Apple	Pomace, peel and seeds	-
2.	Banana	Peel	35
3.	Citrus	Rag, peel and seeds	50
4.	Dragon Fruit	Rind and seeds	30 to 45
5.	Durian	Skin and seeds	60 to 70
6.	Grapes	Skin, stem and seeds	20
7.	Guava	Peel, core and seeds	10
8.	Jackfruit	Rind and seeds	50 to 70
9.	Mango	Peel and stone	45
10.	Mangosteen	Skin and seeds	60 to 75
11.	Onion	Outer leaves	-
12.	Papaya	Rind and seeds	10 to 20
13.	Passion fruit	Skin and seeds	45 to 50
14.	Pea	Shell	40
15.	Pineapple	Core and skin	33
16.	Potato	Peel	15
17.	Rambutan	Skin and seeds	50 to 65
18.	Tomato	Core, skin and seeds	20

7.8.1 DIETARY FIBER

Dietary fiber concentrations in fruit waste. Grape pomace was found to be a rich source of dietary fibers, namely, hemicelluloses, cellulose, and small proportions of pectins. Mango by-products have been shown to possess high amounts of dietary fibers. Ajila and Prasada Rao (2013) analyzed dietary fiber of mango peels and found that the TDF content was in the range of 40.6–72.5%, with galactose, glucose, and arabinose being the major neutral sugars in insoluble and soluble dietary fibers. "Tommy Atkins" mango had 28.05% dietary fibers, including 13.80% insoluble and 14.25% soluble fibers. The kernel has 2% crude fiber. The peel of oranges contains 57% DW TDFs, of which 9.41% DW was the soluble fraction and 47.6% DW the insoluble fraction, and the main components of the fibers were characterized as cellulose and pectin polysaccharides. It has been reported that soluble fraction ranging between 34.5 and 35.8% of the TDF in the peel and pulp, respectively, is optimal for human consumption (Russo et al., 2014). The TDF concentrations in the waste of different fruits and vegetables are summarized in Table 7.3.

7.8.2 PHENOLIC COMPOUNDS

Citrus waste is a rich wellspring of phenolic mixes on the grounds that citrus strip contains a higher amount of polyphenols in correlation with the consumable piece of the organic product. Aside from citrus, the strips of different natural products have additionally been found to contain higher convergences of phenolics in contrasted and the consumable segments. Phenolic mixes are the plant optional metabolites capable of tangible attributes and add to the dietary nature of foods grown from the ground, among different capacities. Phenolic mixes are among the biggest classes of bioactive mixes with assorted and significant natural capacities (Ignat et al., 2011). Polyphenolic mixes are characterized into different classes, for example, flavonoids (subclasses, flavonols, flavanones, flavones, flava-nonols, isoflavones, flavanols, and anthocyanidins), tannins, stilbenes, phenolic acids, and lignans, among different classes. The skin, strip, and seeds of products of the soil have high measures of phenolic compounds. The citrus industry produces significant measures of seeds and strip deposits, which comprise about half of the complete natural product. Extraction of phenolic mixes relies upon the method utilized, and in this way, it is conceivable to expand their extraction from kinnow (Citrus reticulate L.) strip squander by multiple times utilizing the ultrasound-helped extraction than the maceration procedure (Safdar et al., 2016).

TABLE 7.3   Total (TDF), Insoluble (IDF), and Soluble (SDF) Dietary Fiber Contents in the Waste of Different Fruits and Vegetables.

Sr. No.	Commodity	Type of waste	TDF (%)	IDF (%)	SDF (%)
1.	Apple	Peel	0.91	0.46	0.43
2.	Apple	Pomace	88.5	69.9	18.6
3.	Apricot	Seeds	27 to 35	-	-
4.	Banana	Peel	50	-	-
5.	Carrot	Pomace	63.6	50.1	13.5
6.	Cauliflower	Stem	3.11	-	-
7.	Cranberry	Seeds	51.06	45.93	5.13
8.	Dates	Seeds	57.87 to 92.4	-	-
9.	Garlic	Husk	62.23	58.07	4.16
10.	Grapes	Seeds	40	-	-
11.	Grapes	Pomace	77.9	68.4	9.5
12.	Grapes	Pomace	77.2	73.5	3.77
13.	Green chili	Peel and Seeds	80.41	-	-
14.	Kiwifruit	Pomace	25.80	18.70	7.10
15.	Lemon	Peel	14	9.04	4.93
16.	Mango	Peel	51.2	32	19
17.	Onion	Skin	68.3	-	-
18.	Orange	Peel	57	47.6	9.41
19.	Pea	Peel	91.5	87.4	4.1
20.	Peach	Pomace	54.5	35.5	19.1
21.	Pear	Pomace	43.9	36.3	7.6
22.	Potato	Peel	5.6	-	-
23.	Pumpkin	Pomace	76.94	-	-
24.	Raspberry	Pomace	77.5	75	2.5
25.	Tomato	Pomace	50	25	25

7.8.3   FLAVORING AGENTS AND AROMAS

The waste materials of natural products are a significant wellspring of different bioproducts that can fill in as a wellspring of flavors and fragrances.

Strong state aging (SSF) is a change system by which numerous potential items have been disengaged from FW, including flavors, ethanol, catalysts, methane, citrus extract, lactic corrosive, and different nourishment fixings. The market for smells, aromas, and flavors has expanded on account of expanded customer interest for regular, natural, and safe sources. Vanillin (4-hydroxy-3-methoxybenzaldehyde) is delivered from vanillic corrosive. Vanillin is the primary segment of vanilla flavor, which is the most significant and exceptionally utilized flavor in the nourishment, corrective, pharmaceutical, and cleanser enterprises (Tilay et al., 2008). The extraction of normal vanillin is accomplished from the aged cases of vanilla orchids (*Vanilla planifolia*). Pineapple strip squander contains ferulic corrosive, an antecedent for vanillic corrosive. An expansion sought after for normal flavors has activated research on characteristic vanillin generation from common crude materials through microbial biotransformation. Vanillin union from pineapple squander is a 3-advance procedure (Lun et al., 2014). Aside from vanillin, different fragrances are likewise gotten from plant side effects. At the business level, rhamnose is gotten through chemical hydrolysis from rutin or citrus organic products. The pineapple season segment "ethyl butyrate" is delivered with the assistance of a microorganism, *Ceratocystis fimbriata*, from apple pomace. Unpredictable mixes from pineapple preparing deposits (skin and strands abandoned after the juice extraction step) were extricated and 35 unstable mixes were distinguished. This property shows that they have potential for the creation of fragrant common characters, which could later be added to items, for example, pineapple juice condensed to improve its tactile quality (Dorta and Sogi, 2017).

7.8.4 ENZYMES

7.8.4.1 AMYLASES

This gathering is made out of three chemicals, to be specific α-amylase, β-amylase, and glucoamylase. Many organic product buildups are utilized as substrate for the creation of amylases. A few models incorporate citrus squander (Mahmoud, 2015), cassava squander (Selvama et al., 2016), and mango bits (Kumar et al., 2013). In addition, orange waste powder is used to deliver α-amylase with the assistance of *Aspergillus niger*. Amylases are created by an assortment of microorganisms, for example,

A. niger, Aspergillus awamori, Aspergillus oryzae, Aspergillus tamarii, Bacillus subtilis, Bacillus licheniformis, Rhizopus oryzae, Candida guilliermondii, and *Thermomyces lanuginosus.* Among these, *A. niger, B. subtilis,* and *R. oryzae* are the most applied species in the business (Said et al., 2014). Amylases are generally utilized in the nourishment handling enterprises for different items, natural product juices, starch syrup, sodden cakes, chocolate cakes, etc., and various procedures, for example, fermenting, and readiness of stomach-related guides, and preparing.

7.8.4.2 CELLULASES

Cellulases comprise exo-1,4-β-glucanase, endo-1,4-β-D-glucanase, and β-D-glucosidase. They are utilized in the nourishment businesses, in the freedom of fragrance rich mixes, just as in the extraction of phenolic mixes from grape pomaces. Kinnow squander was additionally used to create endo-1,4-β-glucanase (CMCase) with the assistance of *Trichoderma reesei* and wheat grain in the proportion of 3,2 and 4,1, individually (Oberoi et al., 2010).

7.8.4.3 INVERTASE

Invertase is utilized to create transform sugar. Invertase has a low crystallinity level contrasted with sucrose, and in this manner, it keeps the item delicate and new for a more extended time frame (Kumar and Kesavapillai, 2012). Uma et al. (2010) advanced the conditions for the generation of invertase by *Aspergillus flavus.* A more significant level of invertase creation was accounted for under advanced conditions utilizing natural product strip squander as the substrate. In like manner, *A. niger* was blended in with different carbon sources, for example, fructose, organic product strip, lactose, and sucrose to create invertase. Among them, fructose was seen as the best carbon hotspot for the generation of extracellular invertase. Invertase is explicitly used to create confections, jam, and confectionary and pharmaceutical items (Panda et al., 2016).

7.8.4.4 PECTINASES

Pectinases corrupt pectic mixes, in which significant foods are grown from the ground auxiliary parts in cell dividers. Pectate and gelatin lyases can sort the long carbon chain by breaking its glycosidic bonds, while gelatin esterase takes a shot at methoxyl gatherings. The creation of pectinase is finished by solid-state aging procedure from grape pomace utilizing *A. awamori* yeast. Mrudula and Anitharaj (2011) utilized six distinct substrates (lemon strip, orange strip, banana strip, wheat grain, rice wheat, and sugarcane bagasse) for pectinase creation utilizing *A. niger* in solid-state aging. Orange strip indicated the best outcome among all substrates for the creation of pectinase (1224 U/g DMS). Gelatin proteins have different significant applications in the nourishment businesses (organic product squeezes and wines) for extraction, explanation, and fixation. Additionally, the extraction of flavors, shades, and basic oils is accomplished utilizing these chemicals from plant deposits.

7.9   CONCLUSION

Over the top transfer of citrus preparing modern waste into landfill is dangerous to human well-being over the world, and logical valorization of these natural buildups is an appealing idea that has picked up notoriety among specialists. Citrus squander produced from juice preparing plant, that is, strip, mash, and seeds can be reused as crude material in different ventures. Leftover strong buildup can be utilized for extraction of fundamental oils, while fluid can be utilized for creation of proteins. Extraction of hydrophobic material from strip can be utilized for nourishment grade kraft paper, biodegradable polymers, and bundling material from the strip additionally held in decreased utilization of oil-based polyesters. Usage of citrus buildup decreases the ecological contamination just as produces elective fuel as far as bio-oil, biogas, ethanol, and initiated carbons. Expanded extent of item advancement builds the general comes back to producer, business age, and manageable financial improvement and keeps up ecological steadiness. The result of the exploration is beneficial for the future age, contributing toward world's most noteworthy need to focus on supportable improvement.

KEYWORDS

- **citrus fruits**
- **medicinal value**
- **antioxidants**
- **flavonoids**
- **by-products**

REFERENCES

Ajila, C. M.; Aalami, M.; Leelavathi, K.; Rao, U. J. S. P. Mango Peel Powder, A Potential Source of Antioxidant and Dietary Fibre in Macaroni Preparations. *Innov. Food Sci. Emerg.* **2010,** *11* (1), 219–224.

An, S.; Park, H. S.; Kim, G. H. Evaluation of the Antioxidant Activity of Cooked Gomchwi (*Ligularia fischeri*) Using the Myoglobin Methods. *Prevent. Nutr. Food Sci.* **2014,** *19* (1), 34.

Avgouropoulos, G.; Avgouropoulos, G.; Schlicker, S.; Schelihaas, K. P.; Papavasiliou, J.; Papadimitriou, K. D.; Neophytides, S. Performance Evaluation of a Proof-of-Concept 70 W Internal Reforming Methanol Fuel Cell System. *J. Power Sourc.* **2016,** *307,* 875–882.

Alisaraei, A. T.; Hosseini, S. H.; Ghobadian, B.; Motevali, A. Biofuel Production from Citrus Wastes, A Feasibility Study in Iran. *Renew. Sustain. Energy Rev.* **2017,** *69,* 1100–1112.

Arrieta, M. P.; López, J.; Hernández, A.; Rayón, E. Ternary PLA-PHB-Limonene Blends Intended for Biodegradable Food Packaging Applications. *Eur. Polym. J.* **2013,** *49,* 3630–3641.

Ajila, C. M.; Prasada Rao, U. J. S. Mango Peel Dietary Fibre, Composition and Associated Bound Phenolics. *J. Funct. Foods* **2013,** *5,* 444–450.

AL-Juhaimi, F.; Ghafoor, K. Bioactive Compounds, Antioxidant and Physico-Chemical Properties of Juice from Lemon, Mandarin and Orange Fruits Cultivated in Saudi Arabia. *Pak. J. Bot.* **2013,** *45* (4), 1193–1196.

Astell, K. J.; Mathai, M. L.; Su, X. Q. A Review on Botanical Species and Chemical Compounds with Appetite Suppressing Properties for Body Weight Control. *Plant Foods Hum. Nutr.* **2013,** *68,* 213–221.

Assis, C. R. C. L.; Hermsdorff, H. H. M.; Bressan, J. Anti-Inflammatory Properties of Orange Juice, Possible Favorable Molecular and Metabolic Effects. *Plant Foods Hum. Nutr.* **2013,** 68, 1–10.

Alvarez-Gonzales, I.; Madrigal-Bujaidar, E.; Sanchez-Garcia, V. Y. Inhibitory Effect of Grapefruit Juice on the Genotoxic Damage Induced by Ifosfamide in Mouse. *Plant Foods Hum. Nutr.* **2010,** *65,* 369–373.

Arvanitoyannis, I. S., Varzakas, T. H. Vegetable Waste Treatment, Comparison and Critical Presentation of Methodologies. *Crit. Rev. Food Sci.* **2008,** *48* (3), 205–247.

Amitava, D.; Kimberly, K. Chapter 15—Antioxidant Vitamins and Minerals. In *Antioxidants in Food, Vitamins and Supplements,* 2014, pp. 277–294.

Arancon, R. A. D.; Lin, C. S. K. L.; Chan, K. M.; Kwan, T. H.; Luque, R. Advances on Waste Valorization, New Horizons for a More Sustainable Society. *Energy Sci. Eng.* **2013,** *1* (2), 53–71.

Anagnostopoulou, M. A.; Kefalas, P.; Papageorgiou, V. P.; Assimopoulou, A. N.; Boskou, D. Radical Scavenging Activity of Various Extracts and Fractions of Sweet Orange Peel (*Citrus sinensis*). *Food Chem.* **2006,** *94,* 19–25.

Bizzo, H. R. Óleos essenciais no Brasil, aspectos gerais, desenvolvimento e-perspectivas. *Quimica Nova* **2009,** *32* (3), 588–594.

Çelik, S. E.; Özyürek, M.; Güçlü, K.; Apak, R. Determination of Antioxidants by a Novel On-Line HPLC-Cupric Reducing Antioxidant Capacity (CUPRAC) Assay with Post-Column Detection. *Anal. Chim. Acta* **2010,** *674* (1), 79–88.

Chaudhary, P. R.; Jayaprakasha, G. K.; Porat, R.; Patil, B. S. Low Temperature Conditioning Reduces Chilling Injury While Maintaining Quality and Certain Bioactive Compounds of 'Star Ruby' Grapefruit. *Food Chem.* **2014,** *153,* 243–249.

Da Silva, D.; Nogueira, G.; Duzzioni, A.; Barrozo, M. Changes of Antioxidant Constituents in Pineale (*Ananas comosus*) Residue During Drying Process. *Ind. Crop Prod.* **2013,** *50,* 557–562.

Dai, J.; Mumper, R. J. Plant Phenolics, Extraction, Analysis and Their Antioxidant and Anticancer Properties. *Molecules* **2010,** *15* (10), 7313–7352.

Dhelipan, M.; Arunchander, A.; Sahu, A. K.; Kalpana, D. Activated Carbon From Orange Peels as Supercapacitor Electrode and Catalyst Support for Oxygen Reduction Reaction in Proton Exchange Membrane Fuel Cell. *J. Saudi Chem. Soc.* **2017,** *21,* 487–494.

Dorta, E.; Sogi, D. S. Value Added Processing and Utilization of Pineale By-Products. In *Handbook of Pineale Technology, Production, Postharvest Science, Processing and Nutrition.* John Wiley and Sons: Oxford, **2017,** pp. 196–220.

Elleuch, M.; Bedigian, D.; Roiseux, O.; Besbes, S.; Blecker, C.; Attia, H. Dietary Fibre and Fibre Rich By-Products of Food Processing, Characterisation, Technological Functionality and Commercial Applications, A Review. *Food Chem.* **2011,** *4,* 411–421.

Fejzić, A.; Ćavar, S. Phenolic Compounds and Antioxidant Activity of Some Citruses. *Bull. Chem. Technol. Soc. Bosnia Herzegovina* **2014,** *42,* 1–4.

FAO. Statistics Data, **2017.**

Fava, F.; Zanaroli, G.; Vannini, L.; Guerzoni, E.; Bordoni, A.; Viaggi, D.; Robertson, J.; Waldron, K.; Bald, C.; Esturo, A.; Talens, C.; Tueros, I.; Cebrián, M.; Sebők, A.; Kuti, T.; Broeze, J.; Macias, M.; Brendle, H. G. New Advances in the Integrated Management of Food Processing By-Products in Europe, Sustainable Exploitation of Fruit and Cereal Processing By-Products with the Production of New Food Products (NAMASTE EU). *New Biotechnol.* **2013,** *30,* 647–655.

Fang, Z.; Bhandari, B. Encapsulation of Polyphenols, A Review. *Trends Food Sci. Technol.* **2010,** *21,* 510–523.

Galanakis, C. M. Recovery of High Added-Value Components from Food Wastes, Conventional, Emerging Technologies and Commercialized Applications. *Trends Food Sci. Technol.* **2012,** *26,* 68–87.

Helkar, P. B.; Sahoo, A. K.; Patil, N. J. Review, Food Industry By-Products used as a Functional Food Ingredients. *Int. J. Waste Resour.* **2016,** *6,* 248.

Hernandez-Carranze, P.; Ávila-Sosa, R.; Guerrero-Beltran, J. A.; Navarro-Cruz, A. R.; Corona-Jimenezi, E.; Ochoa-Velasco, C. E. Optimization of Antioxidant Compounds Extraction From Fruit By-Products, Ale Pomace, Orange and Banana Peel. *J. Food Proc. Preserv.*, **2016**, *40*, 103–115.

He, W. H.; Liu, X.; Xu, H. G.; Gong, Y.; Yuan, F.; Gao, Y. X. On-Line HPLC-ABTS Screening and HPLC-DAD-MS/MS Identification of Free Radical Scavengers in Gardenia (*Gardenia jasminoides* Ellis) Fruit Extracts. *Food Chem.* **2010**, *123* (2), 521–528.

Ignat, I.; Volf, I.; Popa, V. I. A Critical Review of Methods for Characterisation of Polyphenolic Compounds in Fruits and Vegetables. *Food Chem.* **2011**, *126*, 1821–1835.

Jung, U. J.; Lee, M. K.; Park, Y. B.; Kang, M. A.; Choi, M. S. Effect of Citrus Flavonoids on Lipid Metabolism and Glucose-Regulating Enzyme mRNA Levels in Type-2 Diabetic Mice. *Int. J. Biochem. Cell Biol.* **2006**, *38* (7), 1134–1145.

Kumar, R.; Kesavapillai, B. Stimulation of Extracellular Invertase Production from Spent Yeast When Sugarcane Pressmud Used as Substrate Through Solid State Fermentation. *Springer Plus*, **2012**, *1*, 81.

Koriem, K. M.; Arbid, M. S.; Emam, K. R. Therapeutic Effect of Pectin on Octylphenol Induced Kidney Dysfunction, Oxidative Stress and Apoptosis in Rats. *Environ. Toxicol. Pharmacol.* **2014**, *38* (1), 14–23.

Kumar, D.; Lamers, H.; Singh, I. P.; Ladaniya, M. S.; Sthapitm B. Phytochemical Evaluation of Pummelo Fruits (*Citrus grandis*) in India for Enhancing Marketing Opportunities. *Indian J. Plant. Genet. Resour.*, **2015**, *28* (1), 50–54.

Kumar, D.; Yadav, K. K.; Muthukumar, M.; Garg, N. Production and Characterization of [α]-Amylase from Mango Kernel by *Fusarium solani* NAIMCC-F-02956 using Submerged Fermentation. *J. Environ. Biol.* **2013**, *34*, 1053–1058.

Kasaai, M. R.; Moosavi, A. Treatment of Kraft Paper with Citrus Wastes for Food Packaging Applications, Water and Oxygen Barrier Properties Improvement. *Food Packaging Shelf Life*, **2017**, *12*, 59–65.

Kaderides, K.; Goula, A. M.; Adamopoulos, K G. A Process for Turning Pomegranate Peels into a Valuable Food Ingredient Using Ultrasound-Assisted Extraction and Encapsulation. *Innov. Food Sci. Emerg. Technol.* **2015**, *31*, 204–215.

Lun, O. K.; Wai, T. B.; Ling, L. S. Pineale Cannery Waste as a Potential Substrate for Microbial Biotranformation to Produce Vanillic Acid and Vanillin. *Int. Food Res. J.* **2014**, *21*, 953–958.

Mahmoud, K. Statistical Optimization of Cultural Conditions of an Halophilic Alpha-Amylase Production by Halophilic *Streptomyces* sp. Grown on Orange Waste Powder. *Biocatal. Agric. Biotechnol.* **2015**, *4*, 685–693.

Magiorkinis, E.; Beloukas, A.; Diamantis, A. Scurvy, Past, Present and Future. *Eur. J. Int. Med.* **2011**, *22*, 147–152.

Makris, D. P.; Boskou, G.; Andrikopoulos, N. K. Polyphenolic Content and In Vitro Antioxidant Characteristics of Wine Industry and Other Agri-Food Solid Waste Extracts. *J. Food Compos. Anal.* **2007**, *20*, 125–132.

Moretti, C. L.; Mattos, L. M.; Calbo, A. G.; Sargent, S. A. Climate Changes and Potential Impacts on Postharvest Quality of Fruit and Vegetable Crops, A Review. *Food Res. Int.* **2010**, *43* (7), 1824–1832.

Mandalari, G.; Bennett, R. N.; Bisignano, G.; Trombetta, D.; Saija, A.; Faulds, C. B.; Gasson, M. J.; Narbad, A. Antimicrobial Activity of Flavonoids Extracted From

Bergamot (*Citrus bergamia* Risso) Peel, a Byproduct of the Essential Oil Industry. *J. Appl. Microbiol.* **2007,** *103* (6), 2056–2064.

Mamma, D.; Kourtoglou, E.; Christakopoulos, P. Fungal Multienzyme Production on Industrial By-Products of the Citrus-Processing Industry. *Bioresour. Technol.* **2008,** *99*, 2373–2383.

Martín, M. A.; Siles, J. A.; Chica, A. F.; Martín, A. Biomethanization of Orange Peel Waste. *Bioresour. Technol.* **2010,** *101*, 8993–8999.

Mrudula, S.; Anitharaj, R. Pectinase Production in Solid State Fermentation by *Aspergillus niger* using Orange Peel as Substrate. *Glob. J. Biotechnol. Biochem.* **2011,** *6*, 64–71.

Noor, N.; Sarfraz, R. A.; Ali, S.; Shahid, M. Antitumour and Antioxidant Potential of Some Selected Pakistani Honeys. *Food Chem.* **2014,** *143*, 362–366.

Nakao, K.; Murata, K.; Itoh, K.; Hanamoto, Y.; Masuda, M.; Moriyama, K. Anti-hyperuricemia Effects of Extracts of Immature Citrus Unshiu Fruit. *J. Tradit. Med.* **2011,** *28* (1), 10–15.

Nanthagopal, K.; Ashok, B.; RKR, T.; Jathar, S.; Samuel, J. K.; Krishnan, R.; Logesh, S. Lemon Essential Oil – A Partial Substitute for Petroleum Diesel Fuel in Compression Ignition Engine. *Int. J. Renew. Energy Res.* **2017,** *7* (2), 467–475.

Netzel, M.; Netzel, G.; Tian, Q.; Schwartz, S.; Konczak, I. Native Australian Fruits—A Novel Source of Antioxidants for Food. *Innov. Food Sci. Emerg. Technol.* **2007,** *8* (3), 339–346.

Özyürek, M.; Güngör, N.; Baki, S.; Güçlü, K.; Apak, R. Development of a Silver Nanoparticle-Based Method for the Antioxidant Capacity Measurement of Polyphenols. *Analyt. Chem.* **2012,** *84* (18), 8052–8059.

Oberoi, H. S.; Chavan, Y.; Bansal, S.; Dhillon, G. S. Production of Cellulases Through Solid State Fermentation using Kinnow Pulp as a Major Substrate. *Food Biol. Technol.* **2010,** *3*, 528–536.

Prior, R. L.; Wu, X. Diet Antioxidant Capacity, Relationships to Oxidative Stress and Health. *Am. J. Biomed. Sci.* **2013,** *5*, 126–139.

Pantelidis, G. E.; Vasilakakis, M.; Manganaris, G. A.; Diamantidis, G. Antioxidant Capacity, Phenol, Anthocyanin and Ascorbic Acid Contents in Raspberries, Blackberries, Red Currants, Gooseberries and Cornelian Cherries. *Food Chem.* **2007,** *102* (3), 777–783.

Park, H. Y.; Kim, G. Y.; Choi, Y. H. Naringenin Attenuates the Release of Pro-Inflammatory Mediators from Lipopolysaccharide-Stimulated BV2 Microglia by Inactivating Nuclear Factor-κB and Inhibiting Mitogen-Activated Protein Kinases. *Int. J. Mol. Med.* **2012,** *30* (1), 204–210.

Puril, M.; Kauri, A.; Singhl, R. S.; Kanwa, J. R. Immobilized Enzyme Technology for Debittering Citrus Fruit Juices. In *Food Enzymes, Application of New Technologies.* 2008, pp. 91–103.

Panda, S. K.; Mishra, S. S.; Kayitesi, E.; Ray, R. C. Microbial-Processing of Fruit and Vegetable Wastes for Production of Vital Enzymes and Organic Acids, Biotechnology and Scopes. *Environ. Res.* **2016,** *146*, 161–172.

Qura'n, S. Ethnobotanical and Ecological Studies of Wild Edible Plants in Jordan. *Libyan Agric. Res. Center J. Int.* **2010,** *1* (4), 231–243.

Rapisarda, P.; Bianco, M. L.; Pannuzzo, P.; Timpanaro, N. Effect of Cold Storage on Vitamin C, Phenolics and Antioxidant Activity of Five Orange Genotypes [*Citrus sinensis* (L.) Osbeck]. *Postharvest Biol. Technol.* **2008,** *49* (3), 348–354.

Rodríguez, R.; Jiménez, A.; Fernández-Bolaños, J.; Guillén, R.; Heredia, A. Dietary Fibre from Vegetable Products as Source of Functional Ingredients. *Trends Food Sci. Technol.* **2006,** *17* (1), 3–15.

Rezzadori, K.; Benedetti, S.; Amante, E. R. Proposals for the Residues Recovery, Orange Waste as Raw Material for New Products. *Food Bio-Prod. Process.* **2012,** 90, 606–614.

Raeissi, S.; Diaz, S.; Espinosa, S.; Peters, C. J.; Brignole, E. A. Ethane as an Alternative Solvent for Supercritical Extraction of Orange Peel Oils. *J. Supercri. Fluids* **2008,** *45,* 306–313.

Rekha, C.; Poornima, G.; Manasa, M.; Abhipsa, V.; Devi, P. J.; Kumar, V. H. T. Ascorbic Acid, Total Phenol Content and Antioxidant Activity of Fresh Juices of Four Ripe and Unripe Citrus Fruits. *Chem. Sci. Trans.* **2012,** *1* (2), 303–310.

Rashid U.; Ibrahimc, M.; Yasin, S.; Yunus, R.; Taufiq-Yap, Y. H.; Gerhard, K. Biodiesel from Citrus Reticulata (Mandarin Orange) Seed Oil, A Potential Non-Food Feedstock. *Ind. Crops Prod.* **2013,** *45,* 355–359.

Rudra, S. G.; Nishad, J.; Jakhar, N.; Kaur, C. Food Industry Waste, Mine of Nutraceuticals. *Int. J. Sci. Environ. Technol.* **2015,** *4,* 205–229.

Russo, M.; Bonaccorsi, I.; Torre, G.; Sar`o, M.; Dugo, P.; Mondello, L. Underestimated Sources of Flavonoids, Limonoids and Dietary Fibre, Availability in Lemon's By-Products. *J. Funct. Foods* **2014,** *9,* 18–26.

Selvama, K.; Selvankumarb, T.; Rajiniganthb, R.; Srinivasanb, P.; Sudhakarb, Ch.; Senthilkumara, B.; Govarthanan, M. Enhanced Production of Amylase from *Bacillus* sp. Using Groundnut Shell and Cassava Waste as a Substrate Under Process Optimization, Waste to Wealth Approach. *Biocatal. Agric. Biotechnol.* **2016,** *7,* 250–256.

Said A.; Leila, A.; Kaouther, D.; Sadia, B. Date Wastes as Substrate for the Production of α-Amylase and Invertase. *Iran J. Biotechnol.* **2014,** *12,* 41–49.

Scampicchio, M.; Wang, J.; Blasco, A. J.; Sanchez Arribas, A.; Mannino, S.; Escarpa, A. Nanoparticle-Based Assays of Antioxidant Activity. *Anal. Chem.* **2006,** *78* (6), 2060–2063.

Shen, W.; Xu, Y.; Lu, Y. H. Inhibitory effects of *Citrus* Flavonoids on Starch Digestion and Antihyperglycemic Effects in HepG2 Cells. *J. Agric. Food Chem.* **2012,** *60* (38), 9609–9619.

Sahraoui, N.; Vian, MA.; Maataoui, ME.; Boutekedjiret, C.; Chemat, F. Valorization of Citrus By-Products Using Microwave Steam Distillation (MSD). *Innov. Food Sci. Emerg. Technol.* **2011,** *12,* 163–170.

Sulieman, A. M. E.; Khodari, K. M. Y.; Salih, Z. A. Extraction of Pectin from Lemon and Orange Fruits Peels and Its Utilization in Jam Making. *Int. J. Food Sci. Nutr.* **2013,** 3(5), 81–84.

Sothornvit, R. Effect of hydroxypropyl Methyl Cellulose and Lipid on Mechanical Properties and Water Vapor Permeability of Coated Paper. *Food Res. Int.* **2009,** *42,* 307–311.

Spigno, G.; Donsi, F.; Amendola, D.; Sessa, M.; Ferrari, G.; Faveri, D. M. D. Nanoencapsulation Systems to Improve Solubility and Antioxidant Efficiency of a Grape Marc Extract into Hazelnut Paste. *J. Food Eng.* **2013,** *114,* 207–214.

Safdar, M. N.; Kausar, T.; Jabbar, S.; Mumtaz, A.; Ahad, K.; Saddozai, A. A. Extraction and Quantification of Polyphenols from Kinnow (*Citrus reticulate* L.) Peel Using Ultrasound and Maceration Techniques. *J. Food Drug Anal.* **2016,** *25* (3), 488–500.

Tilay, A.; Bule, M.; Kishenkumar, J.; Annapure, U. Preparation of Ferulic Acid from Agricultural Wastes, Its Improved Extraction and Purification. *J. Agric. Food Chem.* **2008,** *56,* 7644–7648.

Terashima, M.; Kakuno, Y.; Kitano, N.; Matsuoka, C.; Murase, M.; Togo, N. Antioxidant Activity of Flavonoids Evaluated with Myoglobin Method. *Plant Cell Rep.* **2012,** *31* (2), 291–298.

Tiwari, U.; Cummins, E. Factors Influencing Levels of Phytochemicals in Selected Fruit and Vegetables During Pre- and Post-Harvest Food Processing Operations. *Food Res. Int.* **2013,** *50* (2), 497–506.

Uma, C.; Gomathi, D.; Muthulakshmi, C.; Gopalakrishnan, V. K. Production, Purification and Characterization of Invertase by *Aspergillus flavus* Using Fruit Peel Waste as Substrate. *Adv. Biol. Res.* **2010,** *4,* 31–36.

Varzakas, T.; Zakynthinos, G.; Verpoort, F. Plant Food Residues as a Source of Nutraceuticals and Functional Foods. *Foods* **2016,** *5* (4), 88.

Vilari˜no, M. V.; Franco, C.; Quarrington, C. Food Loss and Waste Reduction as an Integral Part of a Circular Economy. *Front Environ. Sci.* **2017,** *5,* 1–5.

Wang, Y. C.; Chuang, Y. C.; Hsu, H. W. The Flavonoid, Carotenoid and Pectin Content in Peels of Citrus Cultivated in Taiwan. *Food Chem.* **2008,** *106* (1), 277–284.

Wadhwa, M.; Bakshi, M. P. S. *Utilization of Fruit and Vegetable Wastes as Livestock Feed and as Substrates for Generation of other Value-Added Products.* Rome, Italy: Food and Agriculture Organization, **2013.**

Wikandari, R.; Nguyen, H.; Millati, R.; Niklasson, C.; Taherzadeh, M. J. Improvement of Biogas Production from Orange Peel Waste by Leaching of Limonene. *Biomed Res. Int.* **2015.**

Yahia, E. M. The Contribution of Fruits and Vegetables to Human Health. In *Fruit and Vegetable Phytochemicals, Chemistry, Nutritional Value and Stability*; De la Rosa, L.; Alvarez-Parrilla, E.; Gonzalez-Aguilar, G.; Eds.; Wiley-Blackwell Publishing: Ames, IA, 2010, pp. 3–51.

Yang, Z.; Zheng, Y.; Cao, S. Effect of High Oxygen Atmosphere Storage on Quality, Antioxidant Enzymes, and DH-Radical Scavenging Activity of Chinese Bayberry Fruit. *J. Agric. Food Chem.* **2008,** *57* (1), 176–181.

Zhou, Z. Q. *Citrus Fruits Nutrition.* Science Press: Beijing, China 2012.

Zhang, Y.; Sun, Y.; Xi, W.; Shen, Y.; Qiao, L.; Zhong, L. Phenolic Compositions and Antioxidant Capacities of Chinese Wild Mandarin (*Citrus reticulata* Blanco) Fruits. *Food Chem.* **2014,** *145,* 674–680.

Zhang, H.; Xi, W.; Yang, Y.; Zhou, X.; Liu, X.; Yin, S. An On-Line HPLCFRSD System for Rapid Evaluation of the Total Antioxidant Capacity of Citrus Fruits. *Food Chem.* **2015,** *172,* 622–629.

CHAPTER 8

Antioxidative Defense System in Plants

RENU YADAV[1], MINERVA SHARMA[1], PORTIA SHARMA[1], and
UDITA TIWARI[2*]

[1]*Department of Botany, St. John's College, Agra, Uttar Pradesh, India*

[2]*Department of Biochemistry, School of Life Sciences,
Khandari Campus, Dr. B. R. Ambedkar University, Agra 282004,
Uttar Pradesh, India*

Corresponding author. E-mail: tiwariudita10@gmail.com

ABSTRACT

Plant cellular metabolism produces reactive oxygen species (ROS) as a normal product. Excessive production of ROS is caused by various environmental stresses that, in turn, lead to oxidative damage and ultimately cell death. This ROS is used as second messenger for various cellular processes; all of these depend on the equilibrium between ROS production and their scavenging. This chapter describes the generation, sites of production of ROS, and the antioxidative defense mechanism operating in the cells for scavenging of ROS overproduced under various environmental stresses, which requires several enzymatic as well as nonenzymatic components that are discussed in detail.

8.1 INTRODUCTION

Production of reactive oxygen species (ROS) is the result of aerobic metabolism that leads to the leakage of electrons onto O_2 from the electron transport chain activities of chloroplasts, mitochondria, and plasma membrane or as a by-product of various metabolic pathways.[1,2] This ROS comprises the following two major components:

- Free radicals have superoxide anion (O_2), hydroxyl radical (OH^-).
- Nonradicals have hydrogen peroxide (H_2O_2), singlet oxygen ($^1O_2$).

The extreme conditions of drought, chilling, UV-B, salinity or metal toxicity, and pathogen attack over a longer period of time play a disturbing role in cellular homeostasis and therefore rise up the production of ROS in the environment.[3] ROS plays the following two distinct roles in the plant metabolism:

- At low concentration: under all such environmental stresses, they mediate various plant responses by behaving as signaling molecules.[4]
- At high concentration: worst effects are caused leading to the damage of cellular factors.[5]

The cell death is often DNA damage, oxidative damage to lipid, protein, and alteration in the membrane properties, including ion transport, fluidity, protein crosslinking, and inhibition in protein synthesis, which are the consequences of advanced level of ROS.[6] A complex antioxidative defense system (including enzymatic and nonenzymatic components) is caused by higher plants to avoid all these types of oxidative hazards.[7]

8.1.1   EFFECTS OF CELLULAR HOMEOSTASIS ON THE LEVELS OF ROS

Disturbance in cellular homeostasis leading to the rise in the level of ROS production in plants is by several environmental stresses such as drought, salinity, chilling, metal toxicity, pathogen effects, and UV-B radiations.[8] This drastic increase in the level of ROS bothers the natural balance of OH, H_2O_2, and O_2^- in the environmental intracellular system.[9]

8.1.1.1   DROUGHT

The drastic drought conditions advance the ROS production levels in various ways. Chloroplast may boost up the generation of ROS in the case of CO_2 assimilation, disturbance in the photosynthetic transport capacity, and photosystem activities.[10] Maximal Ribulose 1,5 –bisphosphate (RUBP) oxygenation by the limitation in the CO_2 fixation may enhance the photorespiratory pathway during drought conditions. Various toxic radical species may rise up by O_2^- initiation damaging the initial reaction products. Generation of •OH in thylakoids by "iron-catalysis" is one of the major threats for chloroplast during drought by the reduction in H_2O_2 of both superoxide dismutase (SOD) and ascorbate (AsA). Oxidative stress is also led by increased ROS in the growing plants and drought tolerance in cotton plants.[11]

8.1.1.2   SALINITY

Excessive ROS production is also caused by salinity stress. Impairment of the cellular electron transport system within various subcellular compartments (such as chloroplasts, mitochondria, and metabolic pathways) results in the overproduction of the ROS such as O_2^-, •OH, H_2O_2, and $^1O_2$, by high salt concentration. High salt stress may result in the stomata closure resulting in the availability of CO_2 gas in the leaves. Therefore, heavy reduction in the photosynthetic electron transport system is recorded to enhance the ROS generation induction in the oxidative stress.[12] Increase in the production of ROS (such as H_2O_2) is also caused by lowering the chloroplast CO_2/O_2 ratio favoring photorespiration. Eliminated CO_2 mitigates the oxidative salinity stress which comprises low ROS production and fine maintenance of redox homeostasis led by high rates of assimilation and low rates of photorespiration. Disturbed metabolism by lipid peroxidation, nucleic acids, and denaturing proteins is led by salinity-induced ROS in many plant species. The indication of damage in oxidation can be noticed by the protein carbonyl content (PCC). PCC was recorded to be increased twice in maize seedlings on the exposure to chilled temperature. On the other hand, activities of lipoxygenase and lipid peroxidation were recorded to be increased during the low temperature in maize leaves.[13]

8.1.1.3   CHILLING

Limitation in the growth and crop production can be highly noticed in the chilling stress of the environment. Chilling effect overproduces the ROS by unbalancing the light absorption as well as the light usage through inhibiting the Calvin–Benson cycle activity of photosynthetic electron flux to the O_2.[14] This results in the overreduction of respiration activity. Conversion of higher electron flux to O_2 is led by RUBISCO. There is a negative correlation between initial RUBISCO activity and photosynthetic rate by the accumulation in chloroplast. Oxidation of protein is a very significant factor showcasing the chilling injury in plants.[15]

8.1.1.4   METAL TOXICITY

Hazardous effect in high level of metal presence in the environment may badly influence the plant growth and development (also the metabolism). Such losses can be recorded as crop yield crises. One of the major issues regarding the presence of toxic metals is the production of ROS (either directly or indirectly) by the metals. This also results in the oxidative damage to various cell components. During metal stress conditions, the rate of net photosynthesis decreases because of the change in photosynthetic metabolism. Later, these changes of metabolism lead to as overgeneration of ROS such as O_2^-, •OH, and H_2O_2. An example for the induced ROS production of metals includes cadmium, nickel, and zinc.[16]

8.1.1.5   PATHOGEN EFFECT

The finest and earliest cellular responses of successful pathogen recognition include the oxidative burst involving the production of ROS. Similarly, recognizing varieties of pathogens leads to the production of O_2^- or other disputative product of H_2O_2 in the apoplast. And also diseases is a major target of environmental pollutants.[17]

8.1.1.6   UV-B RADIATION

According to the plant biologists, UV-B radiations are a matter of great concern, since they are a threat for the global agricultural productivity. Advanced UV-B inhibits the rate of photosynthesis. It has also been recorded that in the UV-B treatment, light-saturated rate of CO_2 declines followed by the decrease in the carboxylation velocity and RUBISCO content. Oxidative damage of plants can also be noticed by the overgeneration of ROS through the limited CO_2 assimilation.[18]

8.2 SITES FOR THE PRODUCTION OF ROS

Both stressed and unstressed cells produce ROS at various locations such as chloroplasts, mitochondria, plasma membrane, peroxisomes, apoplast, endoplasmic reticulum, and cell walls (Fig. 8.1). The inescapable occurrence of electrons on O_2 by the electron transport activities of mitochondria, chloroplast, plasma membrane are the sources of ROS formation as by-product of several metabolic pathways located at different cell components.[19]

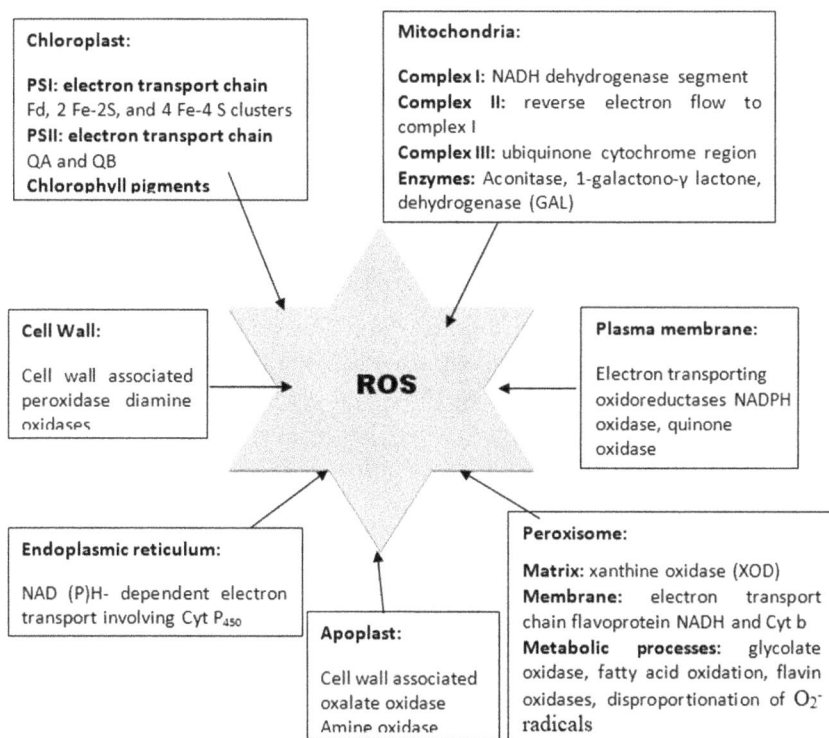

Chloroplast:

PSI: electron transport chain
Fd, 2 Fe-2S, and 4 Fe-4 S clusters
PSII: electron transport chain
QA and QB
Chlorophyll pigments

Mitochondria:

Complex I: NADH dehydrogenase segment
Complex II: reverse electron flow to complex I
Complex III: ubiquinone cytochrome region
Enzymes: Aconitase, 1-galactono-γ lactone, dehydrogenase (GAL)

Cell Wall:

Cell wall associated peroxidase diamine oxidases

ROS

Plasma membrane:

Electron transporting oxidoreductases NADPH oxidase, quinone oxidase

Endoplasmic reticulum:

NAD (P)H- dependent electron transport involving Cyt P$_{450}$

Apoplast:

Cell wall associated oxalate oxidase
Amine oxidase

Peroxisome:

Matrix: xanthine oxidase (XOD)
Membrane: electron transport chain flavoprotein NADH and Cyt b
Metabolic processes: glycolate oxidase, fatty acid oxidation, flavin oxidases, disproportionation of O_2^- radicals

FIGURE 8.1　Sites of production of ROS.

8.2.1 CHLOROPLASTS

There are several factors or locations where the generation of ROS occurs. The main sources may include electron transport chain (ETCs)

in Photosystem I (PSI) and Photosystem II (PSII) to produce ROS in chloroplast. The climatic conditions, including drought, salt, high light stress, and temperature rises, play a vital role for enhancing ROS in plants by limiting CO_2 fixation.[20] During normal situations, the flow of electron from the excited PS centers to the Nicotinamide adenine dinucleotide phosphate (NADP) that later gets reduced to NADPH and enters into the Calvin cycle and then reduces to the final acceptor of electron CO_2.[21]

8.2.1.1   MEHLER REACTION

Sometimes ETC gets overloaded because of the decrement in the NADP supply, which are the results of stressed conditions. It leads to the reduction of O_2 from the leakage of electron from ferredoxin to O_2.

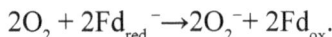

$$2O_2 + 2Fd_{red}{}^- \rightarrow 2O_2{}^- + 2Fd_{ox}.$$

In the ETC of PSI, the leakage of electrons to O_2 can also be observed from the 2Fe–2S and 4Fe–4S clusters. This leakage of electrons from the O_2 site contributes to the production of $O_2{}^-$. This formation of $O_2{}^-$ reduction is known as *rate-limiting step*. Now as the $O_2{}^-$ is formed, it generates ROS more aggressively. In PSII, the acceptor sites of ETC include primary acceptor quinone (QA) and secondary acceptor quinone (QB). In the case of Fe–S centers where Fe^{2+} is available, the transformation of H_2O_2 may also be seen by the *Fenton reaction* into the much more dangerous •OH.[22]

8.2.2   MITOCHONDRIA

Several stages of ETC produce ROS in mitochondria. Here, in the flavoprotein region, reduction directly occurs from oxygen to $O_2{}^-$ in the segment of the respiratory chain (NADH dehydrogenase). Here, the NAD^+ substrates are limited for complex I. Therefore, the electron transport may occur to complex I from complex II (in the reverse flow). This process is regulated by the hydrolysis of ATP and also produces ROS.[23]

The cytochrome region of the complex III (ubiquinone) of ETC produces oxygen to $O_2{}^-$. The ubiquinone in fully reduced stage donates an electron to cytochrome C_1. Later, it leaves an unstable and highly reducing radicle of ubisemiquinone that is favorable during the leakage of electron as O_2

to O_2^- formation. In plants, ETC and ATP syntheses are tightly coupled under the suitable conditions, whereas the stress conditions lead to the inhibition or sometimes modification of the components. This results in the overreduction of the electron carriers and produces ROS. ROS can also be produced by several enzymes present in the mitochondrial region. Some of them may directly produce ROS, such as aconitase.[19]

8.2.3 PEROXISOMES

As a result of the essential oxidative type of metabolism, peroxisomes are one of the major sites of intracellular H_2O_2 production. Here, the major chemical processes involved in the generation are the fatty acid β-oxidation, the enzymatic reaction of flavinoxidases, the glycolate oxidase reaction, and the disproportion of O_2^- radicals. At the time of photorespiration, glycolate oxidation through glycolate oxidase in the peroxisomes leads to the maximum production of H_2O_2.[24]

8.2.4 PLASMA MEMBRANE

Electron transporting oxidoreductases are ubiquitously present in plasma membrane, which results in the production of ROS.[25]

8.2.5 CELL WALL

One of the active sites for the production of ROS is cell wall. There have been evidences that the enzymes located in the cell wall are responsible for the production of apoplastic ROS. On the other hand, cell wall–linked oxalate oxidase releases H_2O_2 and CO_2 to form oxalic acid.[26] ROS are pre-described second messengers under a number of cellular processes, which includes the resistance to extreme climatic conditions.[27]

8.3 ROLES OF ROS AS MESSENGERS

During moderate concentrations, ROS behave as second messengers that mediate various plant reactions in the plant cells, as shown in Figure 8.2.

Some of them are acquisition of tolerance to both biotic and abiotic stresses, the stomata closure, programmed cell death (PCD), and gravitropism.

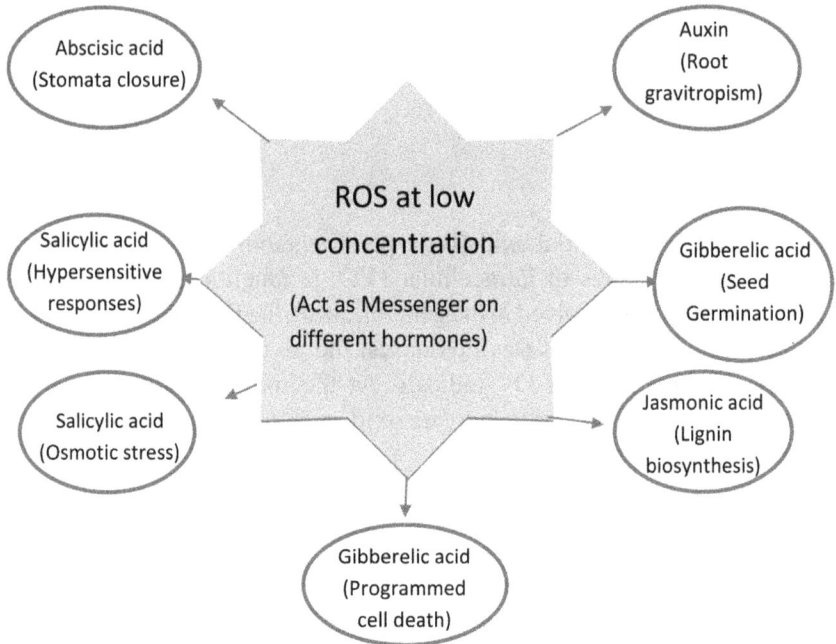

FIGURE 8.2   ROS as second messengers in several plant hormone responses.

Plants have the capacity to transduce and translate ROS signals into the appropriate cell responses with the aid of some calcium mobilization, redox-sensitive proteins, gene expression, and protein phosphorylation. Through proteins key signaling, ROS can be directly sensed such as a tyrosine phosphatase by the oxidation of conserved residues of cysteine.

ROS have also been recorded as modulating activities in signaling such as protein phosphatases, protein kinases, and transcription factors. They help to communicate with various other molecules and form the pathways parting the network of signaling that controls the downstream response of ROS. The goodness in the balance of oxidant production and removal by the antioxidant may decide the strength, life span, and size of ROS. ROS are known as the second messengers in the abscisic acid (ABA) transduction pathway in guard cells. Stomatal closure may reduce water loss by the activation of calcium-permeable channels of the plasma membrane, since ABA-induced H_2O_2 is a mandatory signal in the process. Jannat et al. observed that increase in the level of H_2O_2 has no stomatal closure, the role of ROS as the root gravitropism is seen as second messenger.[28]

8.4 ROS AND OXIDATIVE DAMAGE TO BIOMOLECULES

At high concentration, all the ROS are considered as highly toxic. A cell is said to be in an "oxidative stress" if its level of ROS extends the defense mechanism. The advanced ROS production in the environmental stresses may turn up as a cell threat by causing oxidation of proteins, damage to nucleic acids, enzyme inhibition, peroxidation of lipids, activation of PCD pathway, and finally to the death of the cell.

To avoid severe oxidative stresses, the production of ROS has to be stored at the earliest. Advanced levels of ROS may be toxic to the biomolecules such as proteins, lipids, and DNA. Such reactions can disturb the intrinsic membrane factors such as fluidity, loss of enzymatic activity, ion transport, protein cross-linking and inhibition of protein synthesis, DNA damage, and ultimately the cell death[29] as shown in Figure 8.3.

8.4.1 LIPIDS

Cellular functioning is affected when the level of ROS rises up the threshold and boosts lipid peroxidation in both organellar and cellular membranes. The oxidative stress is aggravated by lipid peroxidation by the generation of lipid-derived radicals that may react and damage DNA and protein. During stressed conditions, the level of lipid peroxidation has been in use broadly as an indicator of ROS-mediated destruction to the cell membrane under different stressful conditions. It has been recorded that increased peroxidation and degradation of lipids in plants grow under stressed conditions of the environment. This lipid peroxidation parallels with the increased ROS production. One of the final products is malondi-aldehyde. There could be chain breakage, increase in membrane fluidity, and permeability through peroxidation of polyunsaturated fatty acid by ROS attack.[30]

Protein: **DNA:**

. Site-specific amino acid modification   . Deoxyribose oxidation

. Enzyme inactivation   . Strand breakage

. Fragmentation of the peptide chain   . Modification of bases

. Increased susceptibility of proteins to   . DNA-protein crosslimks
proteolysis

ROS at high
concentration

(Oxidative damage)

LIPID:

. Chain breakage

. Increase in membrane fluidity and permeability

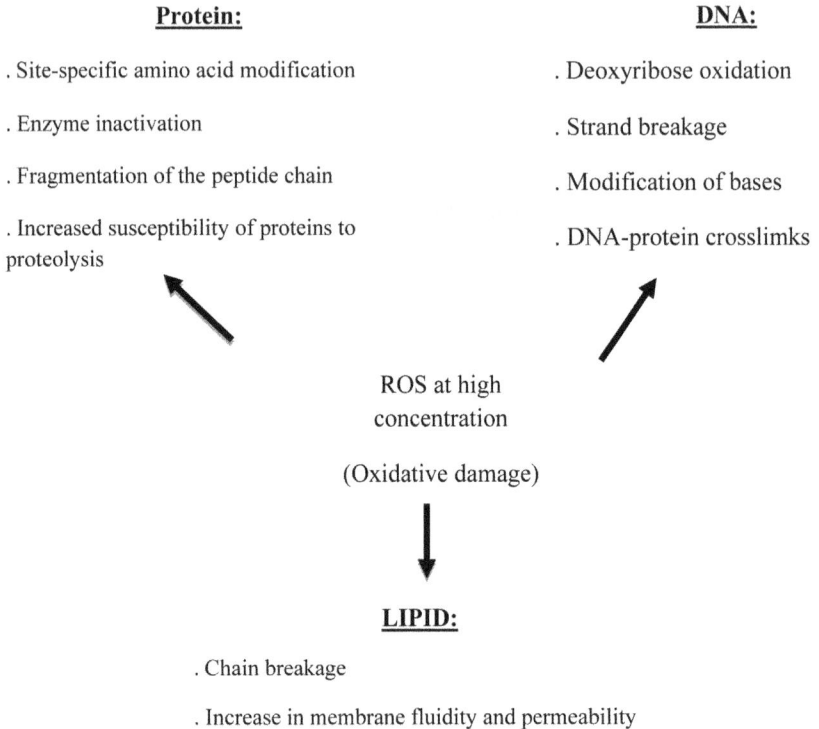

FIGURE 8.3   ROS-induced oxidative damage to lipids, proteins, and DNA.

8.4.2   PROTEINS

Direct or indirect modification of proteins is possible in a variety of ways by the attack of ROS.

- *In direct modification*: Modulation of protein's activity is by nitro-sylation, carbonylation, glutathionylation, and disulphide bond formation.
- *In indirect modification*: Through the conjugation of breakdown products of peroxidation of fatty acid. As a result of extra ROS generation, the site-specific modification of amino acid, aggregation of the cross-linked reaction products, fragmentation of peptide chain, and increased susceptibility of proteins to proteolysis may also occur.[31]

The stress of oxidation injures the tissues and they generally include the concentration of carbonylated proteins that is used as a marker of protein oxidation. In the stressful conditions, plants are noticed to have advanced modification of proteins. DNA damage is majorly done by ROS. ROS may also cause oxidative damage to mitochondria, nuclear, and chloroplast DNA, since DNA is cell's genetic material and so the damage to it may cause change in the entire proteins coding and results in the malfunctions or whole inactivation of the encoded proteins. When the DNA is oxidatively attacked, the DNA outcomes as deoxyribose oxidation, removal of nucleotides, strand breakage, various modifications in the DNA–proteins cross-links, and organic bases of nucleotides as well.[32]

8.5 DNA–PROTEIN CROSS-LINKS

Subsequent mutation can be seen when the nucleotides of one strand may result as the mismatch with nucleotides in other strands. Advanced DNA degradation has been in plants that are exposed to several environmental stresses like salinity and metal toxicity. ROS oxidation makes sugar and moieties of DNA more susceptible.

•OH addition to double bonds may constitute to oxidative attack to DNA bases. On the other hand, sugar damage may result from hydrogen abstraction from deoxyribose. DNA sugar on being attacked by ROS results as single-strand breaks. The hydroxyl radical reacts with all the types of purines and pyrimidine bases and deoxyribose backbone.[33]

8.6 ANTIOXIDATIVE DEFENSE SYSTEM IN PLANTS

Behaving as both damaging and signaling molecule depends on critical equilibrium in between scavenging and ROS production. To rescue from the multifunctional roles of ROS, it has become compulsory to control the level of ROS to avoid injury without eliminating them completely. Through an efficient antioxidative system constituting both nonenzymatic and enzymatic antioxidants, the detoxification or scavenging of data can be easily achieved. Various enzymes have increased their activities in plants to combat the stress introduced by the environment. Plants have specific ROS generating system in various organelles such as chloroplast, mitochondria, or peroxisomes.

8.6.1   ENZYMIC COMPONENTS OF ANTIOXIDATIVE DEFENSE SYSTEM

This category comprises several antioxidant enzymes such as SOD, catalase (CAT), guaiacol peroxidase (GPX), enzymes of ascorbate glutathione (AsA–GSH) cycle ascorbate peroxidase (APX), monodehydroascorbate reductase (MDHAR), dehydroascorbate reductase (DHAR), and glutathione reductase (GR), all of which operate at various compartments and thereby revert as the cell is exposed to the stressful conditions.[34]

8.6.1.1   SUPEROXIDE DISMUTASE

In all the aerobic organisms, SOD plays the central role in defense mechanism under the oxidative stressful conditions and also provides protection against diseases.[35] The enzyme SOD may catalyze the dismuted O_2^- to O_2 and H_2O_2. Also, the SOD enzyme belongs to the metallo-enzyme family. This is found in several subcellular compartments where the generation of activated oxygen takes place.

There are the following three isozymes of SOD, which are observed in subcellular section of plants:

- copper/zinc SOD (Cu/Zn-SOD) in cytosol, chloroplast, peroxisome, and mitochondria;
- manganese SOD (Mn-SOD) in mitochondria; and
- iron SOD (Fe–SOD) in chloroplasts.

All these enzymes are nuclear encoded and trigger their respective parts only through the amino terminal targeting sequence. SOD increases in plants in the stressful conditions, including drought and metal toxicity mainly. Well, increased tolerance of plants is often correlated with the increased SOD activity against the environmental conditions.

8.6.1.2   CATALASE

CAT was the very first enzyme to be discovered and characterized among all other antioxidant enzymes. It is often considered as ubiquitous tetrameric heme-containing enzyme that catalyzes the dismutation of two molecules of H_2O_2 into water and oxygen. They have high certainty for H_2O_2 but weak against organic peroxides. CATs are also known for their quality of not requiring cellular reducing equivalents.[36]

Simultaneously, CAT has a faster turnover rate but higher in APX than H_2O_2. The peroxisomes are the major sites for the H_2O_2 generation. There are various stressful conditions that are implicated on H_2O_2. H_2O_2 is observed to be degraded by CAT in some energy-efficient manner at the time when cells are stressed for energy and gradual generation of H_2O_2 by the catabolic processes. On the basis of intensity, duration, and stress type, enhancement or depletion of CAT can be observed; stress that declines the rate of protein turns over the reduction of CAT activity.

8.6.1.3 GUAIACOL PEROXIDASE

A heme-comprising protein for oxidizing aromatic electron donor such as the guaiacol and pyrogallol at the cost of H_2O_2 is known as GPX that can be observed in all plants, animals, and microbes. These enzymes comprise two structural Ca^{2+} ions and four conserved disulfide bridges. Several isoenzymes of GPX present in the plant tissues are located in vacuoles, cell walls, and cytosols. GPX is associated with several essential biosynthetic processes such as biosynthesis of ethylene, degradation of Indole-3- Acetic Acid (IAA), wound healing, lignification of cell wall, and defense against both abiotic and biotic stresses. GPXs are popularly known as *stress enzyme*. Under the stressful conditions, GPX may work as effective quencher of reactive intermediary forms of peroxy radicals and O_2; this behavior has been shown to induce the activity of GPX.[37]

8.6.2 NONENZYMIC COMPONENTS OF ANTIOXIDATIVE DEFENSE SYSTEM

This category includes the major cellular redox buffers ascorbate (AsA) and glutathione (γ-glutamyl-cysteinyl-glycine) (GSH) as well as tocopherol, carotenoids, and phenolic compounds. They majorly include interaction amid the cellular components. By controlling mitosis, elongation of cell, plant growth, and development may be highly effected leading to the cell death.[38]

8.6.2.1 ASCORBATE (ASA)

AsA is the most widely used antioxidant with low molecular weight. It has recognizable defensive ability against the increased ROS levels. This is due to the nature of donating electrons in both enzymatic and nonenzymatic reactions. In several plant physiologies and metabolisms, AsA plays a vital role that deals with the growth, differentiation, and metabolism. AsA is present in millimolar concentration and about 90% is located in the cytoplasm. Some macromolecules can be secured by AsA from the oxidative damage. In changing climatic conditions, physiological reaction of AsA gives a membrane protection and conserves the activities of the enzymes that contain prosthetic transitional metal ions.[39] AsA also plays a vital role in the removal of H_2O_2 through the AsA–GSH cycle.

8.6.2.2 GLUTATHIONE (GSH)

Tripeptide glutathione plays a very vital role in the intracellular defense mechanism against ROS-induced oxidative damage. Its virtual presence can be seen in all the cell compartments such as cytosol, chloroplasts, and ER. GSH can be generated under the cytosol and chloroplast of plant cells by compartmental peculiar isoforms of γ-ECS and γ-GS. To maintain the cellular redox state, GSH and glutathione disulfide play vital and central component roles. Due to the reducing power, GSH plays an important role in diverse biological processes, including cell growth and division, regulation of sulfate transport, signal transduction, conjugation of metabolites, enzymatic regulation, synthesis of proteins and nucleic acids, synthesis of phytochelatins for metal chelation, detoxification of xenobiotics, and the expression of stress-responsive genes. GSH may react with O_2 and function as free radical scavenger. It may also work as an antioxidant. GSH also protects molecules like protein, lipid, and DNA by proton donation in the presence of free radical or ROS, yielding Glutathione disulfide (GSSG). GSH may also produce another antioxidant AsA by the AsA–GSH cycle.[40] Oxidized AsA is recycled by GSH into the reduced form by the enzyme DHAR. Dehydroascorbic acid (DHA) oxidized product of ascorbic acid in lens epithelium can also be reduced by GSH through a nonenzymic mechanism of pH > 7 at the rate of GSH concentration >1 mM. Proper production and maintenance of reduced GSH by the usage of NADPH (as a cofactor) plays an important role in the cell. GSH provides a rationale for its use as a stress maker in the oxidative defense system. The increment of GSH concentration was the most supported suggestion at the time when apple trees were subject to drought. The degradation of climate could be seen when the stress increases, GSH concentration is dropped and redox state becomes much more oxidized.

8.6.2.3   TOCOPHEROLS

Tocopherols represent a group of lipophilic antioxidants (α, β, γ, and δ) for scavenging of oxygen-free radical. Due to methylation pattern and the amount of methyl groups attached to the phenolic polar head structure, the relative antioxidant behavior of the tocopherol isomers can be observed as $\alpha > \beta > \gamma > \delta$.[3] Tocopherols are generated in the process of photosynthesis and present only in the green parts. Tocopherols are also known as preventives for the chain propagation step under the auto oxidation of lipids that is for the effective free radical trap. The induction of tolerance (for chilling, salinity, and water deficiency) has been seen improving by the accumulation of α-tocopherol depending on the plant species.

8.6.2.4   CAROTENOIDS

They can detoxify ROS and also belong to the lipophilic family of antioxidants. Carotenoids can be seen in both microbes and plants.[41] In the situation of plants, carotenoids absorb light of the visible spectrum (400–550 nm) and pass the energy to the chlorophyll. Plant development and biotic/abiotic stress rate can be highly affected by the presence of carotenoids that are precursors toward the signaling molecules. Their ability to minimize or prevent the generation of triplet chlorophyll depends on the chemical peculiarity. Gomathi and Rakkiyapan[42] noted that higher carotenoids may have greater adaptation under the saline conditions for the sugarcane plantations. Carotenoids often have a chain of isoprene that has numerous conjugated double bonds which allows easy energy uptake from excited molecules and dissipation of excess energy as heat.[43]

8.6.2.5   PHENOLIC COMPOUNDS

Phenolics are the secondary diversified metabolites (including flavonoids, tannins, hydroxycinnamate esters, and lignin) that have the antioxidant properties.[44] They can easily be seen under a plant tissue. Polyphenols comprise an aromatic ring along with -OH and OCH_3 that help in their biological activities. One of the most important radical scavengers is the phenolic antioxidants. They convert peroxy radicals into hydroperoxides and are themselves converted to phenoxy radicals. They do have a strong ability to donate electrons and behave as antioxidants like AsA and α-tocopherol, by trapping the lipid alkoxyl radical, polyphenols may inhibit the lipid peroxidation. This may lead to the decrease in fluidity membrane and enhancement in lipid packing. In later stages, it may not allow the peroxidative reactions and hindrance in the diffusion of free radicals. As an outcome of several stresses, various proves for the induction of phenolic chemical reaction in plants can be noticed. Fruits, vegetables, grains, spices, and herbs are the richest sources of dietary poly phenolic compounds. Intake of these foods in high amount is known to lower the risk of chronic diseases.[45]

KEYWORDS

- **reactive oxygen species (ROS)**
- **antioxidative defense system**
- **nonenzymatic components**
- **enzymatic components**

REFERENCES

1. Nafees, M.; Fahad, S.; Shah, A. N.; Bukhari, M. A. Reactive Oxygen Species in Plant Biology. In *Plant Abiotic Stress Tolerance;* Springer, Cham. 2019; pp 259–272.
2. Kaul, S.; Sharma, S. S.; Mehta, I. K. Free Radical Scavenging Potential of L-Proline: Evidence from In Vitro Assay. *Amino Acids* **2008,** *34* (2), 315–320.
3. Das, K.; Roychoudhary, A. Reactive Oxygen Species (ROS) and Response of Antioxidants as ROS-Scavengers during Environmental Stress in Plants. *Front. Environ. Sci.* **2014,** *2* (53), 1–13.

4. Suzuki, N.; Koussevitzky, S.; Mittler, R.; Miller, G. A. D. ROS and Redox Signaling in the Response of Plants to Abiotic Stress. *Plant Cell Environ.* **2012,** *35* (2), 259–270.

5. Moradi, F.; Ismail, A. M. Responses of Photosynthesis, Chlorophyll Fluorescence and ROS-Scavenging Systems to Salt Stress during Seedling and Reproductive Stages in Rice. *Ann. Bot. Oxf. Acad.* **2007,** *99* (6), 1161–1173.

6. Dandona, P.; Thusu, K.; Cook, S. Oxidative Damage to DNA in Diabetes Mellitus. *Lancet* **1996,** *347* (8999), 444–445.

7. Silva, S. L. F.; Vogit, E. L. Partial Oxidative Protection by Enzymatic and Non-Enzymatic Components in Cashew Leaves under High Salinity. *Biol. Plant.* **2012,** *56* (1), 172–176.

8. Shadel, G. S.; Horvath, T. L. Mitochondrial ROS Signaling in Organismal Homeostasis. *Cell* **2015,** *163* (3), 560–569.

9. Ottavino, F. G.; Handy, D. E. Redox Regulation in the Extracellular Environment. *Circ. J.* **2008,** *72* (1), 1–16.

10. Nxele, X.; Klein, A.; Ndimba, B. K. Drought and Salinity Stress Alters ROS Accumulation, Water Retention and Osmolyte Content in Sorghum Plants. *S. Afr. J. Bot.* **2017,** *108*, 261–266.

11. Aktas, L. Y.; Dagnon, S. Drought Tolerance in Cotton, Involvement of Non-Enzymatic ROS-Scavenging Compounds. *J. Agron. Crop Sci.* **2009,** *195* (4), 247–253.

12. Kurusu, T.; Kazuyuki, K.; Tada, Y. Plant Signaling Networks Involving Ca^{2+} and Rboh/Nox-Mediated ROS Production under Salinity Stress. *Front. Plant Sci.* **2015,** *6*, 427–432.

13. Bose, J.; Rodrigo-Moreno, A.; Shabala, S. ROS Homeostasis in Halophytes in the Context of Salinity Stress Tolerance. *J. Exp. Bot.* **2014,** *65* (5), 1241–257.

14. Elinset, J.; Winge, P. ROS Signaling Pathways in Chilling Stress. *Plant Signaling Behav.* 2007, *2* (5), 365–367.

15. Wise, R. R. Chilling-enhanced Photooxidation, the production, action and study of reactive oxygen species produced during chilling in the light. *Photosynth. Res.* **1995,** *45* (2), 79–97.

16. Gajewska, E. Effect of Nickel on ROS Content and Antioxidative Enzyme Activities in Wheat Leaves. *Biometals* **2007,** *20* (1), 27–36.

17. Bickers, D. R.; Athar, M. Oxidative Stress in the Pathogenesis of Skin Disease. *J. Invest. Dermatol.* **2006,** *126* (12), 2565–2575.

18. Hideg, E.; Jansen, M. A.; Strid, A. UV-B Exposure, ROS and Stress, Inseparable Companions or Loosely Linked Associates. *Trends Plant Sci.* **2013,** *18* (2), 107–115.

19. Chen, Q.; Vazquez, E. J. Production of Reactive Oxygen Species by Mitochondria Central Role of Complex III. *J. Biol. Chem.* **2003,** *278* (38), 36027–36031.

20. Shapiguoz, A.; Julia Vainonen, J. ROS Talk – How the Apoplast, the Chloroplast and the Nucleus Get the Message Through. *Front. Plant Sci.* **2012,** *3*, 292, 1–9.

21. Galvez, G. The Role of Reactive Oxygen Species in Signaling from Chloroplast to the Nucleus. *Physiol. Plant.* **2010,** *138* (4), 430–439.

22. Strizh, I. G. Ontologies for Data and Knowledge Sharing in Biology, Plant ROS Signaling as a Case Study. *BioEssays* **2006,** *28* (2), 199–210.

23. Sabharwal, S. S.; Schumacker, P. T. Mitochondrial ROS in Cancer, Initiators, Amplifiers or a Achilles' Heel? *Nat. Rev. Cancer* **2014,** *14* (11), 709–721.

24. Fransen, M.; Nordgren, M.; Wang, B. Role of Peroxisomes in ROS/RNS-Metabolism, Implications for Human Disease. *Biochim. Biophys. Acta, Mol. Basis Dis.* **2012,** *1822* (9), 1363–1373.

25. Mello, E. O.; Ribeiro, S. F. Antifungal Activity of PvD1 Defensin Involves Plasma Membrane Permeabilization, Inhibition of Medium Acidification and Induction of ROS in Fungi Cells. *Curr. Microbiol.* **2011,** *62* (4), 1209–1217.

26. Tenhhaken, R. Cell Wall Remodeling under Abiotic Stress. *Front. Plant Sci.* **2015,** *5,* 771–779.

27. Das, D. K.; Maulik, N.; Sato. M. ROS Function as Second Messenger during Ischemic Preconditioning of Heart. *Mol. Cell. Biochem.* **1999,** *196* (1–2), 59–67.

28. Reth, M. Hydrogen Peroxide as Second Messenger in Lymphocyte Activation. *Nat. Immunol.* **2002,** *3* (12), 1129–1137.

29. Qisen Xiang, Q. Carnosic Acid Protects Biomolecules from Free Radical-Mediated Oxidative Damage In Vitro. *Food Sci. Biotechnol.* **2013,** *22* (5), 1–8.

30. Wang, J. F.; Azzam, J. E. Valproate Inhibits Oxidative Damage to Lipid and Protein in Primary Cultured Rat Cerebrocortical Cells. *Neuroscience* **2003,** *116* (2), 485–489.

31. Cabiscol, E.; Tamarit, J.; Ros, J. Oxidative Stress in Bacteria and Protein Damage by Reactive Oxygen Species. *Int. Microbiol.* **2000,** *3,* 3–8.

32. Ding, W. Inorganic Arsenic Compounds Cause Oxidative Damage to DNA and Protein by Inducing ROS and RNS Generation in Human Keratinocytes. *Mol. Cell. Biochem.* **2005,** *279* (1–2), 105–112.

33. Barker, S. DNA-Protein Crosslinks, Their Induction, Repair and Biological Consequences. *Mutat. Res.* **2005,** *589* (2), 111–135.

34. Sies, H. Oxidative Stress, Oxidants and Antioxidants. *Exp. Physiol. Transl. Integr.* **1997,** *82* (2), 291–295.

35. Afonso, V. Reactive Oxygen Species and Superoxide Dismutases, Role in Joint Diseases. *Joint Bone Spine* **2007,** *74* (4), 324–329.

36. Nishikawa, M.; Hashida, M. Catalase Delivery for Inhibiting ROS-Mediated Tissue Injury and Tumor Metastasis. *Adv. Drug Deliv. Rev.* **2009,** *61* (4), 319–326.

37. Jebara, S.; Jebara, M.; Limam, F. Changes in Ascorbate Peroxidase, Catalase, Guaiacol Peroxidase and Superoxide Dismutase Activities in Common Bean Nodules under Salt Stress. *J. Plant Physiol.* **2005,** *162* (8), 929–936.

38. Ali, M. B.; Yu, K. W.; Hahn, E. J. Methyl jasmonate and salicylic acid elicitation induces ginsenosides accumulation, enzymatic and non-enzymatic antioxidant in suspension culture *Panax ginseng* roots in bioreactors. *Plant Cell Rep.* **2006,** *25* (6), 613–620.

39. Caverzan, A.; Passaia, G. Plant Responses to Stresses, Role of Ascorbate Peroxidase in the Antioxidant Protection. *Genet. Mol. Biol.* **2012,** *35* (4), 1011–1019.

40. Shao, H. B.; Chu, L. Y.; Shao, M. A. Higher Plant Antioxidants and Redox Signaling under Environmental Stresses. *C. R. Biol.* **2008,** *331* (6), 433–441.

41. Fiedor, J.; Burda, K. Potential Role of Carotenoids as Antioxidants in Human Health and Disease. *Nutrients* **2014,** *6* (2), 466–488.

42. Gomathi, R.; Rakkiyapan, P. Comparative Lipid Peroxidation, Leaf Membrane Thermostability, and Antioxidant System in Four Sugarcane Genotypes Differing in Salt Tolerance. *Int. J. Plant Physiol. Biochem.* **2011,** *3* (4), 67–74.

43. Mittler, R. Oxidative Stress, Antioxidants and Stress Tolerance. *Trends Plant Sci.* **2002,** *7* (9), 405–410.

44. Michalak, A. Phenolic Compounds and Their Antioxidant Activity in Plants Growing under Heavy Metal Stress. *Pol. J. Environ. Stud.* **2006,** *15* (4), 523–530.

45. Zhang, H.; Tsao, R. Dietary Polyphenols, Oxidative Stress and Antioxidant and Anti-Inflammatory Effects. *Curr. Opin. Food Sci.* **2016,** *8*, 33–42.

CHAPTER 9

Bryophytes, An Extensive Source of Antioxidants

PRACHI DIXIT

School of Sciences, ITM University Gwalior, Gwalior, Madhya Pradesh, India

E-mail: prachidixit949@gmail.com

ABSTRACT

From the knowledge of ethno-medicinal uses of bryophytes and the modern research on chemical constituents of some of the plant members, the bryophytes are supposed to have major natural activities. Antioxidant activity is measured as one of the key characteristics of bioactivities and is in focus of attention to pharmacists. Free radicals perform the chief task in the pathogenesis of many diseases. Antioxidative potential of bryophytes can be determined by various methods such as DH radical scavenging assay, ABTS$^{\cdot+}$ radical scavenging assay, hydrogen peroxide radical, metal chelating activity, ferric reducing/antioxidant power assay, and FTIR spectroscopy. The present chapter deals with literature covering the antioxidative aspects of bryophytes. Natural antioxidants form a promising alternative for synthetic ones. Thus, a positive correlation between traditional use and scientific evaluation could create a substitute source of new medicinal compounds, which might overcome the expensive research of synthetic drugs and their detrimental side effects.

9.1 INTRODUCTION

Latest pharmacological investigation of bryophytes has confirmed that the active principles present in these plants are relatively unique and having potential therapeutic applications. Mosses and liverworts are small, low-growing plants and comprise the phylum bryophyta that is phylogenetically positioned between vascular plants and algae. This group of plants possesses strong antioxidative enzymatic mechanism that helps them to cope up with severe climate and stress conditions (Dey and De, 2012). One of the interesting groups of bryophytes, the liverworts are being pharmaceutically used globally, especially in Indian and Chinese cultures, for the treatment of hepatitis and skin diseases due to their antibiotic, anti-inflammatory, and diuretic properties (Friederich, 1999; Gökbulut et al., 2012; Saroya, 2011). Nowadays, the effects of mosses on microorganisms are studied intensively (Basile et al., 1999; Opelt et al., 2007; Singh et al., 2007), but little information exists about other activities, particularly about secondary metabolites with antioxidant properties (Chobot et al., 2006). Among the flavonoids, apigenin, luteolin, kaempferol, and orobol glycosides as well as their dimers are usually found in mosses (Zinsmeister and Mues, 1980; Basile et al., 1999). Although bryophytes are the most ancient earth plants, their value is basically unexplored and quite unidentified.

Specifically, bryophytes exhibit antibacterial, antifungal, antiviral activities, antioxidant, antiplatelet, antithrombin, insecticidal, neuroprotective activities, as well as cytotoxicity in respect to cancer cells (Spjut et al., 1986; Cheng et al., 2012). Bryophytes are supposed to be effective in disease prevention due to their antioxidant properties (Akinmoladun et al., 2007). Antioxidants are substances that can delay or retard lipids, proteins, and nucleic acid oxidation (Zheng and Wang, 2001). From the 1980s to the 1990s, the chemistry of some moss species had been studied by German scientists who established the chemotypes of moss species. Their studies showed that moss species principally contained flavonoids and their derivatives, including biflavonoids and glucosides. They are potential source of bioactive compounds such as secondary metabolites and are commercially used in many therapeutic planning. Flavonoids and phenolic acids are the major sources of secondary metabolites in bryophytes. Flavonoids have demonstrated that antioxidants contain a wide variety of molecules that play an important role in defending biological system against the harmful effects of oxidative processes on macromolecules such as carbohydrates, proteins, lipids, and DNA.

From the research of ethno-medicinal properties of bryophytes and the recent study on chemical constituents of some of the plants, the mosses are supposed to have significant biological activities (Singh et al., 2006).

An evidence of mosses having bioactive phytochemicals has concerned the attention of botanist and pharmaceutical industries. Alkaloids, flavonoids, biflavonoids, and isoflavonoids from bryophyte extract have effective antimicrobial activity against pathogenic microorganisms (Neto et al., 2011; Dan et al., 2008). On the other hand, the existence of flavonoids, tannins, and phenolic compounds of plant systems plays a major role as free radical scavengers, thereby acting as natural antioxidants (Polterait, 1997; Chobot et al., 2006). A variety of compounds isolated from liverworts have high potential as chemotherapeutic agents. It has been reported that marchantin A, isoriccardin C, riccardin B, plagiochin E, and marchantin C isolated from *Reboulia hemisphaerica* were found to display cytotoxicity against EYFP-tubulin HeLa cells with IC50 values of 22.6, 42.2, 41.6, 32.7, and 23.2 mmol/L, respectively (Gao et al., 2009). The antioxidant potential of mosses are using CERAC, CUPRAC, TEAC, DH, TPC, and FRAP (ferric reducing/antioxidant power) methods (Ertürk et al., 2015). The traditional use of bryophytes could be due to certain active compounds having antioxidant capacity. Ethno-medicinal use of different bryophytes should be scientifically investigated for active principles in order to bridge between conventional knowledge and pharmacology (Yayintas et al., 2017). The present chapter deals with literature covering the antioxidative feature of bryophytes.

9.1.1 ANTIOXIDANTS

Antioxidants are man-made or natural substances that may avoid some types of cell damage. Several decades of nutritional research findings recommended that consuming larger amounts of antioxidant-rich diet might help one to defend against various diseases. Because of these results, there has been a lot of study on antioxidant supplements.

The chemical reaction that can generate free radicals and leads to chain reactions that may harm the cells of organisms is known as the oxidation, whereas the substances that inhibit or retard the oxidation of compounds are known as antioxidants (Sindhi et al., 2013). They can be classified into the following three main categories:

- The first line defense antioxidants that include superoxide dismutase (SOD), catalase (CAT), glutathione reductase, and minerals like Se, Cu, and Zn.

- The second line defense antioxidants that include glutathione (GSH), vitamin C, albumin, vitamin E, carotenoids, flavonoids, etc.
- The third line defense antioxidants that include a complex group of enzymes for repairing damaged DNA, damaged proteins, oxidized lipids, and peroxides. Some examples are lipase, protease, DNA-repair enzymes, transferases, and methionine sulfoxide reductase (Irshad and Chaudhuri, 2002).

Antioxidants are any substances that can delay or retard lipids, proteins, and nucleic acid oxidation (Zheng and Wang, 2001). Antioxidants can be classified into two types: primary and secondary antioxidants that are categorized due to their protective properties at different stages of the oxidation process and their action by different mechanisms. Primary antioxidants scavenge free radicals, whereas secondary antioxidants inhibit the oxidative mechanisms that lead to degenerative diseases (Fu et al., 2011). Currently, there has been an upsurge of interest on natural antioxidants in plants to be used in pharmaceutical industry due to carcinogenic properties of some synthetic antioxidants such as butylated hydroxyanisole and butylated hydroxytoluene (Pejin and Bogdanović-Pristov, 2012).

The chemical reaction that can generate free radicals and leads to chain reactions that may harm to the cells of organisms is known as the oxidation, and the substances that inhibit or retard the oxidation of compounds are known as antioxidants (Sindhi et al., 2013). Antioxidants are any substances that can delay or retard lipids, proteins and nucleic acids oxidation (Zheng and Wang, 2001). Antioxidants can be classified into two types known as primary and secondary antioxidants. Primary and secondary antioxidants are categorized due to their protective properties at different stages of the oxidation procedure and their action by various mechanisms. Primary antioxidants scavenge free radicals whereas secondary antioxidants reduce the oxidative mechanisms that lead to degenerative diseases (Fu et al., 2011). Antioxidants can consequently be considered effective in reducing increased blood sugar level (Mousinho et al., 2013). Two enzymes α-amylase and α-glucosidase perform the main function in diabetes. By inhibiting these enzymes, the rate of glucose absorption and postprandial blood sugar levels can be reduced. Researchers have also studied antioxidants in in vivo experiments. These experiments demonstrated that antioxidants interacted with free radicals and stabilized them, thus preventing the free radicals from causing cell damage.

9.1.2 ANTIOXIDATIVE POTENTIAL IN BRYOPHYTES

Bryophytes generate a number of secondary metabolites that strengthen these delicate plants with strong antioxidative mechanism to cope up with a number of both biotic and abiotic stresses (Xie and Lou, 2009; Dey and De, 2012). Antioxidant activity (AA) is considered as one of the major aspects of bioactivities and is in focus of attention to pharmacists. Free radicals play the main role in pathogenesis of various diseases and are important components of stress signal cascades (Castro and Freeman, 2001).

Antioxidants for counteracting oxidative damage have been proven in angiosperms, gymnosperms, and pteridophytes (Bernaert et al., 2011). Antioxidants constitute an endogenous defensive mechanism against reactive oxygen species (ROS) and hence find extensive usage in pharmaceutical industries (Frahm, 2004). A number of earlier researches exhibited antioxidant potential of solvent extracts of different other mosses. Ethanol extracts of *Atrichum undulatum*, *Polytrichum formosum*, and *Pleurozium schreberi* were revealed to have antioxidant properties (Chobot et al., 2006, 2008). The liverworts such as *Marchantia* are the source of natural antioxidant. The presence of flavonoids, tannins, and phenolic compounds plays the chief role as free radical scavengers, thereby performing as natural antioxidants (Polterait, 1997). The methanol and ethyl acetate extracts of *Marchantia polymorpha* L. showed moderate antioxidant potential (Gökbulut et al., 2012). Aqueous extract of moss *Bryum moravicum* was also observed to have good antioxidant potential (Pejin et al., 2013).

A research conducted on antioxidant potential of the Antarctic mosses *Sanionia uncinata* (Hedw.) Loeske and *Polytrichastrum alpinum* (Hedw.) G.L. Sm. var. alpinum has demonstrated their potential to be used as antioxidants for pharmaceutical and cosmetic purpose (Bhattarai et al., 2008, 2009). A research exposed that the antioxidant assets of the aqueous extract of the three mosses, namely, *Brachythecium rutabulum*, *Calliergonella cuspidata*, and *Hypnum mammillatum*, in the context of their ABTS (2,2'-azino-bis(3-ethylbenzothiazoline-6-sulfonic acid)) cation scavenging activities and phenolic content have known to show some positive responses. Out of the three extracts, *B. rutabulum* has shown the highest of the phenolic content that further suggested potential of this extract in search of many other novel antioxidant compounds in this moss (Chandra et al., 2014).

Many phenolic acids are present in *M. polymorpha* such as gallate, vanilate, chlorogenate, cinnamate, protocatechol, coumarate, ferulate, sinapic, caffeate, and hydroxyl benzoate (Krishnan and Murugan, 2013). The AA of three European mosses *B. rutabulum* (Hedw.) Schimp., *C. cuspidata* (Hedw.) Loeske, and *H. mammillatum* (Brid.) Loeske was measured from aqueous extract with the help of ABTS (Pejin et al., 2012). Among all the bryophytes, liverworts, being significant reservoir of natural products, are pharmaceutically used worldwide, especially in Indian and Chinese systems of medicine for the treatment of skin diseases (Friederich et al., 1999; Saroya et al., 2011; Gokbulut et al., 2012).

9.1.3 SOURCE OF ANTIOXIDANT

Table 9.1 enlists defined various medicinal bryophytes having considerable antioxidant potential (preferred on the basis of studied literature) available.

Several natural processes like photosynthesis, respiration, and stress responses generate ROS as a byproduct. These ROS can lead to the disruption of the normal physiological and cellular functions (Asada, 1994) and also damage biomolecules of plasma membranes and cell walls, thus affecting directly the cell survival (Schutzendubel and Polle, 2002). Plants that can respond and adapt to drought stress are equipped with complex and highly efficient antioxidative defense systems composed of protective nonenzymatic as well as enzymatic mechanisms that efficiently scavenge ROS and prevent damaging effects of free radicals (Breusegem et al., 2001). Plants produce antioxidant enzymes such as catalase and peroxidase to get rid of these ROS.

Bryophytes produce a number of secondary metabolites and also possess strong antioxidative machinery that helps them to cope with both biotic and abiotic stresses (Xie and Lou, 2009; Dey and De, 2012). Against oxidative damage, the antioxidant defenses crucially protect cellular membranes and organelles present in plants that are grown under unfavorable conditions. Antioxidant enzymes protect cells against oxidative stress and are associated with stress tolerance and longevity. ROS react with cellular constituents such as protein and lipids, leading to damage and, thus affecting directly the cell survival.

TABLE 9.1 Some Medicinal Bryophytes and Their Decrypted Composites Presenting Antioxidant Potential.

Sr. no.	Name of bryophyte	Antioxidant compound	References
01	*Atrichum undulatum* and *Polytrichum formosum*	Phenolics	Chobot et al. (2008)
02	*Bryum moravicum*	Phenolics	Pejin (2013)
03	*Dumortiera hirsuta*	Riccardin D [macrocyclic bis(bibenzyl)]	Cheng et al. (2001)
04	*Frullania muscicola*	3-Hydroxy-4'-methoxybenzyl, 7,4-dimethyl-apigenin	Lou et al. (2002)
05	*Jungermannia subulata, Lophocolea heterophylla*, and *Scapania parvitexta*	Subulatin	Tazaki et al. (2002)
06	*Marchantia paleacea* var. *diptera*	Superoxide dismutase	Tanaka et al. (1998)
07	*Marchantia polymorpha*	Plagiochin E, riccardin H, marchantin E, neomarchantin A, and marchantins A and B	Niu et al. (2006)
08	*Pallavicinia* sp., *Plagiochila* sp., *Plagiomnium* sp., *Mnium* sp., and *Riccardia* sp.	Bicyclohumulenone, plagiochiline A, plagiochilide, plagiochilal B, menthanemonoterpenoids, triterpenoidal saponins, riccardins A and B, and sacullatal	Azuelo et al. (2011)
09	*Philonotis* sp., *Rhodobryum giganteum*	Triterpenoidal saponins, p-hydroxycinnamic acid, 7,8-dihydroxycoumarin	Asakawa (2007)
10	*Plagiochasma appendiculatum*	Prevent lipid peroxidation and increase antioxidant enzymes	Singh (2006)
11	*Plagiochila beddomei*	Phenolics	Manoj et al. (2012)
12	*Sphagnum magellanicum*	Phenolics	Montenegro et al. (2009)
13	*Mastigophora diclados*	Sesquiterpenoids	Komala et al. (2010)
14	*Thuidium tamariscellum*	Terpenoids	Mohandas et al. (2018)
15	*Thuidium tamariscinum* and *Platyhypnidium riparioides*	Phenolics	Aslanbaba et al. (2017)

9.2 APPLICATIONS OF ANTIOXIDANTS

9.2.1 ANTIOXIDANTS IN DERMATOLOGY

Many inflammation conditions demonstrate redox imbalance and significant consumption of their antioxidant systems in local cells such as atopic dermatitis or burned skin, as well as in the scarring process, in which the excess of ROS hinders dermal and epidermal repair, especially in the moment of acute inflammation (Wagener et al., 2013). The use of oral or topical antioxidants in the treatment of dermatoses basically seeks to neutralize excess free radicals, reducing or preventing the attack on cellular structures (Addor, 2017). In this context, the use of concentrations close to the physiological ones is preferential, since they adjust more easily to the cellular physiology, in addition to reducing risks of toxicity or even of drug interaction with any drugs that the patient uses. Effects of antioxidants can vary considerably depending on the concentrations (Sadowska and Bartosz, 2014).

9.2.2 ANTIOXIDANTS IN FOOD

Antioxidants are essential for animal and plant life since they are involved in complex metabolic and signaling mechanisms. They protect plants by producing phytoalexins, for example, isoflavonoid structures, in response to microbiological and fungal pathogen invasion (Ahuja et al., 2012). Vitamin C, vitamin E, and beta carotene are among the most widely studied dietary antioxidants. Vitamin C is considered the most important water-soluble antioxidant in extracellular fluids. It is capable of neutralizing ROS in the aqueous phase before lipid peroxidation is initiated (Kumar, 2014). Antioxidants are known to play a key role in the protective influence exerted by plant foods (Gey, 1990; Gey et al., 1991; Willett, 1991; Liyana et al., 2006). Regular consumption of vegetables and fruits helps one to reduce the risk of chronic diseases (Dembinska et al., 2008). The recommendations on the basis of epidemiological studies are such that fruits, vegetables, and less-processed staple foods ensure the best protection against the development of diseases caused by oxidative stress such as cancer, coronary heart disease, obesity, type 2 diabetes, hypertension, and cataract (Halvorsen et al., 2002). The explanation consists in the beneficial health effect, due to antioxidants present in fruit and vegetables (Halvorsen et al., 2006). Among food components fighting against chronic diseases, great attention has been paid to phytochemicals, plant-derived molecules endowed with steady antioxidant power. The cumulative and synergistic activities of the bioactive molecules present in plant food are responsible for their enhanced antioxidant properties.

9.2.3 IN PREVENTION OF LIPID PEROXIDATION

Lipid peroxidation refers to the oxidative deterioration of lipids containing any number of carbon–carbon double bonds such as unsaturated fatty acids, phospholipids, glycolipids, cholesterol esters, and cholesterol itself. Radical scavengers can directly react and quench peroxide radicals to terminate the chain reaction. Lipid peroxidation and DNA damage are associated with a variety of chronic health problems such as cancer, ageing, and athero-sclerosis (Marnett, 2000; Shigenaga et al., 1994; Bland, 1995). Antioxidant compounds may scavenge ROS and peroxide radicals, thereby preventing or treating certain pathogenic conditions. Lipid peroxidation has been extensively used as a research model for identifying natural antioxidants as well as the studies of their mechanisms of action (Lü et al., 2010).

9.2.4 IN METAL STRESS TOLERANCE

Antioxidant activities are considered as one of the major aspects of bioactivities and are in focus of interest to pharmacists. Free radicals play the major role in pathogenesis of diseases and are important components of stress signal cascades (Castro and Freeman, 2001). Overproduction of ROS is a common response of plants to stress factors caused by heavy metal (Mittler, 2002; Schützendübel et al., 2002), which could react with lipids, proteins, pigments, and nucleic acids and cause lipid peroxidation, membrane damage, and inactivation of enzymes, thus affecting cell viability (Dixit et al., 2001). To maintain the balance between the generation and degradation of ROS, plants induce a diverse array of enzymes, for example, SOD, peroxidase (POD), catalase (CAT), ascorbate peroxidase (APX), and low molecular weight antioxidants such as ascorbic acid (AsA), glutathione (GSH), nonprotein thiol (NPT), and cysteine (Cys) to scavenge different types of ROS, thereby protecting cells against potential tissue dysfunction (Singh et al., 2006). SOD is a key enzyme in protecting cells against oxidative stress, which could transform superoxide radicals

(O_2) into H_2O_2, a less destructive oxygen species, hence decreasing the risk of hydroxyl radical ($\cdot OH^-$) formation (Foyer et al., 1994). CAT, POD, and APX are involved in the destruction of H_2O_2 (Weckx and Clijsters, 1996), while Cys, NPT, AsA, and GSH could directly interact with and detoxify oxygen free-radicals and thus contribute significantly to nonenzymatic ROS scavenging (Garnczarska, 2005).

Apart from the need of bryophytes to neutralize or remove heavy metals from the cells to avoid harmful effects on cellular structures and processes, they also have to possess an antioxidative system to deal with the overproduction of ROS caused by heavy metals. This system comprises numerous enzymes and compounds of low molecular weight (Zengin and Munzuroglu, 2005). SOD is one of the most important enzymes in the protection of plant cells against oxidative stress, since it transforms superoxide radicals into less destructive H_2O_2 that can further be removed by peroxidase (POD), catalase (CAT), or APX. Additionally, low molecular weight compounds such as ascorbic acid (AsA), glutathione, NPT, cysteine, proline, and others could directly interact with and detoxify these reactive species (Sun et al., 2009). Sun et al. (2009, 2010) treated the moss *Hypnum plumaeforme* with different concentrations of Pb and Ni, singly or combined, to investigate the activity of the ROS scavenging system under heavy metal stress in bryophytes. They discovered that the predominant enzyme involved in the bryophyte protection against the oxidative stress induced by heavy metals was POD, with its activity being dose dependent on the concentrations of the applied metals. Additionally, a synergistic effect of these metals with POD activity was observed. The activity of other enzymes (APX and SOD) was only slightly increased, while the catalase activity actually decreased. On the other hand, the accumulation of both of the investigated components of the nonenzymatic antioxidative system (AsA and proline) has been detected, with Pb and Ni displaying a synergistic effect on their accumulation. This indicated that both AsA and proline could be important superoxide anion scavengers in bryophyte cells, with a significant role in the reduction of the damage to cell membranes under heavy metal stress. The accumulation of these two low molecular weight substances in response to the stress induced by metals other than Ni and Pb has also been observed in other plants, indicating that they could represent significant heavy metal tolerance constituents in other bryophytes (Zengin and Munzuroglu, 2005).

9.3 DETERMINATION OF ANTIOXIDATIVE POTENTIAL

9.3.1 DH RADICAL SCAVENGING ASSAY

2,2'-Diphenyl-L-picryl-hydrazyl-hydrate (DPPH) antioxidant method as explained by Blois (1958) was used to investigate the free radical scavenging capacity of the moss, and the absorbance was measured at 517 nm. Ascorbic acid was used as the standard. AA of the moss extract was evaluated using 2,2'-diphenyl-L-picrylhydrazyl (DH) radical scavenging assay following the method of Khaing (2011). The AA potential was calculated as

$$\text{Scavenging activity}\,(\%) = \frac{\text{A blank} - \text{A sample}}{\text{A blank}} \times 100$$

Where, A is Absorbance

9.3.2 ABTS$^{•+}$ RADICAL SCAVENGING ASSAY

The ABTS assay (Manoj and Murugan, 2012) is based on the oxidation of the ABTS by potassium persulfate to form a radical cation ABTS$^+$. The absorbance was taken at 734 nm, and the activity was expressed as percentage inhibition of ABTS radicals.

9.3.3 HYDROGEN PEROXIDE RADICAL

A solution of 40 mM H_2O_2 was prepared in phosphate buffer (pH 7.4). From the extracts, 1.4 mL of different concentrations was added to 0.6 mL of the H_2O_2 solution. The assay mixture could stand for 10 min at 25°C and the absorbance was measured against a blank solution at 230 nm (Delpour et al., 2009).

9.3.4 METAL CHELATING ACTIVITY

The chelation of ferrous ions by terpenoids extract was estimated. The absorbance of the solution was measured at 562 nm. The percentage inhibition of ferrozine–Fe^{2+} complex formation was calculated as [($A0$ - As)/

$A0] \times 100$, where $A0$ was the absorbance of the control, and As was the absorbance of the extract/standard (Dinis et al., 1994).

9.3.5   FRAP (FERRIC REDUCING/ANTIOXIDANT POWER) ASSAY

The FRAP was assayed as per the protocol of Benzie and Strain (1999). The absorbance of the reaction mixture was read at 593 nm spectrophoto-metrically after incubation at 37°C for 10 min.

9.3.6   FTIR SPECTROSCOPY

FTIR spectrometer was used to collect spectra of different solvent extracts of the moss (Kumar et al., 2012). The sample was mixed with KBr. The IR spectrum gives information about the functional groups. The range of measurements is 4000–300 cm^{-1}. The region above 1200 cm^{-1} shows spectral bands due to vibrations of individual functional groups, whereas the region below 1200 cm^{-1} shows bands due to vibrations of whole molecule and is known as the fingerprint region.

9.4   CONCLUSION

In conclusion, the outcomes of this chapter recommend that phenolics and flavonoids are important compounds in plants that contribute to AA. The significant amount of the antioxidant potential is caused by phenolic substances in mosses formation, and the high antioxidant property shown by the plant is mainly due to the presence of considerable amount of terpenoids. Previous research demonstrated that the extract of the bryo-phytes examined here has immense potential to be used in medicine and agricultural use as well as chemical components can be used in pharma-ceutical laboratories as active ingredients for the curing of cancer, and hepatic, cardiovascular, and skin diseases, and other pathologies. The food and cosmetic industries can also discover a powerful source of active molecules in the bryophyte world, taking into account that only a very limited fraction of existing species have been studied and characterized. At present, only about 5% of liverworts are chemically studied worldwide (Asakawa, 2008).

Natural antioxidants form a promising alternative for synthetic antioxidants. Thus, a positive correlation between traditional use and scientific evaluation could create a substitute source of new medicinal compounds, which might overcome the expensive research of synthetic drugs and their detrimental side effects. Bryophytes play an important role in the development of new drugs. This chapter will help the researchers to facilitate all necessary information about the different species of bryophytes as one of the important medicinal plants and development work should be undertaken for the production of plant-based drugs for their better economic and therapeutic utilization for the betterment of mankind. Further, there is a continuous and urgent need to discover new drugs with diverse chemical structures and novel mechanisms of action because there has been an alarming increase in the incidence of new and reemerging infectious diseases.

KEYWORDS

- **bryophytes**
- **antioxidants**
- **DH**
- **FRAP**
- **FTIR**
- **ABTS**
- **ethno medicinal**

REFERENCES

Ahuja, I.; Kissen, R.; Bones, A. M. Phytoalexins in Defense against Pathogens. *Trends Plant Sci.* **2012,** *17*, 73–90.

Akinmoladun, A. C.; Ibukun, E. O.; Obuotor, E. M.; Farombi, E. O. Phytochemical Constituent and Antioxidant Activity of Extract from the Leaves of *Ocimum gratissimum*. *Sci. Res. Essays* **2007,** *2* (5), 163–166.

Anilkumar, V. S.; Dinesh-Babu, K. V.; Sunukumar, S. S.; Murugan, K. Taxonomic Discrimination of *Solanum nigrum* and *S. giganteum* by Fourier Transform Infrared Spectroscopy Data. *J. Res. Biol.* **2012,** *2*, 482–488.

Asakawa, Y. Biologically Active Compounds from Bryophytes. *Pure Appl. Chem.* **2007**, *79*, 557–580.

Asakawa, Y. Maechantiophyta, a Good Source of Biologically Active Compounds. In *Bryology in the New Millennium*; Mohamed, H., Baki, B. B., Boyce, A. N., Lee, P. K. Y., Eds.; University of Malaya: Kuala Lumpur, 2008; p 367.

Aslanbaba, B.; Yilmaz, S.; Tonguc Yayinta, O.; Ozyurt, D.; Ozyurt, B. D. Total Phenol Content and Antioxidant Activity of Mosses from Yenice Forest (Ida Mountain). *J. Sci. Perspect.* **2017**, *1* (1), 1–12.

Azuelo, A. G.; Sariana, L. G.; Pabulan, M. P. Some Medicinal Bryophytes, Their Ethnomedical Uses and Morphology. *Asian J. Biodivers.* **2011**, *2*, 49–80.

Basile, A.; Giordano, S.; López-Sáez J.-A.; Cobianchi, R. C. Antibacterial Activity of Pure Flavonoids Isolated from Mosses. *Phytochemistry* **1999**, *52*, 1479D1482.

Benzie, I. F.; Strain, J. J. Ferric Reducing/Antioxidant Power Assay, Direct Measure of Total Antioxidant Activity of Biological Fluids and Modified Version for Simultaneous Measurement of Total Antioxidant Power and Ascorbic Acid Concentration. *Methods Enzymol.* **1999**, *299*, 15–27.

Bernaert, N. B.; Van Droogenbroeck, C.; Bouten, D.; De Paepe, E.; Van Bockstaele, H.; De Clercq, D.; Stewert, D.; De Loose, M. The Antioxidant Capacity of Leek (*Allium ampeloprasum* var. *porrum*). *Commun. Agric. Appl. Biol. Sci.* **2011**, *76*, 173–176.

Bhattarai, H. D.; Paudel, B.; Lee, H. K.; Oh, H.; Yim, J. H. In Vitro Antioxidant Capacities of Two Benzonaphthoxanthenones, Ohioensins F and G, Isolated from the Antarctic Moss *Polytrichastrum alpinum*. *J. Nat. Res. C* **2009**, *64*, 197–200.

Bhattarai, H. D.; Paudel, B.; Lee, H. S.; Lee, Y. K.; Yim, Y. Antioxidant Activity of *Sanionia uncinata*, a Polar Moss Species from King George Island, Antarctica. *Phytother. Res.* **2008**, *22*, 1635–1639.

Bland, J. S. Oxidants and Antioxidants in Clinical Medicine, Past, Present and Future Potential. *J. Nutr. Environ Med.* **1995**, *5*, 255–280.

Blois, M. Antioxidant Determinations Using a Stable Free Radical. *Nature* **1958**, *181* (4617), 1199–1200.

Castro, L.; Freeman, B. Reactive Oxygen Species in Human Health and Disease. *Nutrition* **2001**, *17*, 163–165.

Chandra, R.; Mishra, R.; Pandey, V. K. Potential of Bryophytes as Therapeutics. *Int. J. Pharm. Sci. Res.* **2014**, *5* (9), 3584–3593. DOI: 10.13040/IJPSR.0975-8232.5 (9).3584-93.

Cheng, A. L.; Sun, X. W.; Lou, H. The Inhibitory Effect of a Monocyclic Bisbibenzylricardin D on the Biofilms of *Candida albicans*. *Biol. Pharm. Bull.* **2001**, *32*, 1417–1421.

Cheng, X.; Xiao, Y.; Wang, X.; Wang, P.; Li, H.; Yan, H.; Liu, Q. Anti-tumor and Pro-apoptic Activity of Ethanolic Extract and Its Various Fractions from *Polytrichum commune* L. Ex Hedw in L1210 Cells. *J. Ethnopharmacol.* **2012**, *143*, 49–56.

Chobot, V.; Kubicova, L.; Nabbout, S.; Jahodar, L.; Hadacek, F. Evaluation of Antioxidant Activity of Some Common Mosses. *J. Nat. Sci.* **2008**, *63*, 476–482.

Chobot, V.; Kubicova, L.; Nabbout, S.; Jahodar, L.; Vytlacilova, J. Antioxidant and Free Radical Scavenging Activities of Five Moss Species. *Phytotherapy* **2006**, *77*, 598–600.

Delpour, A. A.; Ebrahimzadeh, M. A.; Nabawi, S. F.; Nabavi, S. M. Antioxidant Activity of the Methanol Extract of *Ferula assa-foetida* and Its Essential Oil Composition. *Grasas Aceites* **2009**, *60* (4), 405–412.

Dembinska-Kiec, A.; Mykkanen, O.; Kiec-Wilk, B.; Mykkanene, H. Antioxidant Phytochemicals against Type 2 Diabetes. *Br. J. Nutr.* **2008**, *99*, 109–117.

Dey, A.; De, J. N. Antioxidative Potential of Bryophytes, Stress Tolerance and Commercial Perspectives, a Review. *Pharmacologia* **2012**, *3*, 151–159.

Dinis, T. C. P.; Madeira, V. M. C.; Almeida, L. M. Action of Phenolic Derivatives (Acetaminophen, Salicylate and 5-Aminosalicylate) as Inhibitors of Membrane Lipid Peroxidation and as Peroxyl Radical Scavengers. *Arch. Biochem. Biophys.* **1994**, *315* (1), 161–169.

Erturk, O.; Sahın, H.; Erturk, E. Y.; Hotaman, H. E.; Koz, B.; Özdemr, Ö. The Antimicrobial and Antioxidant Activities of Extracts Obtained from Some Moss Species in Turkey. *Herba Pol.* **2015**, *61* (4), 52–65.

Flavia Alvim, S. A. Antioxidants in Dermatology. *An. Bras. Dermatol.* **2017**, *92* (3), 356–362.

Frahm, J. P. Recent Developments of Commercial Products from Bryophytes. *Bryologist* **2004**, *107* (3), 277–283.

Friederich, S.; Maier, U. H.; Deus-Neumann, B. Biosynthesis of Cyclic Bis (Bibenzyls) in *Marchantia polymorpha*. *Phytochemistry* **1999**, *50*, 589–598.

Fu, L.; Xu, B. T.; Xu, X. R.; Gan, R. Y.; Zhang, Y.; Xia, E. Q.; *et al.* Antioxidant Capacities and Total Phenolic Contents of 62 Fruits. *Food Chem.* **2011**, *129*, 345–350.

Garnczarska, M. Response of the Ascorbate-Glutathione Cycle to Re-Aeration Following Hypoxia in Lupine Roots. *Plant Physiol. Biochem.* **2005**, *43*, 583–590.

Gey, K. F. The Antioxidant Hypothesis of Cardiovascular Disease, Epidemiology and Mechanisms. *Biochem. Soc. Trans.* **1990**, *18*, 1041–1045.

Gey, K. F.; Puska, P.; Jordon, P.; Moser, U. K. Total Antioxidant Capacity of Plant Foods. Inverse Correlation between Plasma Vitamin E and Mortality from Ischemic Heart Disease in Cross-Cultural Epidemiology. *Am. J. Clin. Nutr.* **1991**, *53*, 326–334.

Gökbulut, A.; Satilmiş, B.; Batcioğlu, K.; Cetin, B.; Şarer, E. Antioxidant Activity and Luteolin Content of *Marchantia polymorpha* (L.). *Turk J. Biol.* **2012**, *36*, 381–385.

Halvorsen, B. L.; Carlsen, M. H.; Phillips, K. M.; Bohn, S. K.; Holte, K. Content of Redox-Active Compounds (Antioxidants) in Foods Consumed in the United States. *Am. J. Clin. Nutr.* **2006**, *84*, 95–135.

Halvorsen, B. L.; Holte, K.; Myhrstad, M. C. W.; Barikmo, I.; Hvattum, E. A Systematic Screening of Total Antioxidants in Dietary Plants. *J. Nutr.* **2002**, *132*, 461–471.

Irshad, M.; Chaudhuri, P. S. Oxidant-antioxidant System, Role and Significance in Human Body. *Indian J. Exp. Biol.* **2002**, *40*, 1233–1239.

Khaing, T. A. Evaluation of the Antifungal and Antioxidant Activities of the Leaf Extract of *Aloe vera* (*Aloe barbadensis* Miller). *World Acad. Sci. Eng. Technol.* **2011**, *75*, 610–612.

Komala, I.; Ito, T.; Nagashima, F.; Yagi, Y.; Asakawa, Y. Cytotoxic, Radical Scavenging and Antimicrobial Activities of Sesquiterpenoids from the Tahitian Liverwort *Mastigophora diclados* (Brid.) Nees (Mastigophoraceae). *J. Nat. Med.* **2010**, *64* (4), 417–422.

Krishnan, R.; Murugan, K. Polyphenols from *Marchantia polymorpha* L. A Bryophyta, a Potential Source of Antioxidants. *World J. Pharm. Pharm. Sci.* **2013**, *2*, 5182–5198.

Kumar, S. The Importance of Antioxidant and Their Role in Pharmaceutical Science – A Review. *Asian J. Res. Chem. Pharm. Sci.* **2014**, *1* (1), 27–44.

Liyana-Pathirana, C. M.; Shahidi, F.; Alasalvar, C. Antioxidant Activity of Cherry Laurel Fruit (*Laurocerasus officinalis* Roem.) and Its Concentrated Juice. *Food Chem.* **2006**, *99*, 121–128.

Lou, H. X.; Li, G. Y.; Wang, F. Q. A Cytotoxic Diterpenoid and Antifungal Phenolic Compounds from *Frullania muscicola* Steph. *J. Asian Nat. Prod. Res.* **2002,** *4*, 87–94.

Lü, J.-M, Peter, H. L., Qizhi, Y., Changyi, C. Chemical and Molecular Mechanisms of Antioxidants, Experimental Approaches and Model Systems. *J. Cell. Mol. Med.* **2010,** *14* (4). 840–860.

Manoj, G. S.; Murugan, K. Phenolic Profiles, Antimicrobial and Antioxidant Potentiality of Methanolic Extract of a Liverwort *Plagiochila beddomei* Steph. *Indian J. Nat. Prod. Res.* **2012,** *3* (2), 173–183.

Marnett, L. J. Oxyradicals and DNA Damage. *Carcinogenesis* **2000,** *21*, 361–370.

Mohandas, G. G.; Kumaraswamy, M. Antioxidant Activities of Terpenoids from *Thuidium tamariscellum* (C. Muell.) Bosch. and Sande-Lac. A Moss. *Pharmacogn. J.* **2018,** *10* (4), 645–649.

Montenegro, G.; Portalui, M. C.; Salas, F. A.; Diaz, M. F. Biological Properties of Chilean Native Moss *Sphagnum magellanicum. Biol. Res.* **2009,** *42* (2), 233–237.

Niu, C.; Qu, J. B.; Lou, H. X. Antifungal Bis[Bibenzyls] from the Chinese Liverwort *Marchantia polymorpha* L. *Chem. Biodivers.* **2006,** *3*, 34–40.

Opelt, K.; Chobot, V.; Hadacek, F.; Schönmann, S.; Eberl, L.; Berg, G. Investigations of the Structure and Function of Bacterial Communities Associated with *Sphagnum* Mosses. *Environ. Microbiol.* **2007,** *9*, 2795–2809.

Pejin, B.; Bogdanović-Pristov, J. ABTS Cation Scavenging Activity and Total Phenolic Content of Three Moss Species. *Hem. Ind.* **2012,** *66* (5), 723–726.

Pejin, B.; Bogdanovic-Pristov, J.; Pejin, I.; Sabovljevic, M. Potential Antioxidant Activity of the Moss *Bryum moravicum. Nat. Prod. Res.* **2013,** *27*, 900–902.

Polterait, O. Antioxidants and Free-Radical Scavengers of Natural Origin. *Curr. Org. Chem.* **1997,** *1*, 415–440.

Sadowska-Bartosz, I.; Bartosz, G. Effect of Antioxidants Supplementation on Aging and Longevity. *Biomed. Res. Int.* **2014,** *2014*, 404680.

Saroya, A. S. *Herbalism, Phytochemistry, and Ethnopharmacology.* Science Publishers: Punjab, 2011; pp 286–293.

Shigenaga, M. K.; Hagen, T. M.; Ames, B. N. Oxidative Damage and Mitochondrial Decay in Aging. *Proc. Natl. Acad. Sci. U.S.A.* **1994,** *91*, 10771–10778.

Singh, M.; Govindrajan, R.; Nath, V.; Rawat, A. K. S.; Mehrotra, S. Antimicrobial, Wound Healing and Antioxidant Activity of *Plagiochasma appendiculatum* Lehm. et Lind. *J Ethnopharmacol.* **2006,** *107*, 67–72.

Singh, M.; Rawat, A. K. S.; Govindarajan, R. Antimicrobial Activity of Some Indian Mosses. *Phytotherapy* **2007,** *78*, 156–158.

Spjut, R. W.; Suffness, M.; Cragg, G. M.; Norris, D. H. Mosses, Liverworts and Hornworts Screened for Antitumor Agents. *Econ. Bot.* **1986,** *40* (3), 310–338.

Tanaka, K. S.; Takio, S.; Yamamoto, I.; Satoh, T. Characterization of a cDNA Encoding CuZn-superoxide dismutase from the liverwort *Marchantia paleacea* var. diptera. *Plant Cell Physiol.* **1998,** *39*, 235–240.

Tazaki, H.; Ito, M.; Miyoshi, M.; Kawabata, J.; Fukushi, E.; Fujita, T.; et al. Subulatin, an Antioxidic Caffeic Acid Derivative Isolated from the In Vitro Cultured Liverworts, *Jungermannia subulata, Lophocolea heterophylla*, and *Scapania parvitexta. Biosci. Biotechnol. Biochem.* **2002,** *66* (2), 255–261.

Wagener, F. A.; Carels, C. E.; Lundvig, D. M. Targeting the Redox Balance in Inflammatory Skin Conditions. *Int. J. Mol. Sci.* **2013,** *14*, 9126–9167.

Weckx, J. E. J.; Clijsters, H. M. M. Oxidative Damage and Defense Mechanisms in Primary Leaves of *Phaseolus vulgaris* as a Result of Root Assimilation of Toxic Amounts of Copper. *Physiol. Plant.* **1996,** *96*, 506–512.

Willett, W. C. Micro-nutrients and Cancer Risk. *J. Am. Med. Assoc.* **1991,** *53*, 265–269.

Xie, C. F.; Lou, H. X. Secondary Metabolites in Bryophytes, an Ecological Aspect. *Chem. Biodivers.* **2009,** *6*, 303–312.

Yayintas Tonguc, O.; Alpaslan, D.; Yuceer Karagul, Y.; Yilmaz, S.; Sahiner, N. Chemical Composition, Antimicrobial, Antioxidant and Anthocyanin Activities of Mosses (*Cinclidotus fontinaloides* (Hedw.) P.Beauv. and *Palustriella commutata* (Hedw.) Ochyra) Gathered from Turkey. *Nat. Prod. Res.* **2017,** *31* (18), 2169–2173.

Zheng, W.; Wang, S. Y. Antioxidant Activity and Phenolic Compounds in Selected Herbs. *J. Agric. Food Chem.* **2001,** *49*, 5165–5170.

Zinsmeister, H. D.; Mues, R. The Flavonoid Chemistry of Bryophytes. *Rev. Latinoam. Quim.* **1980,** *11*, 23–29.

CHAPTER 10

Natural Antioxidants in the Management of Alzheimer's Disease

EKTA KHARE

School of Pharmacy, ITM University, Gwalior, Madhya Pradesh, India

E-mail: ektakhare23@gmail.com

ABSTRACT

Alzheimer's disease is a neurodegenerative one characterized by gradual changes in behavior because of aggregation of amyloid β protein and tau (τ) protein which blocks signal transduction pathway. There is one hypothesis that accounts for the heterogeneous nature of Alzheimer in the involvement of free radicals. The probability of this involvement includes oxidative stress that accumulates free radicals and leads to excessive lipid peroxidation and neuronal degeneration in certain brain regions. Our brain utilizes more oxygen than other tissues and undergoes mitochondrial respiration, which increases the potential for reactive oxygen species (ROS) exposure. In this way, oxidative imbalance and stress play a crucial role in the pathogenesis of neuron degeneration and it remains as a challenge to design some sort of treatment intervention because it lacks typical treatment target. In this chapter, we will describe natural antioxidants that are capable of scavenging free radicals, donating hydrogen and electrons, and providing reducing activity.

10.1 INTRODUCTION

10.1.1 ALZHEIMER'S DISEASE

Alzheimer's disease (AD) is neurodegenerative one characterized by gradual changes in behavior because of aggregation of amyloid β protein and tau (τ) protein which blocks signal transduction pathway. There is one hypothesis that accounts for the heterogeneous nature of Alzheimer in the involvement of free radicals. The probability of this involvement includes oxidative stress that accumulates free radicals and leads to excessive lipid peroxidation and neuronal degeneration in certain brain regions. Our brain utilizes more oxygen than other tissues and undergoes mitochondrial respiration, which increases the potential for ROS exposure. In this way, oxidative imbalance and stress play a crucial role in the pathogenesis of neuron degeneration, and it remains as challenge to design some sort of treatment intervention because it lacks typical treatment target. In this chapter, we will describe natural antioxidants that are capable of scavenging free radicals, donating hydrogen and electrons, and providing reducing activity.

Nowadays, the problem of this neurodegenerative disorder is common. Early scientist was thinking that it occurs after the age of 60 but in todays' generation it spreads. Even a woman, who is diseased, is characterized by typical neuropathology, impaired synaptic function, and massive cell loss. The patho-biochemistry of this disorder involves oxidative stress that accumulates free radicals leading to excessive lipid peroxidation and neuronal degeneration in certain brain regions. Moreover, radical-induced disturbances of DNA, proteins, and lipid membranes have been measured. The hypothesis has been proposed that cellular events involving oxidative stress may be one basic pathway leading to neurodegeneration in AD. In this work, there is evidence for increased oxidative stress and disturbed defense mechanisms in AD, which may result in a self-propagating cascade of neurodegenerative events. Furthermore, it is evident from experimental data that aggregation of amyloid is favorably caused by oxidative stress. Therefore, oxidative stress plays a key role in the conversion of soluble to unsoluble amyloid, suggesting that oxidative stress is primary to the amyloid cascade.

10.1.2   OXIDATIVE DAMAGE

Oxidative stress can attack on brain cells by chemicals called free radicals. Free radical–induced oxidative damage may play a role for neurodegeneration of AD. Free radicals are reactive oxygen compounds that may damage lipids and proteins. As per literature review, evidence for oxidative damage has been obtained from postmortem brain tissue as well as from living patients with AD. It is caused when the brain utilizes more oxygen than other tissues and undergoes mitochondrial respiration that increases the potential for ROS exposure (Fig. 10.1). AD is also associated with the augmentation of protein oxidation, protein nitration, glycoloxidation, and lipid peroxidation as well as the accumulation of Aβ protein. The treatment with antioxidant compounds would provide protection against oxidative stress and Aβ toxicity.

However, oxidative stress is only a single feature of AD; therefore, antioxidant strategy was challenged for its potency to stop the progression of AD. Various natural antioxidants show promising activity in treating the disease.

Oxidative stress is caused mainly by the following:

- Mutation or decreased activity of catalase and glutathione peroxidase enzyme
- Decreased intake of exogenous antioxidants from food
- Increased amount of metal ion like Fe, Cu, and Cr
- Easily peroxidized amino acids like lysine
- Increased triplet oxygen ($3O_2$) concentration
- Increased physical activity of an untrained individual
- ROS from ionizing radiation, air pollution, and smoking
- Chronic inflammation (Poljsak, 2013)

Excessive generation of free radicals may overwhelm natural cellular antioxidant defenses, which may lead to oxidation and further functional impairment. These reductions of oxidative stress can be achieved by the three following levels:

I.   By lowering exposure to environmental pollutants.
II. By increasing the level of endogenous and exogenous antioxidants to scavenge ROS before causing any damage.
III. By stabilizing mitochondrial energy production and reducing amount of ROS formed per amount of oxygen consumed (Xiaoguang, 2018).

10.1.3   FREE RADICALS INVOLVED IN ALZHEIMER'S AND RADICAL SCAVENGERS

Various free radicals are involved in AD. Due to toxicity and its role in chemical reactions, these free radicals are suspected to be the cause of

Alzheimer's. Hydroxyl, super oxide radical hydrogen peroxide, and peroxynitrile may be formed by combining superoxide and nitric oxide. These peroxynitrites can react with carbon dioxide to form unstable transmitters that may act as free hydroxyl radical.

Radical scavengers are the agents that interact directly with the free radicals and thus reduce oxidative stress. A considerable number of substances with radical scavenging properties are known and evaluated in pharmacological trials. From a clinical point of view, the following should be mentioned: Gingko biloba, vitamin A, vitamin C, vitamin E, and idebenone.

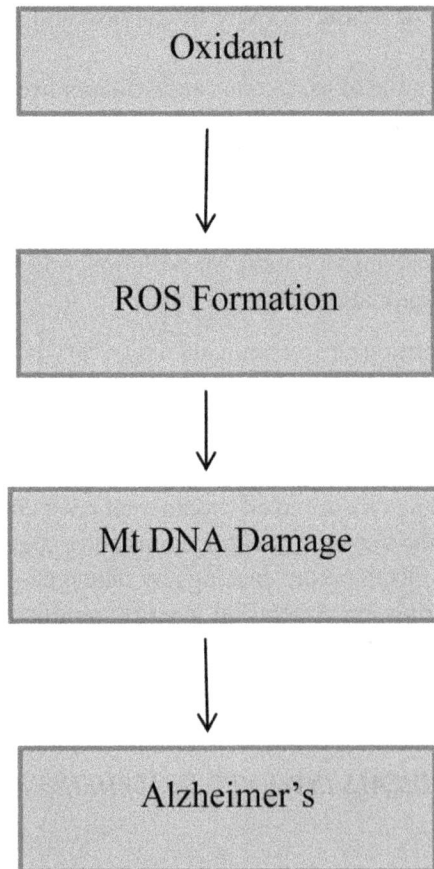

FIGURE 10.1   Pathway of showing how free radicals are causing Alzheimer's.

10.2 DEFENCES AGAINST ROS AND STRATEGIES TO REDUCE OXIDATIVE STRESS

Generation of ROS and the activity of antioxidant defenses are balanced in vivo. The balance may be slightly tied in favor of ROS so that there is continuous low-level oxidative damage in the human body. In addition to the endogenous and exogenous antioxidative protection, the second category of defense is repair processes that remove the damaged biomolecules before they accumulate to cause altered cell metabolism or viability.

10.2.1 PRIMARY ANTIOXIDANT DEFENSES

I. **Superoxide dismutase (SOD)**
    Superoxide dismutases (SODs) are a group of metalloenzymes which catalyze the conversion of superoxide anion to hydrogen peroxide and dioxygen. This reaction is a source of cellular hydrogen peroxide.

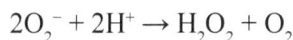

    $$2O_2^- + 2H^+ \rightarrow H_2O_2 + O_2$$

II. **Catalase**
    Hydrogen peroxide formed is scavenged by heme protein catalase. It catalyzes the dismutation of hydrogen peroxide into water and molecular oxygen.

    $$2H_2O_2 \rightarrow O_2 + 2H_2O$$

    One antioxidative role of catalases is to lower the risk of hydroxyl radical formation from H_2O_2 via Fenton reaction catalyzed by chromium or ferrous ions.

III. **Glutathione peroxidase (GPx)**
    All glutathione peroxidases may catalyze the reduction of H_2O_2 using glutathione (GSH) as a substrate. They can also reduce other peroxides (e.g., lipid peroxides in cell membranes) to alcohols.

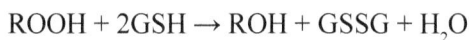

    $$ROOH + 2GSH \rightarrow ROH + GSSG + H_2O$$

    It is responsible for the detoxification of low H_2O_2 amounts, while in higher H_2O_2 amounts, catalase takes the leading part in cellular detoxification.

IV. Glutathione-related systems

GSH is the most abundant intracellular thiol-based antioxidant, present in millimolar concentrations in all aerobic cells. It is a sulfhydryl buffer that detoxifies compounds through conjugation reactions catalyzed by glutathione-*S*-transferases, directly with peroxide in the GPx-catalyzed reaction.

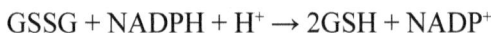

$$GSSG + NADPH + H^+ \rightarrow 2GSH + NADP^+$$

The NADPH required is from several reactions, the best known from the oxidative phase of pentose phosphate pathway. Both glutathione reductase and glucose-6-phosphate dehydrogenase are involved in the glutathione recycling system (Poljsak, 2013).

10.2.2   SECONDARY ANTIOXIDANT DEFENSES

The antioxidant enzymes do not prevent the oxidative damage completely. Age-related oxidative changes are most common in nonproliferating cells as there is no dilution effect of damaged structures through cell division.

There is an age-related decline in proteasome activity and proteasome content in different tissues which leads to the accumulation of oxidatively modified proteins. Proteosomes are a part of the protein-removal system in eukaryotic cells. In addition to elevated levels of oxidized proteins, oxidized lipids, advanced DNA oxidation, and glycol-oxidation end products have shown that proteasome inhibition is a mediator of oxidative stress and ROS production and is affecting mitochondrial function.

An important player in the immediate cellular response to ROS-induced DNA damage is the enzyme polymerase. It recognizes DNA lesions and flags them for repair. Lipid peroxides or damaged lipids are metabolized by peroxidases or lipases. An antioxidant defense seems to be approximately balanced with the generation of ROS in vivo (Poljsak, 2013).

10.3   ANTIOXIDANT

On account of their pharmacological point of attack, these substances intervene in the process of the emergence of oxidative stress, prevent the production of free radicals or reduce them. The best known substance from this group is *selegiline*. A further drug with possible antioxidative effects in Alzheimer's dementia is *tenilsetam*. Future candidates may arrive from the group of antiphlogistics.

Huge numbers of different substances can act as antioxidants. Some of the most well known include vitamin C, vitamin E, beta-carotene and other related carotenoids, flavonoids, phenols, and many more. Putting all these chemicals into one large group is actually quite misleading.

Each antioxidant has a different chemical composition, behaves slightly different, and has a slightly different role. This makes it difficult to examine antioxidants as a general and single aspect in dementia risk. Brains of people with AD appear to have higher levels of natural antioxidants responsible for "clearing up" excess free radicals, suggesting that the body is trying to combat this damage.

10.3.1 NATURAL ANTIOXIDANT

10.3.1.1 VITAMIN-E (α-TOCOPHEROL)

A powerful, lipid-soluble antioxidant is found in lipid membranes, circulating lipoproteins and low-density lipoprotein particles. It has been shown to decrease free radical–mediated damage caused by toxic chain reactions in neuronal cells and helps to inhibit dementia pathogenesis in mammalian cells.

The biological function of vitamin E (Fig. 10.2) may be related to its membrane localization property. Generation of superoxide radicals may be enhanced during vitamin E deficiency. Thus, vitamin E may modulate xenobiotic metabolism by altering the activities of microsomal enzymes. Vitamin E may regulate immune response or cell-mediated immunity by modulating the generation of prostaglandins and other lipid peroxidation products (Ching kuano, 1991).

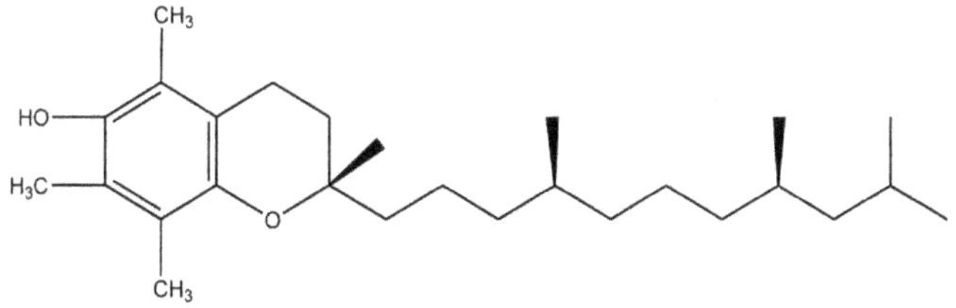

FIGURE 10.2   Vitamin-E (α-tocopherol).

10.3.1.2   VITAMIN C

It is a water-soluble antioxidant and an inhibitor of lipid peroxidation which acts as a major defense against free radicals in whole blood and plasma. This antioxidant is hydrophilic because p*K*a of ascorbic acid is 4.25; the ascorbate anion is the predominant form existing at physiological pH in the blood. Vitamin C (Fig. 10.3) can act directly scavenging superoxide, hydroxyl, and lipid hydroperoxide radicals, playing an important role in recycling of vitamin E. The most striking chemical activity of ascorbic acid is its ability to act as a reducing agent, implicated in detoxifying various oxygen radicals in vivo. The donation of one electron by ascorbic acid produces semidehydro ascorbate radical, which can be further oxidized to DHA. The change in DHA/Asc ratio is commonly used for the estimation of antioxidant role of ascorbic acid (Popovic, 2015).

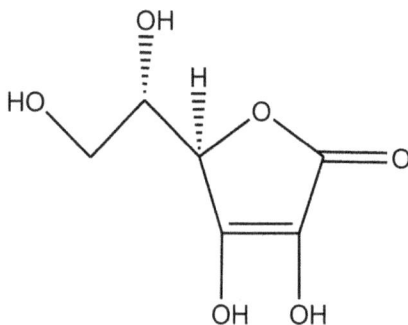

FIGURE 10.3   Structure of vitamin C.

10.3.1.3   CURCUMIN

Curcumin is a yellow pigment of turmeric, a spice manufactured from the root of *Curcuma longa*. Turmeric is one of the major spices in certain Asian cuisines. An antioxidant that has antioxidant, anti-inflammatory and anti-amyloid pathology activity in an Alzheimer's which makes curcumin a superb antioxidant. In the keto form of curcumin, the heptadienone linkage between the two methoxyphenolrings contains a highly activated carbon atom. It is obvious that the C–H bonds on this carbon should be very weak, due to the delocalization of the unpaired electron on the adjacent oxygens. If this is the case, this group can serve as an H-atom donor (Jovanovic, 1999).

The antioxidant activity of curcumin (1,7-bi(4-hydroxy-3-meth-oxyphenyl)-1,6-heptadiene-3,5-dione) was determined by the inhibition of controlled initiation of styrene oxidation. Synthetic nonphenolic curcuminoids exhibited no antioxidant activity; therefore, curcumin is a classical phenolic chain-breaking antioxidant, donating H atoms from the phenolic groups, not the CH_2 group, as has been suggested. The antioxidant activities of *o*-methoxyphenols are decreased in hydrogen bond accepting media (Ross, 2000).

10.3.1.4 VITAMIN B_{12}

In vitro evidence in human aortic endothelial cells showed that supplementation of physiologically relevant concentrations of cyanocobalamin (Fig. 10.4) decreases superoxide levels in the cytosol and the mitochondria. If subclinical B_{12} deficiency indeed mediates oxidative stress through any of the proposed mechanisms, oxidative by-products may, in turn, impair cellular B_{12} uptake. This theory concerns advanced glycation end products (AGEs) that constitute proteins or lipids that are glycated by sugar molecules. It has been posited that AGEs can induce oxidative stress and impair cellular B_{12} uptake and that oxidative stress can likewise contribute to AGE formation. This would create a positive feedback cycle where (subclinical) B_{12} deficiency mediates oxidative stress, and oxidative stress impairs cellular B_{12} uptake through AGE formation, thus perpetuating the B_{12} deficiency.

An overview of the potential role of subclinical B_{12} deficiency in oxidative stress and the onset of age-related diseases results suggest that B_{12} might protect against inflammation-induced oxidative stress by modulating the expression of cytokines and growth factors. It is hypothesized that B_{12} might achieve this by modifying the activity of transcription factors. An antioxidant that increases choline acetyltransferase activity in cholinergic neurons in cats and improves cognitive functions in AD patients (Van de Lagemaat et al., 2019).

10.3.1.5 B-CAROTENE

A lipid-soluble antioxidant that may reduce lipid peroxidation and improve antioxidant status. β-Carotene (Fig. 10.5) scavenges radical species by at least two independent pathways: electron transfer and radical-addition. The antioxidant properties of β carotene perhaps in combination with its immunomodulating properties are believed to play an important role in preventing disease initiation and progression (Steven, 1995).

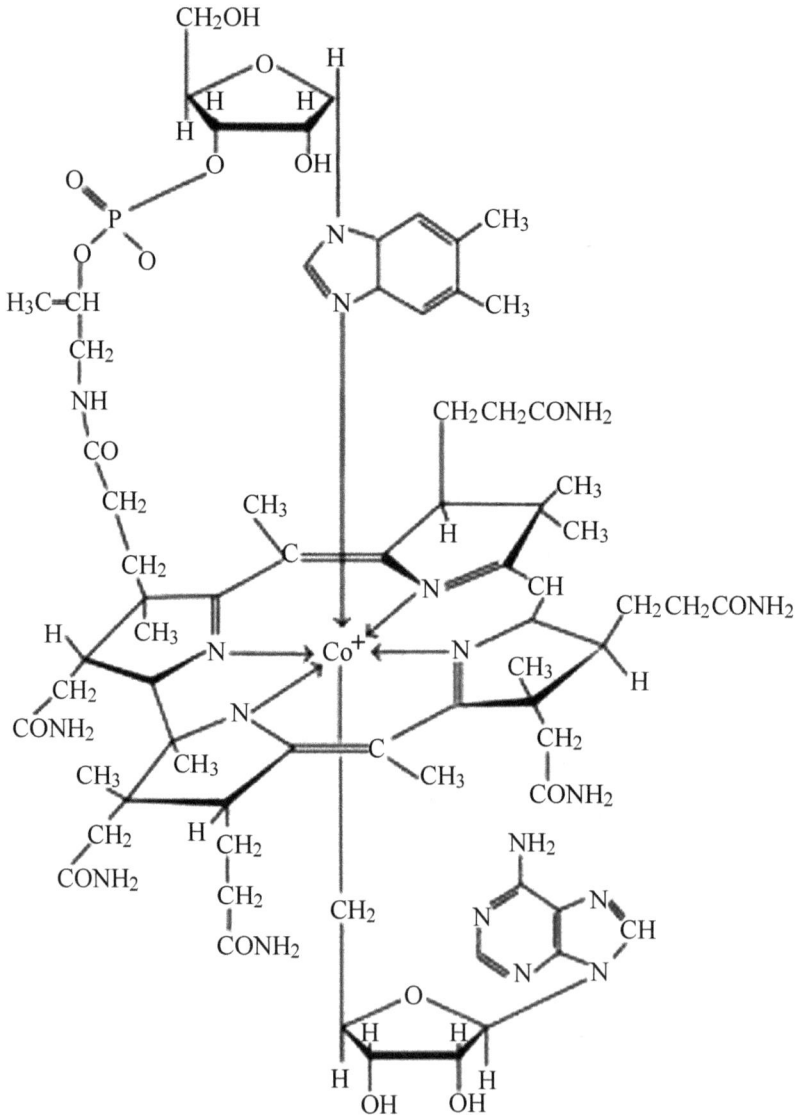

FIGURE 10.4   Structure of vitamin B^{12}.

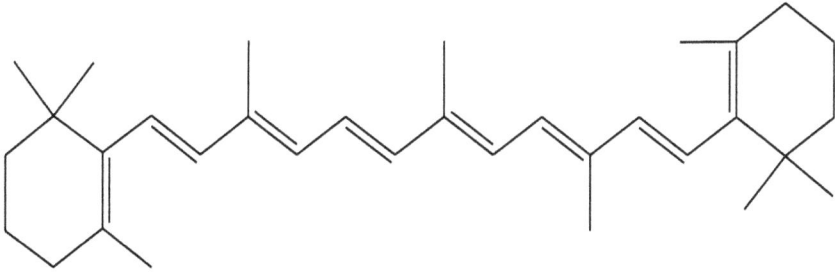

FIGURE 10.5   Structure of *β-carotene*.

10.3.1.6   CAFFIENE

Coffee (Fig. 10.6) is a rich source of dietary antioxidants that can inhibit Aβ production and reduce Aβ levels in brain for early onset familiar AD.

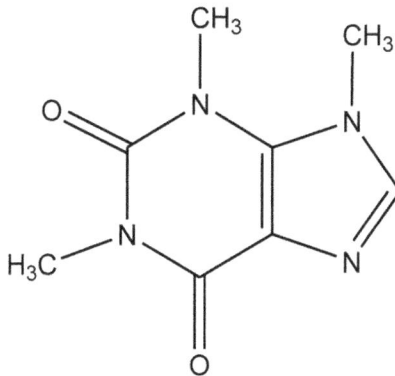

FIGURE 10.6   Structure of Caffiene.

10.3.1.7   CoQ10 (UBIQUINONE)

CoQ10 is a cofactor of the electron transportchain (Fig. 10.7). It preserves mitochondrial membrane potential during oxidative stress and protects neuronal cells through attenuating Aβ overproduction and intracellular Aβ plaque deposits.

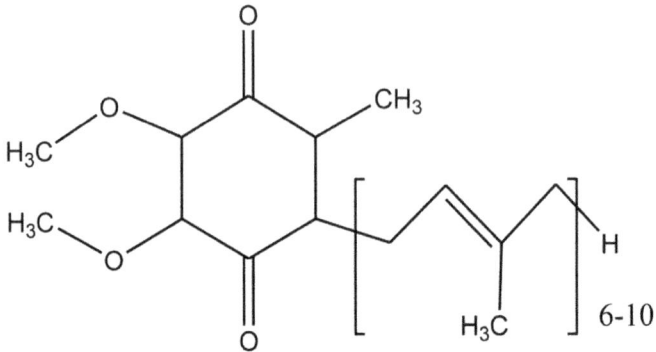

FIGURE 10.7   Structure of CoQ10 (ubiquinone).

10.3.1.8 POLYPHENOLS

Polyphenols are secondary metabolites of plants, and they are found largely in fruits, vegetables, cereals, and beverages. The phenolic compounds of wine can be divided into flavonoids and nonflavonoids. Flavanoid quercetin is an antioxidant agent present in wine that has been shown to prevent or delay the initiation of Alzheimer's through different biological effects (Ilaria, 2018).

10.4 CONCLUSION

Excessive production of ROS and reduced antioxidant defense with age significantly. Genetic, medical, environmental, and lifestyle-related factors for AD are associated with increased oxidative stress. At the preclinical stage of AD, there is consistent evidence that oxidative insult is a significant early event in the pathologic cascade of AD. It is important to note that these were trials on supplements increasing levels of antioxidants by increasing fresh fruit and vegetable consumption which is associated with many long-term benefits. Focusing on recently reported modifiable risk factors for AD, daily diet and physical activity may be important targets in the antioxidative strategy for the prevention and treatment of AD. Natural antioxidant supplements may help to correct the high levels of oxidative stress that cannot be controlled by the synthetic or endogenous antioxidant systems.

KEYWORDS

- **Alzheimer's disease**
- **oxidative stress**
- **free radicals**
- **radical scavengers**
- **defenses against ROS and strategies to reduce oxidative stress**
- **natural antioxidants**

REFERENCES

Adair, J. C.; Knoefel, J. E.; Morgan, N. Controlled Trial of *N*-Acetylcysteine for Patients with Probable Alzheimer's Disease. *Neurology* **2001**, *57* (8), 1515–1517.

Ahmed, T.; Javed, S.; Javed, S.; et al. Resveratrol and Alzheimer's Disease, Mechanistic Insights. *Mol. Neurobiol.* **2017**, *54* (4), 2622–2635.

Andrade, S.; Ramalho, M. J.; Loureiro, J. A.; Pereira, M. C. Natural Compounds for Alzheimer's Disease Therapy, A Systematic Review of Preclinical and Clinical Studies. *Int. J. Mol. Sci.* **2019**, *20*, 2313.

Badia, M.; Giraldo, E.; Dasi, F.; et al. Reductive stress in Young Healthy Individuals at Risk of Alzheimer Disease. *Free Radical Biol. Med.* **2013**, *63*, 274–279.

Baldeiras, I.; Santana, I.; Proenca, M. T.; et al. Peripheral Oxidative Damage in Mild Cognitive Impairment and Mild Alzheimer's Disease. *J. Alzheimer's Disease,* **2008**, *15* (1), 117–128.

Beckman, K. B.; Ames B.N. The Free Radical Theory of Aging Matures. *Physiol. Rev.* **1998**, *78*, 547–581.

Behrens, M. I.; Silva, M.; Salech, F.; et al. Inverse Susceptibility to Oxidative Death of Lymphocytes Obtained from Alzheimer's Patients and Skin Cancer Survivors, Increased Apoptosis in Alzheimer's and Reduced Necrosis in Cancer. *J. Gerontol. Ser. A* **2012**, *67* (10), 1036–1040.

Bermejo, P.; Martin Aragon, S.; Benedi, J. et al. Peripheral Levels of Glutathione and Protein Oxidation as Markers in the Development of Alzheimer's Disease from Mild Cognitive Impairment. *Free Radical Res.* **2009**, *42* (2), 162–170.

Bjertness, E.; Candy, J. M.; Torvik, A. et al. Content of Brain Aluminum is not Elevated in Alzheimer Disease. *Alzheimer Dis. Assoc. Disord.* **1996**, *10*, 171–174.

Bulteau, M.; Ikeda-Saito, L.; Szweda, I. Redox-Dependent Modulation of Aconitase Activity in Intact Mitochondria. *Biochemistry* **2003**, *42* (50), 14846–14855.

Calabrese, V.; Sultana, R.; Scapagnini, G.; et al. Nitrosative Stress, Cellular Stress Response, and Thiol Homeostasis in Patients with Alzheimer's Disease. *Antioxidants Redox Signal.* **2006**, *8* (11–12), 1975–1986.

Cardinali, D. P.; Furio, A. M.; Brusco, L. I. Clinical Aspects of Melatonin Intervention in Alzheimer's Disease Progression. *Curr. Neuropharmacol.* **2010**, *8* (3), 218–227.

Casteilla, L., Rigoulet, M., Penicaud L. Mitochondrial ROS Metabolism, Modulation by Uncoupling Proteins. *Life,* **2001**, *52*, 181–188.

Cataldo, A. M.; Hamilton, D. J.; Nixon, R. A. Lysosomal Abnormalities in Degenerating Neurons Link Neuronalcompromise to Senile Plaque Development in Alzheimer Disease. *Brain Res.* **1994**, *640*, 68–80.

Cataldo, A. M.; Paskevich, P. A.; Kominami, E.; Nixon, R. A. Lysosomal Hydrolases of Different Classes are Abnormally Distributed in Brains of Patients with Alzheimer Disease. *Proc. Natl. Acad. Sci. U.S.A.* **1991,** *88*, 10998–11002.

Cataldo, A. M.; Thayer, C. Y.; Bird, E. D.; Wheelock, T. R.; Nixon, R. A. Lysosomal Proteinase Antigens are Prominently Localized Within Senile Plaques of Alzheimer's Disease, Evidence for a Neuronal Origin. *Brain Res.* **1990,** *513*, 181–192.

Chaturvedi, R. K.; Flint Beal, M. Mitochondrial Diseases of the Brain. *Free Radic. Biol. Med.* **2013,** *63*, 1–29.

Ching kuano, C. Vitamin E and Oxidative Stress. *Free Radical Biol. Med.* **1991,** *1* (1), 215–232.

Choi, H., Park, H. H.; Koh, S. H.; et al. Coenzyme Q10 Protects Against Amyloid Beta-Induced Neuronal Cell Death by Inhibiting Oxidative Stress and Activating the P13K Pathway. *Neurotoxicology* **2012**, *33* (1), 85–90.

Cornelius, C.; Trovato Salinaro, A.; Scuto, M.; et al. Cellular Stress Response, Sirtuins and UCP Proteins in Alzheimer Disease, Role of Vitagenes. *Immun. Ageing,* **2013,** *10* (1), 41–45.

Craer, D. R.; Quittkat, S.; Krishnan, S. S.; Dalton, A. J.; De Boni, U. Intranuclear Aluminum Content in Alzheimer's Disease, Dialysis Encephalopathy, and Experimental Aluminum Encephalopathy. *Acta Neuropathol.* **1980,** *50*, 19–24.

Davies, K. J. Oxidative Stress, the Paradox of Aerobic Life. *Biochem. Soc. Symp.* **1995,** *61*, 1–31.

Di Domenico, F.; Barone, E.; Perluigi, M.; Butterfield, D. A. Strategy to Reduce Free Radical Species in Alzheimer's Disease, An Update of Selected Antioxidants. *Exp. Rev. Neurotherapeutics* **2015**, *15* (1), 19–40.

Dorszewska, J.; Jaroszewska Kolecka J.; et al. Expression and Polymorphisms of Gene 8-Oxoguanine Glycosylase 1 and the Level of Oxidative DNA Damage in Peripheral Blood Lymphocytes of Patients with Alzheimer's Disease. *DNA Cell Biol.* **2009**, *28* (11), 579–588.

Du, X.; Wang, X.; Geng, M. Alzheimer's Disease Hypothesis and Related Therapies. *Transl. Neurodegener.* **2018**, *7*, 2–7.

Everett, S. A.; Kundu, S. C.; Willson, R. Mechanism of Free Radical Scavenging by the Nutritional Antioxidant β-Carotene. *Biochem. Soc. Trans.* **1995**, *23*, 230–247.

Fata, G.; Weber, P.; Mohajeri, M. Effects of Vitamin E on Cognitive Performance During Ageing and in Alzheimer's Disease. *Nutrients* **2014**, *6* (12), 5453–5472.

Feldhaus, P.; Fraga, D. B.; Ghedim, F. V.; et al. Evaluation of Respiratory Chain Activity in Lymphocytes of Patients with Alzheimer Disease. *Metabolic Brain Dis.* **2011**, *26* (3), 229–236.

Fontana, L.; Klein, S. Aging, Adiposity and Calorie Restriction. *JAMA* **2007,** *297*, 986–994.

Gabbita, S. P.; Aksenov, M. Y.; Lovell, M. A.; Markesbery, W. R. Decrease in Peptide Methionine Sulfoxide Reductase in Alzheimer's Disease Brain. *J. Neurochem.* **1999,** *73* (4), 1660–1666.

Galasko, D. R.; Peskind, E.; Clark, C. M. et al. Antioxidants for Alzheimer Disease, A Randomized Clinical Trial with Cerebrospinal Fluid Biomarker Measures. *Arch. Neurol.* **2012**, *69* (7), 836–841.

Gatta, L.; Cardinale, A.; Wannenes, F.; et al. Peripheral Blood Mononuclear Cells from Mild Cognitive Impairment Patients Show Deregulation of Bax and Sod1 mRNAs. *Neurosci. Lett.* **2009**, *453* (1), 36–40.

Gilca, M.; Stoian, I.; Atanasiu, V.; Virgolici B. The Oxidative Hypothesis of Senescence. *J. Postgrad. Med.* **2007**, *53* (3), 207–213.

Grimm, M. O.; Mett, J.; Hartmann, T. The Impact of Vitamin E and Other Fat-Soluble Vitamins on Alzheimer's Disease. *Int. J. Mol. Sci.* **2016**, *17* (11), 234–237.

Hajipour, M. J.; Santoso, M. R.; Rezaee, F.; Aghaverdi, H.; Mahmoudi, M.; Perry, G. Advances in Alzheimer's Diagnosis and Therapy, the Implications of Nanotechnology. *Trends Biotechnol.* **2017**, *35* (10), 937–953.

Hansford, R. G.; Hogue, B. A.; Mildaziene, V. Dependence of H_2O_2 Formation by Rat Heart Mitochondria on Substrate Availability and Donor Age. *J. Bioenerg. Biomembr.* **1997**, *29*, 89–95.

Hargreaves. Coenzyme Q_{10} as a Therapy for Mitochondrial Disease. *Int. J. Biochem. Cell Biol.* **2014**, *49*, 105–111.

Harman, D. A Biologic Clock, the Mitochondria. *J. Am. Geriatrics Soc.* **1972**, *20*, 145–147.

Harman, D. Aging, a Theory based on Free Radical and Radiation Chemistry. *J. Gerontol.* **1956**, *11*, 298–300.

Ishizuka, K.; Kimura, T.; Yoshitake, J.; et al. Possible Assessment for Antioxidant Capacity in Alzheimer's Disease by Measuring Lymphocyte Heme Oxygenase-1 Expression with Real-Time RT-PCR. *Ann. N. Y. Acad. Sci.* **2002**, *977* (1), 173–178.

Jiang, T.; Sun, Q.; Chen, S. Oxidative Stress, A Major Pathogenesis and Potential Therapeutic Target of Antioxidative Agents in Parkinson's Disease and Alzheimer's Disease. *Progr. Neurobiol.* **2016**, *147*, 1–19.

Jovanovic, S. V.; Steenken, S.; Boone, C. W.; Simic, M. G. H-Atom Transfer Is A Preferred Antioxidant Mechanism of Curcumin. *J. Am. Chem. Soc.* **1999**, *121*, 9677–9681.

Kennard, M. L.; Feldman, H.; Yamada, T.; Jefferies, W. A. Serum Levels of the Iron Binding Protein p97 are Elevated in Alzheimer's Disease. *Nat. Med.* **1996**, *2*, 1230–1235.

Khan, T. K.; Alkon, D. L. Peripheral Biomarkers of Alzheimer's Disease. *J. Alzheimer's Dis.* **2015**, *44* (3), 729–744.

Kirkwood, B.; Mathers, J. C. The Basic Biology of Aging. In *Healthy Aging—The Role of Nutrition and Lifestyle*; Stanner, S., Thompson, R., Buttriss, J., Eds.; Wiley_Blackwell, 2009, vol. 1, 667–1698.

Kravitz, S.; Mawal, Y.; et al. Characterization of α_1-Antitrypsin as a Heme Oxygenase-1 Suppressor in Alzheimer Plasma. *Neurobiol. Disease* **2006**, *24* (1), 89–100.

Kryscio, R. J.; Abner, E. L.; Caban-Holt, A.; et al. Association of Antioxidant Supplement Use and Dementia in the Prevention of Alzheimer's Disease by Vitamin E and Selenium Trial. *Neurology* **2017**, *74* (5), 567–573.

Lee, J. M.; Johnson, J. A. An Important Role of Nrf_2-ARE Pathway in the Cellular Defense Mechanism. *J. Biochem. Mol. Biol.* **2004**, *37* (2), 139–143.

Liu, Y.; Ai, K.; Ji, X.; et al. Comprehensive Insights into the Multi-Antioxidative Mechanisms of Melanin Nanoparticles and their Application to Protect Brain from Injury in Ischemic Stroke. *J. Am. Chem. Soc.* **2017**, *139* (2), 856–862.

Lovell, M. A.; Xie, C.; Gabbita, S. P.; Markesbery, W. R. Decreased Thioredoxin and Increased Thioredoxin Reductase Levels in Alzheimer's Disease Brain. *Free Radical Biol. Med.* **2000,** *28* (3), 418–427.

Luth, H. J.; Holzer, M.; Gartner, U.; Staufenbiel, M.; Arendt, T. Expression of Endothelial and Inducible NOS-Isoforms is Increased in Alzheimer's Disease, in A23transgenic Mice and after Experimental Brain Lesion in Rat, Evidence for an Induction by Amyloid Pathology. *Brain Res.* **2001,** *913,* 57–67.

Luth, H. J.; Munch, G.; Arendt, T., Aberrant Expression of NOS Isoforms in Alzheimer's Disease is Structurally Related to Nitrotyrosine Formation. *Brain Res.* **2002,** *953,* 135–143.

Mandal, P. K.; Saharan, M.; Tripathi, G.; Murari. Brain Glutathione Levels – A Novel Biomarker for Mild Cognitive Impairment and Alzheimer's Disease. *Biol. Psychiatry* **2015,** *78* (10), 702–710.

Mangialasche, F.; Baglioni, M.; Cecchetti, R.; et al. Lymphocytic Mitochondrial Aconitase Activity is Reduced in Alzheimer's Disease and Mild Cognitive Impairment. *J. Alzheimer's Dis.* **2015,** *44* (2), 649–660.

Markesbery, W. R. Oxidative Stress Hypothesis in Alzheimer's Disease. *Free Radic. Biol. Med.* **1997,** *23,* 134–147.

Martin, G. M. Interaction of Aging and Environmental Agents, The Gerontological Perspective. *Prog. Clin. Biol. Res.* **1995,** *228,* 25–80.

Martin, G. M.; Austad, S. N.; Johnson, T. E. Genetic Analysis of Ageing, Role of Oxidative Damage and Environmental Stress. *Nat. Genet.* **1996,** *13,* 25–34.

Mazzanti, G.; Di Giacomo, S. Curcumin and Resveratrol in the Management of Cognitive Disorders, what is the Clinical Evidence. *Molecules* **2016,** *21* (9), 345–357.

Mecocci, P.; Polidori, M. C.; Ingegni, T.; et al. Oxidative Damage to DNA in Lymphocytes from AD Patients. *Neurology* **1998,** *51* (4), 1014–1017.

Miller, E. R.; Pastor-Barriuso, R.; Dalal, D.; Riemersma, R. A.; Ael, L. J.; Guallar, E. Meta-Analysis, High-Dosage Vitamin E Supplementation may Increase All-Cause Mortality. *Ann. Internal Med.* **2005,** *142* (1), 37–46.

Mooijaart, S. P.; Van Heemst, D.; Schreuder, J.; Van Gerwen, S.; Beekman, M.; Brandt, B. W. Variation in the SHC_1 Gene and Longevity in Humans. *Exp. Gerontol.* **2009,** *39,* 263–268.

Multhaup, G. Amyloid Precursor Protein, Copper and Alzheimer's Disease. *Biomed. Pharmacother.* **1997,** *51,* 105–111.

Multhaup, G.; Schlicksu, A.; Hesse, L.; et al. The Amyloid Precursor Protein of Alzheimer's Disease in the Reduction of Copper (II) to Copper (I). *Science* **1996,** *271,* 1406–1409.

Muthukumaran, K.; Kanwar, A.; Vegh, C.; et al. Ubisol-Q_{10} (A Nanomicellar Water-Soluble Formulation of Co-Q_{10} Treatment Inhibits Alzheimer-Type Behavioral and Pathological Symptoms in a Double Transgenic Mouse Model of Alzheimer's Disease. *J. Alzheimer's Dis.* **2017,** *61* (1), 221–236.

Nazıroglu, M.; Muhamad, S.; Pecze, L. Nanoparticles as Potential Clinical Therapeutic Agents in Alzheimer's Disease, Focus on Selenium Nanoparticles. *Exp. Rev. Clin. Pharmacol.* **2017,** *10* (7), 773–782.

Poljsak, B.; Milisav, I. *Aging, Oxidative Stress and Antioxidants,* IntechOpen, 2013, pp. 346–367.

Ponce, D. P.; Salech, F.; Martin, C. et al. Increased Susceptibility to Oxidative Death of Lymphocytes from Alzheimer Patients Correlates with Dementia Severity. *Curr. Alzheimer Res.* **2014,** *11* (9), 892–898.

Popovic, L. M.; Mitic, N. R.; Miric, D.; Bisevac, B.; et al. *Influence of Vitamin C Supplementation on Oxidative Stress and Neutrophil Inflammatory Response in Acute and Regular Exercise Oxidative Medicine and Cellular Longevity*. Hindawi Publishing Corporation, 2015.

Ramsey, C. P.; Montgomery, M. B.; et al. Expression of Nrf2 in Neurodegenerative Diseases. *J. Neuropathol. Exp. Neurol.,* **2007,** *66* (1), 75–85.

Reddy, V. P.; Obrenovich, M. E.; Atwood, C. S.; Perry, G.; Smith, M. A. Involvement of Maillard Reactions in Alzheimer Disease. *Neurotox. Res.* **2002,** *4,* 191–209.

Reynolds, W. F.; Rhees, J.; Maciejewski, D.; Paladino, T.; Sieburg, H.; Maki, R. A.; Masliah, E. Myeloperoxidase Polymorphism is Associated with Gender Specific Risk for Alzheimer's Disease. *Exp. Neurol.* **1999,** *155,* 31–41.

Rosales Hernandez, M. C.; Hernandez Rodriguez, M.; Mendieta, J. E.; et al., *Involvement of Free Radicals in the Development and Progression of Alzheimer's Disease*; 2016, Intech Publisher, pp. 247-275

Ross Barclay, L.; Melinda, R. Vinqvist, On the Antioxidant Mechanism of Curcumin, Classical Methods Are Needed To Determine Antioxidant Mechanism and Activity. *Org. Lett.* **2000,** *2* (18), 2841–2843.

Sawda, C.; Moussa, C.; Turner, R. S. Resveratrol for Alzheimer's Disease. *Ann. N. Y. Acad. Sci.* **2017,** *1403* (1), 142–149.

Sayre, L. M.; Zelasko, D. A.; Harris, P. L.; Perry, G.; Salomon, R. G. 4-Hydroxynonenal-Derivedadvanced Lipid Peroxidation End Products are Increased in Alzheimer's Disease. *J. Neurochem.* **1997,** *68,* 2092–2097.

Schier, H. M. Hemeoxygenase Role in Brain Aging and Neurodegeneration. *Exp. Gerontol.* **2000,** *35* (6), 821–830.

Schier, H. M.; Cisse, S.; Stopa, E. G. Expression of Heme Oxygenase-1 in the Senescent and Alzheimer-Diseased Brain. *Ann. Neurol.* **1995,** *37* (6), 758–768.

Schier, H.; Bennett, D.; Liberman, A.; et al. Glial Heme Oxygenase-1 Expression in Alzheimer Disease and Mild Cognitive Impairment. *Neurobiol. Aging* **2006,** *27* (2), 252–261.

Schier, H.; Song, W. A Heme Oxygenase-1 Transducer Model of Degenerative and Developmental Brain Disorders. *Int. J. Mol. Sci.* **2015,** *16* (3), 5400–5419.

Senin, U.; Parnetti, L.; Barbagallo-Sangiorgi, G.; et al. Idebenone in Senile Dementia of Alzheimer Type, a Multicentre Study. *Arch. Gerontol. Geriatrics* **1992,** *15* (3), 249–260.

Smith, C. D.; Carney, J. M.; Starke-Reed, P. E.; Oliver, C. N.; Stadtman, E. R.; Floyd, R.; Markesbery W. R. Excess Brain Protein Oxidation and Enzyme Dysfunction in Normal Aging and in Alzheimer Disease. *Proc. Natl. Acad. Sci. U.S.A.* **1991,** *88* (23) 10540–10543.

Smith, M. A.; Richey Harris, P. L.; Sayre, L.; Perry, G. Iron Accumulation in Alzheimer Disease is a Source of Redox-Generated Free Radicals. *Proc. Natl. Acad. Sci. U.S.A.* **1997,** *94,* 9866–9868.

Smith, R. A.; Porteous, C. M.; Gane, A. M.; Murphy, M. P. Delivery of Bioactive Molecules to Mitochondria In Vivo. *Proc. Natl. Acad. Sci. U.S.A.,* **2003,** *100* (9), 5407–5412.

Speakman, J. R.; Selman, C.; McLaren, J. S.; Harper, E. J. Living Fast, Dying When? The Link Between Aging and Energetics. *J. Nutr.* **2002,** *132,* 1583–1597.

Sperling, R.A.; Aisen, P. S.; Beckett, L. A.; et al. Toward Defining the Preclinical Stages of Alzheimer's Disease, Recommendations from the National Institute on

Aging-Alzheimer's Association Workgroups on Diagnostic Guidelines for Alzheimer's Disease. *Alzheimers Dementia* **2011**, *7* (3), 280–292.

Staniek, K.; Nohl, H. H_2O_2 Detection from Intact Mitochondria as a Measure for One-Electron Reduction of Dioxygen Requires a Non-Invasive Assay System. *Biochim. Biophys. Acta* **1999**, *1413* (2), 70–80.

Sultana, R.; Baglioni, M.; Cecchetti, R.; et al. Lymphocyte Mitochondria, Toward Identification of Peripheral Biomarkers in the Progression of Alzheimer Disease. *Free Radic. Biol. Med.* **2013**, *65*, 595–606.

Sultana, R.; Mecocci, P.; Mangialasche, F.; Cecchetti, R.; Baglioni, M.; Butterfield, D. A. Increased Protein and Lipid Oxidative Damage in Mitochondria Isolated from Lymphocytes from Patients with Alzheimer's Disease, Insights into the Role of Oxidative Stress in Alzheimer's Disease and Initial Investigations into a Potential Biomarker for this Dementing Disorder. *Journal of Alzheimer's Disease,* **2011**, 24(1),77-84.

Tamaoka, A.; Miyatake, F.; Matsuno, S.; Ishii, K.; Nagase, S.; Sahara, N.; Ono, S.; Mori, H.; Wakabayashi, K.; Tsuji, S. Apolipoprotein E Allele-Dependent Antioxidant Activity in Brains with Alzheimer's Disease. *Neurology* **2000**, *54*, 2319–2321.

Trnka, J.; Blaikie, F. H.; Smith, R. A. J.; Murphy, M. P. A Mitochondria-Targeted Nitroxide is Reduced to its Hydroxylamine by Ubiquinol in Mitochondria. *Free Radic. Biol. Med.* **2008**, *44* (7), 1406–1419.

Turunen, M.; Olsson, J.; Dallner, G. Metabolism and Function of Coenzyme Q. *Biochim. Biophys. Acta (BBA) – Biomembranes* **2004**, *1660*, 171–199.

Ullah, R.; Khan, M.; Shahid, A. S.; Kamran, S.; Myeong, K. Natural Antioxidant Anthocyanins—A Hidden Therapeutic Candidate in Metabolic Disorders with Major Focus in Neurodegeneration. *Nutrients,* **2019**, 11, 1195.

Valla, J.; Schneider, L.; Niedzielko, T.; et al. Impaired Platelet Mitochondrial Activity in Alzheimer's Disease and Mild Cognitive Impairment. *Mitochondrion* **2006**, *6* (6), 323–330.

Van de Lagemaat, E. E.; Lisette. C. P., de Groot, G. M. Vitamin B12 in Relation to Oxidative Stress: A Systematic Review. *Nutrients* **2019**, *11*, 482–501.

Vignini, A,; Nanetti, L.; Moroni, C.; et al. Modifications of Platelet from Alzheimer Disease Patients, A Possible Relation Between Membrane Properties and NO Metabolites. *Neurobiol. Aging* **2007**, *28* (7), 987–994.

Wang, J.; Tan, L.; Yu, J. T. Prevention Trials in Alzheimer's Disease, Current Status and Future Perspectives. *J. Alzheimer's Dis.* **2016**, *50* (4), 927–945.

Wang, Y. Y.; Zheng, W.; Ng, C. H.; Ungvari, G. S.; Wei, W.; Xiang, Y. T. Meta-analysis of Randomized, Double-Blind, Placebo-Controlled Trials of Melatonin in Alzheimer's Disease. *Int. J. Geriatric Psychiatry* **2017**, *32* (1), 50–57.

Weyer, G.; Babej Dolle, R. M.; Hadler, D.; Hofmann, S.; Herrmann, W. M. A Controlled Study of 2 Doses of Idebenone in the Treatment of Alzheimer's Disease. *Neuropsychobiology* **1997**, *36* (2), 73–82.

Wojsiat, J.; Laskowska-Kaszub, K.; Mietelska Porowska, A.; Wojda, U. Search for Alzheimer's Disease Biomarkers in Blood Cells, Hypotheses-Driven Approach. *Biomarkers Med.* **2017**, *11* (10), 917–931.

Zhao, B. Natural Antioxidants Protect Neurons in Alzheimer's Disease and Parkinson's Disease. *Neurochem. Res.* **2009**, *34* (4), 630–638.

CHAPTER 11

Oxidative Stress and Parkinson's Diseases, A Role of Current Therapies

KAVITA SINGH[1*], AARSHI VASHISTHA[2], and GBKS PRASAD[1]

[1]*Centre for Translational Research, School of studies in Biochemistry, Jiwaji University, Gwalior, Madhya Pradesh, India*

[2]*Health Centre, Jiwaji University, Gwalior 474011, MP, India*

Corresponding author. E-mail: kavita.kushwaha786@gmail.com

ABSTRACT

Ageing is considered as the marker for a number of neurodegenerative diseases; second most prevalent in this array is Parkinson's disease (PD). The neuropathological characteristic of PD is dopaminergic neuronal loss and impairments in motor ability. Recently, various reports suggested the link between increased oxidative stresses and PD. The increased overload of ROS in term of upregulated oxidative stress is emerging as the key regulator in the progression of neurodegenerative conditions. Oxidative stress is generated due to the overexpression of reactive oxygen species (ROS) and nitrogen (NOS), which affects the normal brain functioning like alterations in neuron metabolism, glucose metabolism, calcium signaling, transport of neurotransmitters, and crucial mitochondrial dysfunction can obstruct the enzymatic antioxidant defense machinery, as neurons are completely dependent on the mitochondrial functioning for their high energy requirement for synaptic and neurotransmission. This makes brain predominantly susceptible toward the oxidative stress produce by the imbalance of redox potential. Therefore, the intent of this chapter is to illustrate the current considerate and management therapies used for Parkinsonism, which could be of high perspective value for translational health research. Hence, studying molecular mechanism connecting mitochondria and oxidative stress in the progression of PD could be helpful in exploring the new stratagem for recuperating the oxidative strategies as a promising treatment for PD.

Graphical Abstract

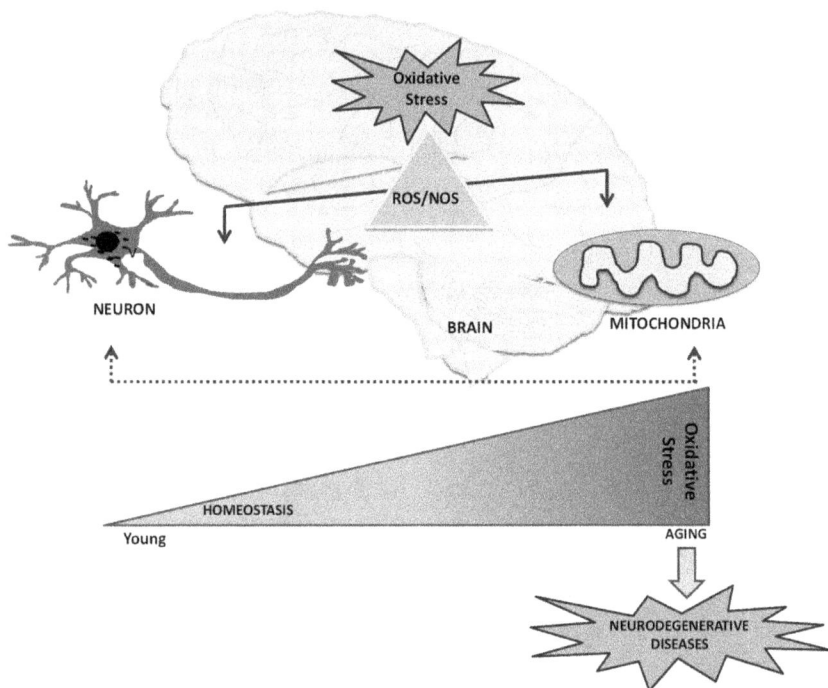

Pictorial representation of homeostasis imbalance in age-dependent manner due to increase in oxidative stress results into neurodegenerative conditions in aged people

11.1 INTRODUCTION

11.1.1 PARKINSON'S

Globally, enhanced age expectancy and declined mortality rates in the elder population, recorded in the latter half of the 20th century, has led to a huge rise in diseases particularly of old population, including Parkinson's diseases (PDs). In current scenario, PD emerges as the most common neurodegenerative disease in the central nervous system (CNS). Parkinson's influences approximately 2% of the population over the age of 65 years and 5% over the age of 85 years. Furthermore, the increased number of PD patients is estimated through many recent studies. The Global Burden of Disease reports PD as the second most devastating neurodegenerative disease (Rijkde et al., 2000; Bekris et al., 2010; Farrer, 2006).

Although PD was discovered 200 year ago, its persistence and increment are taking place in an exponential rate, and hence, its pathogenesis needs mechanistic exploration. Due to lack of knowledge of PD pathogenesis, the diagnosis is not possible before it is established. This is the most crucial point as these neurodegenerative diseases have tendency to exaggerate with age. So the promising, steadfast, and reliable analysis of PD is only possible with the more illustration of neuropathological alterations in the brain that are archetypal for these diseases. It is well known that there is a scarcity of data regarding early and late onset of PD, making it more complicated to provide effectual therapy to inhibit the succession of the disease and eventually promote healthy ageing.

PD is named after its discoverer James Parkinson (1755–1824) who first called it shaking palsy. Primarily, he described the PD as a devastating motor condition of limbs and organs correlated with it (Goedert et al., 2017).

11.1.2 PD

It is a well-established fact that the neurodegenerative process in PD takes place several years prior to the appearance of clinical indications. There are various hypothetical concepts to explain the processes in PD. One strong concept points toward the involvement of reactive oxygen species (ROS) during neurodegeneration, which deleteriously affects the dopaminergic (DA) neurons. In oxidative neuron damage, the metabolic imbalance between homocysteine (Hcy) and other biothiols, including methionine (Met), Cysteine (Cys), and glutathione (GSH), might be involved. Furthermore, the by-product of homocysteinic acid may upregulate the productive activity via agnostic pathway interaction to NMDA receptors. Hence, various studies have reported that the pathogenesis of PD is strongly linked with cell death or cellular degeneration. Medically, PD is characterized by cellular death of dopaminergic neurons, resulting in motor deficits gradually.

Clinically, it is characterized by apoptotic loss of dopaminergic neurons, resulting in subsequent and gradual loss of muscle control. This disease is diagnosed by resting tremors, rigidity of muscle, change in gait and speech, postural instability, depression, fatigue, anxiety, sleep disturbances, decline in cognition, and dementia. Premature death of patients occurs due to complications such as pneumonia and injuries. PD is prevalent in the adult population, usually in people over the age of 65 years. The male population is approximately 1.5–2 times more susceptible to this disease than the female population.

11.1.3   POTENTIAL THERAPY FOR PARKINSON TARGETED TO OXIDATIVE STRESS

11.1.3.1   ANTIOXIDANT SYSTEM

Normally, the human body has its own regulation system for cellular metabolism, which has to maintain a balance between the production of ROS and antioxidants molecules to defend its own system. The metabolic homeostasis is particularly important for survival and optimum functioning of neuronal cells. Due to their enormous oxygen consumption, long life span, and continuous liberation of nitric oxide (NO) in the metabolic signaling, neurons are extremely vulnerable to oxidative stress (Uttara et al., 2009; Gandhi et al., 2012). The human body has its own antioxidant system to cope up with the redox potential imbalance.

In brain particularly, the prime sites for ROS production are mitochondria in neuronal as well as glial cells. The accumulation of these free reactive species of oxygen and nitrogen is even acerbated in PD conditions due to neuroinflammation, dopamine deprivation, mitochondrial dysfunction, ageing, GSH depletion, and high levels of heme or calcium (). The build-up of ROS may be more damaging when the individuals are exposed to environmental factors such pesticides, neurotoxins, and dopamine (). This is substantiated by the link between enhanced risk of PD incidence and pesticides exposures. ROS has been reported to contribute significantly to dopaminergic neuron loss. Some studies also reported that the functional loss of dopaminergic neurons is more dangerous (Perfeito et al., 2012).

11.1.3.2   THE BIOCHEMISTRY OF OXIDATIVE STRESS

Oxidative stress is identified as a disequilibrium between the levels of reactive oxygen and nitrogen species generated and the capacity of a natural system to calibrate the reactive intermediates, mounting a frightening condition for cell survival. ROS can be produced via various pathways including direct reaction between redox-active metals and oxygen species via reactions including the Fenton and Haber–Weiss reaction, or through indirect approach that engages the transition and activation of enzymes like NADPH oxidizes or NO syntheses (NOS). Generally, the biochemical starting point of the key free radicals necessitates the activation of molecular oxygen (Smith et al., 1990). There are various types of ROS containing superoxide anion radical (O_2^{2-}), hydrogen peroxide (H_2O_2), and hydroxyl radical (OH). Superoxide anion produced by mitochondrial complexes I and II via electron transport chain presents highest toxicity and has high permeability through the inner mitochondrial membrane and reduced to H_2O_2, whereas H_2O_2, chiefly by mitochondrial but second big producer for H_2O_2 are peroxisomes since they contain catalase enzyme which converts H_2O_2 into water ant accumulation of H_2O_2 is prohibited.

Along with the ROS, there are several reports stating the engrossment of nitrogen (RNS) in generating nitrosative stress. RNS are engendered by the speedy reaction of superoxide ion with NO, resulting into the secretion of enormous amounts of peroxynitrite ($ONOO^-$). The enzyme responsible for the high secretion of NO is NOS, a synthesis that occurs in three isoforms, endothelial NOS (eNOS), neuronal (nNOS) recognized in neurons, and inducible form recognized in glial cells (Malkus et al., 2006; Vincent et al., 1998; Murphy et al., 1993; Hirsch et al., 2003). NO is located inside and outside the cellular space enveloping dopaminergic neurons determined by whether it is eNOS or iNOS. Furthermore, during the glial activation phenomenon, iNOS expressing glial cells also secretes huge amount of NO, and the level of NO is upregulated. The NO shows inhibitory action on the several mitochondrial enzymes contributing to electron transport chain, which ultimately results into ROS production. Also, NO reacts with proteins to form *S*-nitrosothiols, thus altering functionality of protein structures with heir lipid counterparts. This phenomenon is known as peroxidation (). For instance, an oxidizing agent known as peroxynitrite is a very vigorous and powerful oxidizing agent causing DNA fragmentation and lipid peroxidation. It also promotes a dose-dependent destruction in dopamine self-governing synthesis of dopamine oxidation or cellular degeneration (Carr et al., 2000; Szabo et al., 2007). Tyrosine hydroxylase (TH) is the initial and rate-limiting enzyme in the biosynthesis of dopamine (DA). TH activity is significantly diminished in Parkinson's disease (PD) and by the neurotoxic amphetamines, thereby accentuating the reductions in DA associated with these conditions (Park et al., 2003; Ara et al., 1998). The function of NO in PD is proofed through postmortem brain sections, presenting enhanced expression of *iNOS* in different region of brains including basal ganglia through in situ hybridization and immunocytochemical examinations. In MPTP (1-methyl-phenyl 4-phenyl-1,2,3,6-tetrahydropyridine) animal model study, the gliosis is reported to be associated with significant increase of *iNOS* (Liberatore et al., 1999).

11.1.3.3   NEUROPROTECTIVE ACTION OF VITAMIN

Vitamin E comes under the lipid-soluble endogenous antioxidants that have a capacity of scavenging several ROS, including hydroxyl and peroxyl radicals, thereby restricting the lipid peroxidation process. The natural vitamin E, α-tocotrienol, acts on key molecular checkpoints to protect against glutamate- and stroke-induced neurodegeneration. Primarily, a combo therapy of ascorbic acid and α-tocopherol was given to PD patients in open-labeled pilot trial. These results evidently present that the antioxidants may promote the development of the diseases. More-over, a big cohort study confirmed that nutritional ingestion of vitamin E reduces the risk of PD irrespective of the gender (46–47), whereas other data put forth issues on the efficiency of Vitamin E in slow progress of PD. Particularly, in the follow-up study of antioxidant intake, it was found that there was no positive outcome regarding the PD development irrespective of age, education, living status, etc. (48). Also, two other double-blind clinical trial studies reported neutral effect of vitamin E on PD pathogenesis. The MPTP animal model study strongly linked the glial activation in SN region with elevated levels of iNOS, whereas the reticence of nNOS protects against it.

Experimentally in the MPTP model, the gliosis in the SN is associated with significant upregulation of iNOS, while inhibition of nNOS protects against MPTP toxicity. Together, these observations are taken.

All kinds of living organisms have evolved the adaptive mechanism to cope up with the detrimental oxidative stress that comes through upregulated production of defensive enzymes, molecular chaperons, heat shock proteins, and most importantly antioxidant molecules. In normal physiological conditions, ROS are encompassed in signaling mechanism arbitrate by thiol residues in a protein structure that is capable of regulating transcription. On the other side, when oxidative stress is high, free radicals show damaging effect on almost each and every cellular process leading to the cellular damage (Fomenko et al., 2011). This includes the peroxidation process of cell membrane lipids, which generates the toxic by-products such as HNE and malondialdehyde (), cross-linking and scattering of proteins, and formation of carbonyl group (Floor et al., 1998; Yoritaka et al., 1996).

11.2   ANTIOXIDANTS TO COUNTERBALANCE OXIDATIVE STRESS

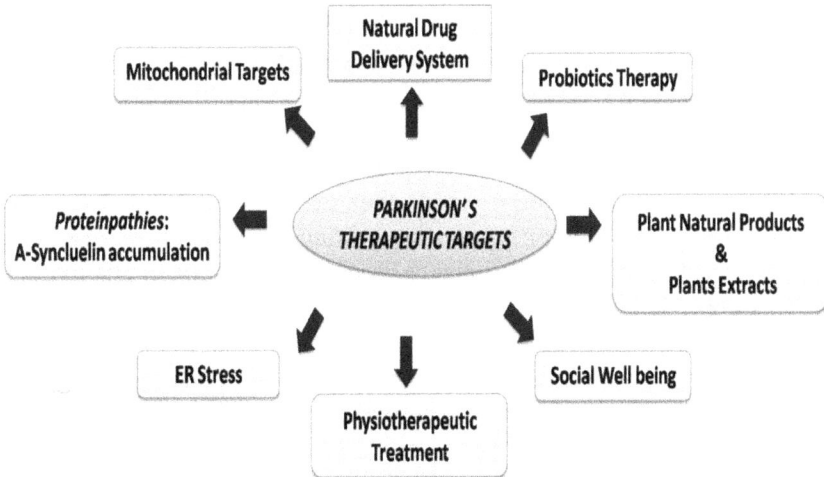

FIGURE 11.1   Different types of alterations in Parkinson's used as the therapeutic target points.

There is a plethora of evidence that associate the functional disorders of mitochondrial complexes with dopaminergic neurons in PD. The most compliant model for PD in this context was first reported in the 20th century, which demonstrates how MPTP of the mitochondrial is conscientious for

PD (Hu et al., 2016; Langston et al., 1983; Carreras et al., 2004). Afterwards, several studies independently reported that sporadic PD patients present decline in mitochondrial complex 1 activity in different regions of brain including peripheral, neural, and extraneural tissues and in cells (Haas et al., 1998; Parker et al., 2008)

Later on, several researchers independently discovered that sporadic PD patients have reduced complex I in different brain areas, peripheral cells, and neural and extraneural tissues and in cells (cytoplasmic hybrid), which are derived from PD patients. Another study on hybrid cell lines showed that complex I deficiency is correlated with the increased ROS generation. Furthermore, many studies based on model organs and human neuroblastoma cells showed that in some patients, the disorder may reflect exposure to the plant-extracted insecticide rotenone (complex I inhibitor). Rotenone induces apoptosis in SH-SY5Y cells At concentrations equal to or lower than 150 nM in serum-free medium, or up to 250 nM in serum-containing medium, rotenone treatment caused condensation of the cell body, nuclear fragmentation, and condensation into discrete dense chromatin clumps. The binding site for rotenone appears to be irrefutably defined as mitochondrial complex I. It seems that injury of cells is not simply caused metabolic machinery inefficiency, as similar levels of ATP suppression stimulated by other poisonous chemicals such as glycolysis inhibition by 2-deoxyglucose completely failed to cause approximately the same cell injury. Rather, cells protect themselves using their antioxidant protection system, suggesting that oxidative stress is the primary mechanism for cell injury. Mitochondrial complex I is particularly susceptible to modification caused by oxidative stress and thereby is a potential producer of ROS.

A recent study on cell lines, human brain tissues, and mice suggests that mutations in α-synuclein are associated with the pathogenesis and progression of PD. Furthermore, point mutations in α-synuclein are responsible for its decreased association with mitochondria-associated membranes, coincidence with a lower degree of apposition of endoplasmic reticulum with mitochondria, a reduction in mitochondria-associated membranes function, and increase in fragmentation of mitochondria. Mutations in Parkin and PINK1 also contribute in the progression of different types of PDs. The Parkin gene is highly expressed in brain tissues, including the substantia nigra, and contains 12 exons, of which five (exons 3–7) are generally deleted and cause the pathogenesis and progression of disease. Likewise, PINK1 (PTEN-induced kinase 1) is a mitochondrially located molecule and has a protective impact on a cell. A mutation in its kinase domain can make cells susceptible to oxidative stress and is thereby involved in the progression of disease.

Besides the factors mentioned before, many others have been reported to be involved in dysfunction of mitochondria-associated membranes. However, these factors were identified in other brain-associated disorders, which is beyond the scope of our review. In short, c-secretase activity itself is highly enriched in a subcompartment of the endoplasmic reticulum that is biochemically and physically connected to mitochondria. Mutation in the catalytic components of c-secretase (Presenilin-1 and -2) increases mitochondria-associated membranes functions and communication between endoplasmic reticulum and mitochondria, which is the prominent characteristic of the familial and sporadic forms of Alzheimer's disease. These results will help to understand calcium deregulation, mitochondrial dysfunction, and oxidative stress in this disease and explore the contribution of this mutant in other brain-associated diseases. Similarly, Sigma 1 receptor plays a crucial biological role in the protection of motor neurons, and its mutation leads to degeneration of motor neurons and cause amyotrophic lateral sclerosis. A recent study reported that mutation occurs in highly conserved amino acid reside in the sigma receptor of *SIGMAR1* gene. The neuronal cells that express this mutant protein are less resistant to apoptosis stimulated by cellular stress. Here, we garnered different contributing factors that are responsible for neurodegenerative diseases, for example, Alzheimer's disease, and that should be the focus of future studies to determine the biological role of these factors in brain-associated diseases.

As a whole, cellular viability depends on the biological functions of mitochondria, and alterations in its biological functions can lead to cell functional abnormality and even cell death. Neuronal cells are especially susceptible to mitochondrial dysfunction due to their dependence for energy requirement on the mitochondrial metabolism. Dysfunction of mitochondrial respiration has been demonstrated to be involved in the pathogenesis of neurodegenerative diseases. Genetic mitochondrial defects are also a probable primary pathogenic cause of some neurodegenerative conditions.

KEYWORDS

- ageing
- mitochondrial dysfunction
- oxidative stress
- neurodegenerative diseases

REFERENCES

Ara, J.; Przedborski, S.; Naini, A.; Jackson-Lewis, V.; Trifiletti, R.; Horwitz, J.; Ischiropoulos, H. Inactivation of Tyrosine Hydroxylase by Nitration Following Exposure to Peroxynitrite and 1-Methyl-4-Phenyl-1236-Tetrahydropyridine (MPTP). *Proc. Natl. Acad. Sci. U.S.A.* **1998**, *95*, 7659–7663.

Bal-Price, A.; Brown, G. C. Inflammatory Neurodegeneration Mediated by Nitric Oxide from Activated Glia-Inhibiting Neuronal Respiration Causing Glutamate Release and Excitotoxicity. *J. Neurosci.* **2001**, *21*, 6480–6491.

Beal, M. F.; Matthews, R. T.; Tieleman, A.; Shults, C. W. Coenzyme Q10 Attenuates the 1-Methyl-4-Phenyl-123Tetrahydropyridine (MPTP) Induced Loss of Striatal Dopamine and Dopaminergic Axons in Aged Mice. *Brain Res.* **1998**, *783* (1), 109–114. doi, 10.1016/S0006-8993(97)01192-X.

Bekris, L. M.; Mata, I. F.; Zabetian, C. P. The Genetics of Parkinson Disease. *J. Geriatric Psychiatry Neurol.* **2010**, *23*, 228–242.

Bové, J.; Prou, D.; Perier, C.; Przedborski, S. Toxin-Induced Models of Parkinson's Disease. *NeuroRx* **2005**, *2* (3), 484–494. doi, 10.1602/neurorx.2.3.484.

Carr, A. C.; McCall, M. R.; Frei, B. Oxidation of LDL by Myeloperoxidase and Reactive Nitrogen Species, Reaction Pathways and Antioxidant Protection. *Arterioscler. Thromb. Vasc. Biol.* **2000**, *20*, 1716–1723.

Carreras, M.; Franco, M. C.; Peralta, J. G.; Poderoso, J. J. Nitric Oxide Complex I and the Modulation of Mitochondrial Reactive Species in Biology and Disease. *Mol. Aspects Med.* **2004**, *25*, 125–139. doi, 10.1016/j.mam.2004.02.014.

Eve, D. J. N. A.; Kingsbury, A. E.; Hewson, E. L.; Daniel, S. E.; Lees, A. J.; Marsden, C. D.; Foster, O. J. Basal Ganglia Neuronal Nitric Oxide Synthase mRNA Expression in Parkinson's Disease. *Brain Res. Mol. Brain Res.* **1998**, *63*, 62–71.

Farrer, M. J. Genetics of Parkinson Disease, Paradigm Shifts and Future Prospects. *Nat. Rev. Genetics* **2006**, *7*, 306–318.

Floor, E.; Wetzel, M. Increased Protein Oxidation in Human Substantia Nigra Pars Compacta in Comparison with Basal Ganglia and Prefrontal Cortex Measured with an Improved Dinitrophenylhydrazine Assay. *J. Neurochem.* **1998**, *70*, 268–275.

Fomenko, D. E.; Koc, A.; Agisheva, N.; Jacobsen, M.; Kaya, A.; Malinouski, M.; Ruthetford, J. C.; Siu, K. L.; Winge, D. R.; Gladyshev, V. N. Thiol Peroxidases Mediate

Specific Genome-Wide Regulation of the Gene Expression in Response to Hydrogen Peroxide. *Proc. Natl. Acad. Sci. U.S.A.* **2011**, *198*, 2729–2734.

Fujino Noguchi, T.; Matsuzawa, A.; Yamauchi, S.; Saitoh, M.; Takeda, K.; Ichijo, H. G. Thioredoxin and TRAF Family Proteins Regulate Reactive Oxygen Species-Dependent Activation of ASK1 Through Reciprocal Modulation Of the N-Terminal Homophilic Interaction of ASK1. *Mol. Cell Biol.* **2007**, *27*, 8152–8163.

Gandhi, S.; Abramov, A. Y. Mechanism of Oxidative Stress in Neurodegeneration. *Oxid. Med. Cell. Longev.* **2012**, *2012*, 428010.

Global Regional and National Burden of Parkinson's Disease 1990–2016, A Systematic Analysis for the Global Burden of Disease Study 2016. *Lancet Neurol.* **2018**, *17*, 939–935.

Gong, L.; Daigneault, E. A.; Acuff, R. V.; Kostrzewa, R. M. Vitamin E Supplements Fail to Protect Mice from Acute MPTP Neurotoxicity. *Neuroreport* **1991**, *2* (9), 544–546. doi, 10.1097/00001756-199109000-00012.

Hirsch, E. C.; Breidert, T.; Rousselet, E.; Hunot, S.; Hartmann, A. M.. The Role of Glial Reaction and Inflammation in Parkinson's Disease. *Ann. N. Y. Acad. Sci.* **2003**, *991*, 214–228.

Horstink, M. W.; van Engelen, B. G. The Effect of Coenzyme Q10 Therapy in Parkinson Disease Could Be Symptomatic. *Arch. Neurol.* **2003**, *60* (8), 1170–1172. doi, 10.1001/archneur.60.8.1170-b.

Horvath, T. L.; Diano, S.; Leranth, C.; Garcia-Segura, L. M.; Cowley, M. A.; Shanabrough, M.; Elsworth, J. D.; Sotonyi, P.; Roth, R. H.; Dietrich, E. H.; Matthews, R. T.; Barnstable, C. J.; Redmond, D. E. Jr. Coenzyme Q Induces Nigral Mitochondrial Uncoupling and Prevents Dopamine Cell Loss in a Primate Model of Parkinson's Disease. *Endocrinology* **2003**, *144* (7), 2757–2760. doi, 10.1210/en.2003-0163.

Hu, Q.; Wang, G. Mitochondrial Dysfunction in Parkinson's Disease. *Transl. Neurodegener.* **2016**, *5*, doi, 10.1186/s40035-016-0060-6.

Hunot, S.; Boissièrs, F.; Faucheux, B.; Brugg, B.; Mouatt-Prigent, A.; Agid, Y.; Hirsch, E. Nitric Oxide Synthase and Neuronal Vulnerability in Parkinson's Disease. *Neuroscience* **1996**, *72*, 355–363.

Lan, J.; Jiang, D. H. Desferrioxamine and Vitamin E Protect Against Iron and MPTP-Induced Neurodegeneration in Mice. *J. Neural Transm. (Vienna)* **1997**, *104* (4–5), 469–481. doi, 10.1007/BF01277665.

Langston, J. W.; Ballard, P.; Tetrud, J. W.; Irwin, I. Chronic Parkinsonism in Humans Due to a Product of Meperidine-Analog Synthesis. *Science* **1983**, *219*, 979–980. doi, 10.1126/science.6823561.

Liberatore, G. T.; Jackson-Lewis, V.; Vukosavic, S.; Mandir, A. S.; Vila, M.; McAuliffe, W. G.; Dawson, V. L.; Dawson, T. M.; Przed-borski, S. Inducible Nitric Oxide Synthase Stimulates Dopaminergic Neurodegeneration in the MPTP Model of Parkinson Disease. *Nat Med.* **1999**, *5*, 403–409.

Malkus, K. A.; Tsika, E.; Ischiropoulos, H. Oxidative Modifications Mitochondrial Dysfunction and Impaired Protein Degradation in Parkinson's Disease, How Neurons Are Lost in the Bermuda Triangle. *Mol. Neurodegene.* **2009**, *4*, 24.

Mander, P.; Borutaite, V.; Moncada, S.; Brown, G. C. Nitric Oxide from Inflammatory-Activated Glia Synergizes with Hypoxia to Induce Neuronal Death. *J. Neurosci. Res.* **2005**, *79*, 208–215.

Martinovits, G.; Melamed, E.; Cohen, O.; Rosenthal, J.; Uzzan, A. Systemic Administration of Antioxidants Does Not Protect Mice Against the Dopaminergic Neurotoxicity of 1-Methyl-4-Phenyl-1256-Tetrahydropyridine (MPTP). *Neurosci. Lett.* **1986,** *69* (2), 192–197. doi, 10.1016/0304-3940(86)90602-6.

Muller, F. L.; Liu, Y.; Van Remmen, H. Complex III Releases Superoxide to Both Sides of the Inner Mitochondrial Membrane. *J. Biol. Chem.* **2004,** *279*, 49064–49073.

Müller, T.; Büttner, T.; Gholipour, A. F.; Kuhn, W. Coenzyme Q10 Supplementation Provides Mild Symptomatic Benefit in Patients with Parkinson's Disease. *Neurosci. Lett.* **2003,** *341* (3), 201–204. doi, 10.1016/S0304-3940(03)00185-X.

Murphy, S.; Simmons, M. L.; Agullo, L.; Garcia, A.; Feinstein, D. L.; Galea, E.; Reis, D. J. Minc-Golomb, D.; Schwartz, J. P. Synthesis of Nitric Oxide in CNS Glial Cells. *Trends Neurosci.* **1993,** *16*, 323–328.

Park, S.; Geddes, T. J.; Javitch, J. A.; Kuhn, D. M. Dopamine Prevents Nitration of Tyrosine Hydroxylase by Peroxynitrite and Nitrogen Dioxide, Is Nitrotyrosine Formation an Early Step in Dopamine Neuronal Damage? *J. Biol. Chem.* **2003,** *278*, 28736–28742.

Goedert, M. and Compston, A., 2018. Parkinson's disease—the story of an eponym. *Nat. Rev. Neurol.* **2018,** *14* (1), 57–62.

Ray Huang, B. W.; Tsuji, Y. P. D. Reactive Oxygen Species (ROS) Homeostasis and Redox Regulation in Cellular Signaling. *Cell Signal.* **2012,** *24*, 981–990.

Rijkde, M. C.; Launer, L. J.; Berger, K. et al. Prevalence of Parkinson's Disease in Europe, A Collaborative Study of Population-Based Cohorts. *Neurology* **2000,** *54*, S21–SS3.

Roghani, M.; Behzadi, G. Neuroprotective Effect of Vitamin E on the Early Model of Parkinson's Disease in Rat, Behavioral and Histochemical Evidence. *Brain Res.* **2001,** *892* (1), 211–217. doi, 10.1016/S0006-8993(00)03296-0.

SeoAhn, Y.; Lee, S. R.; Yeo, C. Y.; Hur, K. C. J. H. The Major Target of the Endogenously Generated Reactive Oxygen Species in Response to Insulin Stimulation Is Phosphatase and Tensin Homolog and Not Phosphoinositide-3 Kinase (PI-3 kinase) in the PI-3 Kinase/Akt Pathway. *Mol. Biol. Cell.* **2005,** *16*, 348–357.

Shults, C. W.; Beal, M. F.; Fontaine, D.; Nakano, K.; Haas, R. H. Absorption Tolerability and Effects on Mitochondrial Activity of Oral Coenzyme Q10 in Parkinsonian Patients. *Neurology* **1998,** *50* (3), 793–795. doi, 10.1212/WNL.50.3.793.

Shults, C. W.; Oakes, D.; Kieburtz, K.; Beal, M. F.; Haas, R.; Plumb, S.; Juncos, J. L.; Nutt, J.; Shoulson, I.; Carter, J.; Kompoliti, K.; Perlmutter, J. S.; Reich, S.; Stern, M.; Watts, R. L.; Kurlan, R.; Molho, E.; Harrison, M.; Lew, M. Parkinson Study Group Effects of Coenzyme Q10 in Early Parkinson Disease, Evidence of Slowing of the Functional Decline. *Arch. Neurol.* **2002,** *59* (10), 1541–1550. doi, 10.1001/archneur.59.10.1541.

Silvade, H. R.; Khan, N. L.; Wood, N. W. The Genetics of Parkinson's Disease. *Curre. Opin. Genet. Dev.* **2000,** *10*, 292–298.

Smith, D. G.; Caai, R.; Barnham, K. J. The Redox Chemistry of the Alzheimer's Disease Amyloid Beta Peptide. *Biochim. Biophys. Acta* **2007,** *1768*, 1976–1990.

Szabo, C.; Ischiropoulos, H.; Radi, R. Peroxynitrite, Biochemistry Pathophysiology and Development of Therapeutics. *Nat. Rev. Drug Discov.* **2007,** *6*, 662–680.

Terzioglu, M.; Galter, D. Parkinson's Disease, Genetic Versus Toxin-Induced Rodent Models. *FEBS J.* **2008,** *275* (7), 1384–1391. doi, 10.1111/j.1742-4658.2008.06302.x.

Tieu, K.; Ischiropoulos, H.; Przedborski, S. Nitric Oxide and Reactive Oxygen Species in Parkinson's Disease. *IUBMB Life* **2003**, *55*, 329–335.

Uttara, B.; Singh, A. V.; Zamboni, P.; Mahajan, R. T. Oxidative Stress and Neurodegenerative Diseases, A Review of Upstream and Downstream Antioxidant Therapeutic Options. *Curr. Neuropharmacol.* **2009**, *7*, 65–74.

Valko, M.; Leibfritz, D.; Moncol, J.; Cronin, M. T.; Mazur, M.; Telser, J. Free Radicals and Antioxidants in Normal Physiological Functions and Human Disease. *Int. J. Biochem. Cell Biol.* **2007**, *39*, 44–84.

Vincent, V. A.; Tilders, F. J.; Van Dam, A. M. Production Regulation and Role of Nitric Oxide in Glial Cells. *Mediators Inflamm.* **1998**, *7*, 239–255.

Yoritaka, A.; Hattori, N.; Uchida, K.; Tanaka, M.; Stadtman, E.; Mizuno, Y. Immunohistochemical Detection of 4-Hydroxynonenal Protein Adducts in Parkinson Disease. *Proc. Natl. Acad. Sci. U.S.A.* **1996**, *93*, 2696–2701.

CHAPTER 12

Solanum lycopersicum, a Reservoir of Antioxidants

MADHU PARMAR,[1] HRADESH RAJPUT,[2] and SONIA JOHRI[1]

[1]Department of Life Sciences ITM University Gwalior, MP, India

[2]Department of Food Technology ITM University Gwalior, MP, India

*Corresponding author. E-mail: madhu.sos@itmuniversity.ac.in

ABSTRACT

Solanum lycopersicum (tomato) fruit and its products are consumed by humans all over the world. Tomatoes are rich source of nutrients, vitamins, and minerals. Tomato is a good dietary source of vitamin C and other vitamins found in tomato are vitamin A, vitamin E, vitamin B, (B1, B2, B3, B5, B6, B9) and vitamin K. It has high vitamin C content. Tomato fruit is source of sugars, organic acids, amino acids, proteins, fats, fibers, terpenoids, and minerals (potassium, magnesium, calcium, iron, sodium, phosphate). Tomato fruit is rich in phytochemicals comprising of numerous bioactive compounds. Secondary metabolites include carotenoids, polyphenols, flavonoids, and steroidal glycoalkaloids. Nutritional value, flavor, and color of tomato fruit and their products depends on carotenoids (lycopene, β-carotene), vitamin C, glutamic acid, sugars, and flavonoids (naringenin chalcone, quercetin). Tomato fruit and its products have high antioxidant activity due to variety of bioactive compounds it possesses. The antioxidant activity of tomato cultivars is 48–118 μmol TEAC/100g. High antioxidant capacity of tomato is ascribed to vitamin C, vitamin E, lycopene, beta-carotene, polyphenols, flavonoids, and other bioactive phytochemicals present in it. In general, quantum of antioxidant activity depends on concentration of antioxidant compounds. During various ripening stages in tomato, antioxidant activity was correlated with bioactive compounds in the following order phenols>carotenes>flavonoids. Vitamin C contributed more to antioxidant activity than phenolic compounds. Different antioxidants act synergetically. In tomatoes, antioxidants scavenge peroxy radical and singlet molecular oxygen. All parts of tomato fruit have antioxidant activity and the antioxidant activity of skin and seeds together is almost equal to antioxidant activity of pulp. Consumption of tomato products relieves oxidative stress; prevents many chronic diseases including cancer, diabetes, respiratory disorder, cardiovascular diseases, and neurodegenerative disorder in humans. It stimulates immune system and has chemopreventive potential. The tomato is considered as a functional healthy food.

12.1   INTRODUCTION

Tomato (*Solanum lycopersicum* L.) fruit is popular edible vegetable all over world. Tomato is the world's third largest vegetable crop; however, it is largest canned vegetable in the world. The production of tomato in world was 182 million tons in 2017 (FAOSTAT, 2019). In India, tomato production in 2018–2019 was 19.37 million tons (DACFW, 2019).

Tomato fruits are consumed raw or cooked. They are processed into juices, purees, and ketchup. Canned tomato products are economically viable. About 40–50% of tomatoes in various countries are used as raw/cooked, and rest are processed for commercial use. All nutritional characteristics are retained in processed tomato products (Salles et al., 2003; Viskelis et al., 2005).

Hybrid tomato cultivar development programs have been initiated in last three decades to enhance nutritional value, quality, antioxidant activity, and resistance to environmental stresses (Atanassova and Georgiev, 2006). In most countries, hybrid cultivars of tomato are grown (Duvick, 1997). Tomato has unique flavor characteristics. In recent years, multidisciplinary approach in tomato research focuses on both nutritive and sensory quality parameters in breeding programs (Paolo et al., 2018).

Tomatoes have low carbohydrate and fat content, high fiber content, and are cholesterol free (Paolo et al., 2018) and thus is considered as healthy food. Tomatoes provide carbohydrates, proteins, amino acids, vitamins, minerals, dietary fibers to human diet (Januskevicius et al., 2005; Olmos et al., 2014), and other health benefitting phytochemicals carotenoids, polyphenols, flavonoids, chlorophyll, organic acids (Giovanelli and Paradise, 2002) and glycoalkaloids. Important carotenoids in it are lycopene and beta-carotene (Nguyen and Schwartz, 1999). Tomato contains glutamate in sufficient quantity which along with adenosine 5-monophosphate (AMP) present in tomato imparts umami taste to tomato, increases palatability and flavor, and is traditionally used in savory dishes (Ghirri and Bignetti, 2012). Composition of phytochemicals, flavor, and stage of ripeness are correlated (Kadar et al., 1977).

The tomato has high antioxidant activity, chiefly ascribed to vitamin C, vitamin E, carotenoids (lycopene, beta-carotene), polyphenols, flavonoids, and other phytochemicals. In human diet, raw or processed tomatoes can provide substantial proportion of the total antioxidants (Martinez-Valverde et al., 2002). All parts of tomato fruit, skin, pulp, and seeds contribute to antioxidant activity of tomato fruit (Elbadrawy and Sello, 2011).

Tomatoes contain many biologically active compounds which promote good health and play a role in disease prevention. Epidemiological studies have concluded that tomato phytochemicals have a potential role in prevention of respiratory disorders, blindness (Agarwal and Rao, 2000), cardiovascular diseases (Sesso et al., 2004), and cancer (Tan et al., 2010). Tomatoes have antioxidant, immunostimulating, anti-inflammatory, anti-diabetic activity, (Friedman, 2013) and chemopreventive activity (Feng et al., 2010).

12.2 CHEMISTRY OF TOMATOES

Composition of tomato fruit depends upon variety, cultivation technologies, and environmental conditions (Heyles et al., 2006). Both volatile and nonvolatile compounds are present in tomatoes, and flavor of tomatoes is due to both. The volatiles present include hydrocarbons (heterocyclic, cyclic, and acyclic), alcohols, phenols, esters, ethers, carboxylic acids, aldehydes, ketones, lactones, and halogen compounds. Some common volatile compounds are wine lactone, geranial, geranylacetone (Buttery et al., 1987). Fatty acid derivatives include C_6 alcohols and aldehydes, and they also contribute to aroma. Amino acid derivatives are mainly phenolic compounds such as phenylethanol and benzaldehyde which have aroma (Baldwin et al., 2008). Terpenoids in ripe fruit include terpineol, linalool, etc.

The nonvolatiles present in tomato are sugars, organic acids, proteins, amino acids, and their salts. They contribute to sensory quality. Sugar accounts for about 50–65% of total soluble solids in tomato fruit (Zhao et al., 2016). Major sugars present are glucose and fructose. The sugar content of ripe tomatoes is 3% (Jones and Scott, 1983), 2.6% (USDA, 2016) and is an important contributor to taste.

Organic acids are another major contributor to soluble solids. Citric acid is most abundant organic acid present in tomatoes (Davies et al., 1981). Other organic acids present in tomatoes include malic acid, acetic acid, fumaric acid, and lactic acid. Sugars and organic acids contribute to sweetness and sourness, respectively, and flavor acceptability of fresh tomatoes is also based on sugar and citric acid content (Malundo et al., 1995; Stevens et al., 1979). Tomatoes contain less oxalic acid than other vegetables such as potatoes, red beet, and lettuce. Oxalic acid affects metabolism adversely.

Major amino acid found in mature and ripe tomatoes is glutamic acid. Free glutamic acid content is higher in tomatoes than many vegetables and glutamic acid imparts umami taste to tomatoes (Ghirri and Bignetti, 2012). In tomatoes, major nucleotide present is AMP and it is also umami compound. Glutamic acid and AMP had synergistic effect in developing umami characteristics in tomatoes (Behrens et al., 2011).

Minerals including nitrates are important nutrients. Humans obtain it through food especially vegetables and to lesser extent through water. Tomatoes are rich in minerals. Tomato has high potassium content 237 mg/100g FW (USDA, 2016). Calcium, magnesium, phosphorus, iron, and zinc in tomatoes is 10 mg, 11 mg, 24 mg, 0.27 mg, and 0.17 mg per 100 g FW, respectively (USDA, 2016). Tomato is non-accumulative selenium plant. Reactive oxygen species (ROS) production in tomato fruits was reduced substantially on application of 1mg/L Na_2SeO_4 (Narvez-Ortiz et al., 2018).

12.3   SECONDARY METABOLITES

Tomato fruits produce large number of secondary metabolites. In ripe tomatoes, main secondary metabolites are polyphenols, carotenoids, alkaloids, and vitamins. It is rich source of carotenoids, and these plant pigments are produced through isoprenoid biosynthetic pathway and they have role in antioxidant activity. Carotenoid content in tomato is higher than polyphenols. The major carotenoids present in tomatoes are lycopene, carotenes, lutein, phytoene, neurosporene. Oxygenated derivatives of carotenes present in tomatoes are violaxanthin and neoxanthin (Perveen et al., 2015). Red color of tomatoes is mainly due to lycopene and to a lesser extent by carotenes and lutein. Phytoene and neurosporene are colorless. Carotenoids including lycopene are found in matrix of chloroplasts and chromoplasts are tightly bound due to which availability of lycopene from raw tomatoes is low (Shi and Maguer, 2000). Three main groups of pigments in tomato fruit include carotenoids, anthocyanins, and chlorophylls. Fruit color is governed by presence of pigments of terpenoid and phenylpropanoid classes.

Phenolics contribute to color, aroma, and taste in tomatoes. Phenolic compounds are present in abundance in tomato fruit. More than 170 phenolic compounds have been identified in tomato fruit (Paolo et al., 2018). Phenolics vary from simple phenolic compounds to complex polyphenols. Phenolic acids found in tomato are caffeic acid, ferulic acid, chlorogenic acid, coumaric acid. Phenolic acids are potent antioxidants. Phenolic acids defend plants against microbial and insect pathogens (Bravo, 1998). Common flavonoids found in tomato are quercetin, naringenin, rutin, myricetin, and kaempferol.

Tomato fruit is a rich source of vitamins chiefly vitamin C and other vitamins present in tomatoes include vitamin A, vitamin B1, vitamin B2, vitamin B6, folic acid, niacin, pantothenic acid, vitamin K, and vitamin E (Souci et al., 1996). The vitamin content in tomatoes depends upon genotype of cultivar, harvest time, maturation, ripeness, and supplementation of ethylene for ripening (Watada et al., 1976). The vitamin C, vitamin E, and vitamin K contents in tomato fruit were 25, 0.8, and 0.008 mg/100g, respectively (Souci et al., 1996).

Steroidal glycoalkaloids are present in all parts of tomato plant including fruit. Over 100 SGAs have been found in tomatoes (Moco et al., 2006). Number of aglycone structures (alkamines) have been identified and sugar moieties included oligosaccharides. The tomatine was first glycoalkaloid isolated from tomato, and it comprises of mixture of two SGA's alpha-tomatine and dehydrotomatine. The tomatine content in ripe fruit was 5mg/kg, while in early development stages of tomato fruit its concentration could be as high as 500mg/kg DW. SGA's have antipathogenic activity and offers protection to plants (Friedman, 2015).

Structure of Lycopene

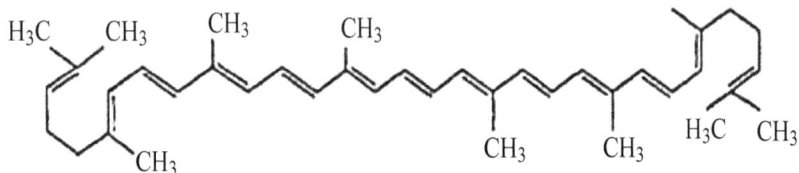

Structure of Beta-Carotene

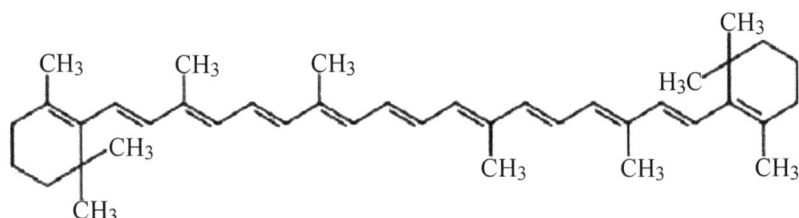

12.4 ANTIOXIDANT ACTIVITY

The antioxidant activity of tomato cultivars was 48–118 µmol TEAC/100g FW (Erge and Karadeniz, 2011), 1400–2730 µmol/100gDW (Khachik et al., 1992; Toor and Savage, 2005a). Widely used method for evaluating antioxidant activity is based on scavenging of DPPH radical capacity. The DPPH radical scavenging activity was variable in different cultivars of tomato, and it was 97–98% (Chang et al., 2006), 72–94% (Erge and Karadeniz, 2011). Value of DPPH essay was in range of 42–58% µmol TE /100g with mean of 52 µmol TE/100g (Erge and Karadeniz, 2011). DPPH activity at 0–50 µg/ml concentration was 20.04–63.80% inhibition (Balaswamy et al., 2015). Scavenging effect of tomato peel extract of 100 µg/ml and 200 µgml concentration was 44.3–81.03% and 86.40–97.32%, respectively, and range in scavenging was due to different solvents used for extraction (Elbadrawy and Sello, 2011).

Tomatoes cultivated in organic systems had higher ascorbic acid and phenolic contents due to it these organically cultivated tomatoes had higher antioxidant activity (Borguini, 2013).

Antioxidant activity of tomato fruits increased on irrigation of tomato plants with saline water (Pascale et al., 2015).

In tomato cultivars, the skin and seeds together contributed to 52% of total antioxidant activity, while antioxidant activity of pulp was 48% of total antioxidant activity and to derive optimum health benefits consuming of all parts of tomato fruit is of significance (Toor and Savage, 2005b).

In fresh tomatoes, antioxidant activity of hydrophilic fraction was more than lipophilic fraction, while in processed tomatoes antioxidant activity of lipophilic fraction was more in comparison to hydrophilic fraction (Lavelli et al., 2000). In general, quantum of antioxidant activity depended on concentration of antioxidant compounds (Elkhatim et al., 2018; Bhandari and Lee, 2016). During various ripening stages in tomato antioxidant activity was correlated with quantum of bioactive compounds in following order phenolics>carotenes>flavonoids (Bhandari and Lee, 2016). Arena et al. (2001) reported that vitamin C contributed more to antioxidant activity than phenolic compounds and other compounds. Carotenoids and vitamin C have synergistic antioxidant activity (Kritchevski, 1999).

Vitamin C is water-soluble antioxidant, removes free oxygen radical, and superoxide radicals. Humans do not synthesize vitamin C, so it has to be obtained through food. Tomato fruit has high vitamin C content. Vitamin C is reducing agent, donates two electrons from double bond between 2nd and 3rd carbons of six carbon molecule. By donating its electrons, it oxidizes ROS; thereby it prevents oxidation of other compounds. Ascorbate is a good scavenger (Bielski et al., 1975). Ascorbyl radical as compared to other free radicals is relatively stable and is relatively unreactive, thus ascorbate is a good antioxidant. The vitamin C content in tomato fruit reported by researchers was 25 mg/100g (Souci et al., 1996), 23 mg/100g (Belitz et al., 2004), 13.7mg/100g (USDA, 2016), 23.5mg/100g FW (Parmar et al., 2019). Vitamin C in tomato is a natural antioxidant and plays role in various biochemical processes including enhancement of immunity, collagen formation, and iron absorption.

Phenolic acids are well known antioxidants. Flavonoids constitute largest family among phenolics in tomatoes, and are found in all parts of tomato fruit; however, the major flavonoid content is found in tomato peel. Polyphenols and flavonoids are exogenous natural antioxidants. They (1) scavenge ROS (Silva et al., 2002); (2) chelate metal ions involved in free radical generation processes by donating single electron or a hydrogen atom (Prochazkova et al., 2011); (3) inhibits activity of enzymes involved in generation of ROS. They inhibit activity of xanthine oxidase, an oxidase of NADPH, involved in generation of super oxide anion radical (Harborne and

Williams, 2000). Other enzymes which polyphenols and flavonoids inhibit are ascorbic acid oxidase, protein kinase, lipoxygenases, cyclooxygenases, Na/K ATPase (Pietta, 2000); and (4) stimulates other antioxidant enzymes and are compatible with other oxidants, exhibits synergistic ROS scavenging activity with other antioxidants. Phenolic content in tomato fruit reported was 23.0 mg GAE/100g (Lutz et al., 2015), 16.0–17.8mg GAE/100g (George et al., 2011), 29.6mg GAE/100g (Parmar et al., 2019). Flavonoid content in tomato was 1.7–20.3 mg QE/100g (Crozier et al., 1997), 4–26 mg/100g (Slimestad et al., 2018), 6.4 mg QE/100g (Parmar et al., 2019).

Vitamin E is a lipid-soluble antioxidant. It acts as peroxyl radical scavenger. It protects polyunsaturated fatty acids in the cell membranes and maintains their bioactivity. Four tocopherols alpha, beta, omega, gamma have antioxidant activity, among them in humans alpha-tocopherol chiefly functions as antioxidant (Taber and Atkinson, 2007). In tomato, vitamin E content was 2–10mg/Kg FW (Lenucci et al., 2006).

Carotenoids are efficient antioxidants scavenging two types of ROS, peroxy radicals and singlet molecular oxygen. Mixture of carotenoids has more effective antioxidant capacity than individual carotenoid compound. Carotenoids interact with other antioxidants synergetically (Stahl and Sies, 2003). The main carotenoids found in tomatoes are lycopene, carotenes, phytoene, and lutein. Beta-carotene is strong antioxidant and had higher antioxidant activity than vitamin C (Lustgarten et al., 2011). It scavenges singlet oxygen. High doses of carotene had adverse effects; at high doses it expressed prooxidant action. Lycopene, beta-carotene, and phytoene content in tomatoes were 7.8–18.1 mg/100g, 0.1–1.2mg/100g, and 1.0–2.9 mg/100g, respectively (Marti et al., 2016). Beta-carotene in cherry tomato was 1.2mg/100g FW (Padmanabhan et al., 2016). Lycopene, beta-carotene, and lutein content was 9.25mg/100g, 0.41mg/100g, and 0.07 mg/100g, respectively (Perveen et al., 2015). Lycopene scavenges singlet oxygen. Lycopene has high antioxidant activity and alpha-tocopherol and beta-carotene have 100 fold and twofold lower antioxidant activity, respectively, in comparison to lycopene (Di Mascio et al., 1989).

12.5   HEALTH BENEFITS

Tomato and its products are functional foods. Tomatoes are beneficial for health, its several bioactive compounds have antioxidant activity, immunostimulating activity, anti-inflammatory activity, and have potential to reduce/prevent diseases such as diabetes, cancer, and cardiovascular diseases (Friedman, 2013; Rao et al., 1999), prevents blindness, modulates respiratory disorders (Chaudhary et al., 2018), and reduces hypertension. Epidemiological and animal studies have shown that regular intake of tomato in diet reduces cardiovascular diseases and cancer risk (Canene-Adams et al., 2005). Tomato is a low glycemic food laden with high antioxidants having antidiabetic potential (Upritchard et al., 2000).

Carotenoids comprise of group of vital micronutrients found in tomatoes and their dietary consumption resulted in lower frequency of cardiovascular diseases and cancer (Kritchevski, 1999; Kiokas and Gordon, 2004).

Red pigment lycopene is principal pigment present in tomato and lycopene exhibits antioxidant activity (Tonucci et al., 1995). Beneficial health effects of lycopene are ascribed to its high antioxidant potential. It oxidizes singlet oxygen and prevents oxidation of lipids. Lycopene intake reduced lipoprotein oxidative damage (Hadley et al., 2003). Half-life of lycopene in blood is 10–14 days, and tomato product consumption for 15 days significantly increased protection against oxidative damage (Hadley et al., 2003). It protects cardiovascular system. Cardiovascular disease risk is mitigated by high concentration of lycopene in blood serum (Cheng et al., 2017). Increased lycopene concentration in fatty tissues had protective effect against cardiac dysfunction (Knekt et al., 2002). Lycopene mitigates chronic neoplastic diseases (Przybylska, 2020). Rich lycopene diet is associated with lower risk of cancers (prostrate, lung, and breast cancer) (Giovannucci, 1999). Epidemiological evidence suggested inverse relationship of prostate cancer risk with intake of tomato consumption and lycopene content in blood (Rowles et al., 2018). Lycopene inhibits proliferation of epithelial cancer cells (Rajoria et al., 2010).

Lycopene reduces blood pressure and cholesterol. Tomato rich diet increased concentration of lycopene and beta-carotene in blood and simultaneously total cholesterol and LDL cholesterol decreased by 5.9% and 12.9%, respectively (Silaste et al., 2007). Lycopene has beneficial effects on skeletal system and neurodegenerative diseases. Lycopene reduces oxidative stress; thereby ROS effect on bone cells is reduced and also down regulates pro-inflammatory cytokines (Markovits et al., 2009) and mitigates osteoporosis (Sahni et al., 2009). Lycopene reduces risk of neurodegenerative disease such as Alzheimer disease and Parkinson's disease. Lycopene oxidizes ROS and mitigates neurotoxicity caused by presence of beta-amyloid and alpha-synuclein deposits (Rahman and Rhim, 2017). Higher lycopene level in blood has been achieved by intake of raw tomatoes/processed tomatoes rather than through intake of purified lycopene (Giovannucci, 1999).

Bioavailability of lycopene cis isomers is more than trans isomers. Processing of tomato enhances lycopene availability (Bates, 2005). Processing breaks down tissue matrix releasing lycopene and enhances cis isomerization (Shi and Maguer, 2000). Processing (heat and homogenization treatments) increased carotenoid availability from vegetables (Van Het Hof et al., 2000). Pressure–temperature treatment for processing tomato juice is a suitable method since both trans and cis isomers are stable in this process. Pressure–temperature method may be alternative to thermal sterilization (Gupta et al., 2010). During processing and storage, (1) lycopene isomerization from trans to cis isomers occurs due to light and thermal energy, and (2) it also reduced total biological properties (Preedy and Watson, 2008). Roldan-Gutierrez and de Castro (2007) opined that better methods of extraction and characterization of lycopene are needed.

Lycopene is lipophilic having hydrophobic characteristics and is soluble in organic solvents. Lycopene-rich tomato extract in vegetable oil can be used as a food product and intake of this product increases absorption in intestine (Urbonaviciene et al., 2015). Lycopene separates from food matrix in stomach and duodenum and thereafter dissolves in lipid phase. Interaction of lipid phase with bile salts and pancreatic lipase occurs, cis isomers are more soluble and in duodenum multilamellar lipid vesicles are formed, and in small intestines these lipids molecules are absorbed (Krinsky and Johnson, 2005). Beta-carotene caused increase in the absorption of lycopene (Bates, 2005).

Lutein is carotenoid synthesized in plants and is found in moderate quantities in tomato. Lutein helps in preservation of visual functions specifically it prevents macular degeneration (Buscemi et al., 2018). Phenolic acids are beneficial for mitigating many chronic diseases including cancer (Prasad et al., 2011).

KEYWORDS

- tomato
- oxidative stress
- lycopene
- sugar
- vitamin C

REFERENCES

Agarwal, S.; Ra, A. V. Tomato Lycopene and its Role in Human Health and Chronic Diseases. *Can. Med. Assoc. J.* **2000,** *163*(6), 739–744.

Arena, E.; Fallico, B.; Maccarone, E. Evaluation of Antioxidant Capacity of Juices as Influenced By Constituents, Concentrations, Process and Storage. *Food Chem.* **2001,** *74*, 423–427.

Atanassova, B.; Georgiev, H. Expression of Heterosis by Hybridization. In *Genetic Improvement in Solanaceous Crop*; Razdan, M. K., Mattoo, A. K., Eds.; CRC Press: Boca Raton, FL, USA, 2006; Vol. 2, pp 113–151.

Balaswamy, K.; Prabhakara-Rao, P. G.; Yadav, P.; Narsing-Rao, G.; Sulochanamma, G.; Satyanarayana A. Antioxidant Activity of Tomato (*Lycopersicon esculentum* L.) of Low Soluble Solids and Development of Shelf Stable Spread. *Int. J. Food Sci. Nutr. Dietetics* **2015,** *4*(4), 202–207.

Baldwin, E. A.; Goodner, K.; Plotto, A. Interaction of Volatiles, Sugars and Acids on Perception of Tomato Aroma and Flavor Descriptors. *J. Food Sci.* **2008,** *73*, S294–S307.

Bates, J. C. Lycopenes and Related Compounds. In *Encyclopedia of Human Nutrition*; Caballero, B., Allen, I., Prentice, A., Eds.; Elsevier: London, 2005; pp 184–190.

Behrens, M.; Meyerhof, W.; Hellfritsch, C.; Hofmann, T. Sweet and Umami Taste: Natural Products, their Chemosensory Targets, and Beyond. *Angew. Chem. Int. Ed.* **2011,** *50*, 2220–2242.

Belitz, H. D.; Grosch, W.; Schieberle, P. *Food Chemistry*, 3rd ed.; Springer: Berlin, 2004.

Bhandari, S. R.; Lee, J. G. Ripening-Dependent Changes in Antioxidants, Color Attributes, and Antioxidant Activity of Seven Tomato (*Solanum lycopersicum* L.) Cultivars. *J. Anal. Methods Chem.* **2016,** *5498618*, 1–13.

Bielski, B. H.; Richter, H. W.; Chan, P. C. Some Properties of the Ascorbate Free Radical. *Ann. N.Y. Acad. Sci.* **1975,** *258*, 231–237.

Borguini, R. G.; Bestos, D. H. M.; Moita-Neto, J. M.; Capasso, F. S.; Torres, A. F. D. S. Antioxidant Potential of Tomatoes Cultivated in Organic and Conventional Systems. *Braz. Archives Biol. Technol.* **2013,** *56*(4), 521–529.

Bravo, L. Polyphenols: Chemistry, Dietary Sources, Metabolism, and Nutritional Signifi-cance. *Nutr. Rev.* **1998,** *56*(11), 317–333.

Buscemi, S.; Corleo, D.; Marchesini, G. The Effect of Lutein on Eye and Extra-Eye Health. *Nutrients* **2018,** *10*(9), 1321.

Buttery, R. G.; Teranishi, R.; Ling, L. C. Fresh Tomato Aroma Volatiles: A Quantity Study. *J. Agric. Food Chem.* **1987,** *3*, 540–544.

Canene-Adams, K.; Campbell, J. K.; Zaripheh, S.; Jeffery, E. H.; Erdan, J. W. The Tomato as a Functional Food. *J. Nutr.* **2005**; 135(5): 1226 -1230.

Chang, C. H.; Lin, H. Y.; Chang, C. Y.; Liu, Y. C. Comparisons on the Antioxidant Properties of Fresh, Freeze-Dried and Hot-Air-Dried Tomatoes. *J. Food Eng.* **2006,** *77*, 478–485.

Chaudhary, P.; Sharma, A.; Singh, B.; Nagpal, A. K. Bioactivities of Phytochemicals Present in Tomato. *J. Food Sci. Technol.* **2018,** *55*(8), 2833–2849.

Cheng, H. M.; Koutsidis, G.; Lodge, J. K.; Ashor, A.; Siervo, M.; Lara, J. Tomato and Lycopene Supplementation and Cardiovascular Risk Factors: A Systematic Review and Meta-Analysis. *Atherosclerosis* **2017,** *257*, 100–108.

Crozier, A.; Michael, E.; Lean, J. Quantitative Analysis of Flavonoid Content of Commercial Tomatoes, Onion, Lettuce and Celery. *J. Agric. Food Chem.* **1997,** *45*(3), 590–595.

DACFW. Department of Agricultural Cooperation & Farmers Welfare. Ministry of Agriculture, Government of India. Horticulture Reports. Monthly Report Tomato (November, 2019).

Davies, J. N.; Hobson, J. E.; McGlasson, W. B. The Constituents of Tomato Fruit- the Influence of Environment, Nutrition and Genotype. *Crit. Rev. Food Sci. Nutr.* **1981,** *15*(3), 205–280.

Di-Mascio, P.; Kaiser, S.; Sies, H. Lycopene as the Most Efficient Biological Carotenoid Singlet Oxygen Quencher. *Arch. Biochem. Biophys.* **1989,** *274*, 532–538.

Duvick, D. N. In *Commercial Strategies for Exploiting Heterosis*, Proceedings of the International Symposium "The Genetics and Exploitation of Heterosis in Crops", Mexico City, Aug 17–22, 1997; pp 206–207.

Elbadrawy, E.; Sello, A. Evaluation of Nutritional Value and Antioxidant Activity of Tomato Peel Extracts. *Arab. J. Chem.* **2011,** *9*, S1010–S1018.

Elkhatim, K. A.; Elagib, R. A. A.; Hassan, A. B. Content of Phenolic Compounds and Vitamin C and Antioxidant Activity in Wasted Parts of Sudanese Citrus Fruits. *Food Sci. Nutr.* **2018,** *6*(5), 1214–1219.

Erge, H. S.; Karadeniz, F. Bioactive Compounds and Antioxidant Activity of Tomato Cultivars. *Int. J. Food Prop.* **2011,** *14*(5), 968–977.

FAOSTAT Crops 2019. http//www.fao.org/faostat/en/home (accessed Aug 25, 2019).

Feng, D.; Ling, W. H.; Duan, R. D. Lycopene Suppresses LPS-Induced NO and IL-6 Production by Inhibiting the Activation of ERK, p38MAPK, and NF-kB in Microphages. *Inflamm. Res.* **2010,** *59*(2), 115–121.

Friedman, M. Anticarcinogenic, Cardioprotective and Other Health Benefits of Tomato Compounds Lycopene. Alpha-Tomatine, and Tomatidine in Pure Form and in Fresh and Processed Tomatoes. *Agric. Food Chem.* **2013,** *61*(40), 9534–9550.

Friedman, M. Chemistry and Anticarcinogenic Mechanisms of Glyalkaloids Produced by Eggplants, Potatoes and Tomatoes. *J. Agric. Food Chem.* **2015,** *63*, 3323–3337.

George, S.; Tourniaire, F.; Gautier, H; et al. Changes in the Contents of Carotenoids, Phenolic Compounds and Vitamin C During Technical Processing and Lyophilisation of Red and Yellow Tomatoes. *Food Chem.* **2011,** *124*, 1603–1611.

Ghirri, A.; Bignetti, E. Occurrence and Role of Umami Molecules in Foods. *Int. J. Food Sci. Nutr.* **2012,** *63,* 871–881.

Giovanelli, G.; Paradise, A. Stability of Dried and Intermediate Moisture Tomato Pulp During Storage. *J. Agric. Food Chem.* **2002,** *50,* 7277–7281.

Giovannucci, E. Tomatoes, Tomato-Based Products, Lycopene, and Cancer: Review of the Epidemiologic Literature. *J. Natl. Cancer Inst.* **1999,** *91*(4), 317–331.

Gupta, R.; Balasubramaniam, V. M.; Schwartz, S. J.; Francis, D. M. Storage Stability of Lycopene in Tomato Juice Subjected to Combined Pressure-Heat Treatments. *J. Agric. Food Chem.* **2010,** *58*(14), 8305–8313.

Hadley, C. W.; Clinton, S. K.; Schwartz, S. J. The Consumption of Processed Tomato Products Enhances Plasma Lycopene Concentrations in Association with Reduced Lipoprotein Sensitivity to Oxidative Damage. *J. Nutr.* **2003,** *133,* 727–732.

Harborne, J. B.; Williams, C. A. Advances in Flavonoid Research. *Phytochemistry* **2000,** *55,* 481–504.

Helyes, L.; Dimeny, J.; Pek, Z.; Lugasi, A. Effects of the Variety and Growing Methods as Well as Cultivation Conditions on the Composition of Tomato (*Lycopersicon lycopersici*). *Acta Horticulturae* **2006,** *712,* 511–516.

Januskevicius, A.; Vaiciulaitiene, O.; Serenas, K. Nutritional Value of Lithuanian Vegetables. *Veterinarija ir Zootechnija* **2005,** *31*(53), 1392–2130.

Jones, A.; Scott, S. J. Improvement of Tomato Flavor by Genetically Increasing Sugar and Acid Contents. *Biomed. Life Sci.* **1983,** *32*(3), 845–855.

Kadar, A. A.; Stevens, M. A.; Albright-Holton, M.; Morris, L.; Algazi, M. Effect of Fruit Ripeness When Picked on Flavor and Composition in Fresh Market Tomatoes. *J. Am. Soc. Hortic. Sci.* **1977,** *102,* 724–731.

Khachik, F.; Goli, M. B.; Beecher, G. R.; Holden, J.; Lusby, W. R.; Tenorio, M. D.; Barrera, M. R. Effect of Food Preparation on Qualitative and Quantitative Distribution of Major Carotenoid Constituents of Tomatoes and Several Green Vegetables. *J. Agric. Food Chem.* **1992,** *40,* 390–398.

Kiokias, S.; Gordon, M. Antioxidant Properties of Carotenoids In Vitro and In Vivo. *Food Rev. Int.* **2004,** *20,* 99–121.

Knekt, P.; Kumpulainen, J.; Jarvinen, R.; Rissanen, H.; Heliovaara, M.; Reunanen, A. Flavonoid Intake and Risk of Chronic Disease. *Am. J. Clin. Nutr.* **2002,** *76,* 560–568.

Krinsky, N. I.; Johnson, E. J. Carotenoid Action and their Relation to Health and Disease. *Mol. Aspects Med.* **2005,** *26,* 459–516.

Kritchevski, S. B. β-Carotene, Carotenoids and the Prevention of Coronary Heart Disease. *J. Nutr.* **1999,** *129,* 5–8.

Lavelli, V.; Peri, C.; Rizzolo, A. Antioxidant Activity of Tomato Products as Studied by Model Reactions Using Xanthine Oxidse, Myeloperoxidase and Copper-Induced Lipid Peroxidation. *J. Agric. Food Chem.* **2000,** *48*(5), 1442–1448.

Lenucci, M. S.; Cadinu, D.; Taurino, M.; Piro, G.; Dalessandro G. Antioxidant Composition in Cherry and High Pigment Tomato Cultivars. *J. Agric. Food Chem.* **2006,** *54,* 2606–2613.

Lustgarten, M.; Muller, F. L.; Remmen, H. V. An Objective Appraisal of the Free Radical Theory of Aging. In *Handbook of the Biology of Aging,* 7th ed.; 2011; pp 177–202.

Lutz, M.; Hernandez, J.; Henriquez, C. Phenolic Content and Antioxidant Capacity in Fresh and Dry Fruits and Vegetables Grown in Chile. *J. Food* **2015,** *13*(4), 541–547.

Malundo, T. M. M.; Shewfelt, R. L.; Scott, J. W. Flavor Quality of Fresh Tomato (*Lycopersicon esculentum* Mill.) as Affected by Sugar and Acid Levels. *Postharvest Biol. Technol.* **1995**, *6*(1–2), 103–110.

Marti, R.; Rosello, S.; Cebolla-Cornejo, J. Tomato as a Source of Carotenoids and Polyphenols Targeted to Cancer Prevention. *Cancers* **2016**, *8*(6), 58.

Martinez-Valverde, I.; Periage, M. J.; Provan, G.; Chesson, A. Phenolic Compounds, Lycopene and Antioxidant Activities in Commercial Varieties of Tomato (*Lycopersicon esculentum*). *J. Sci. Food Agric.* **2002**, *82*, 323–330.

Moco, S. I. A.; Bino, R. J.; Vorst, O. F. J.; Verhoeven, H. A.; et al. A Liquid Chromatography-Mass Spectrometry Based Metabolome Database for Tomato. *Plant Physiol.* **2006**, *141*, 1205–1218.

Narvaez-Ortiz, W. A.; Becvort-Azcurra, A. A.; Funtes-Lara, L. O.; et al. Mineral Composition and Antioxidant Status of Tomato with Application of Selenium. *Agronomy* **2018**, *8*, 185.

Nguyen, M. L.; Schwartz, S. J. Lycopene: Chemical and Biological Properties. *Food Technol.* **1999**, *53*, 38–45.

Markovits, N.; Amotz, A. B.; Levy, Y. The Effect of Tomato-Derived Lycopene on Low Carotenoids and Enhanced Systemic inflammation and Oxidation in Severe Obesity. *ISR Med. Assoc. J.* **2009**, *11*(10), 598–601.

Olmos, C. C.; Leiva-Brondo, M.; Rosello, J.; Raigon, M. D. Cebolla-Cornejo, J. The Role of Traditional Varieties of Tomato as Sources of Functional Compounds. *J. Sci. Food Agric.* **2014**, *94*(14), 2888–2904.

Padmanabhan, P.; Cheema, A.; Paliyath, G. Solanaceous Fruits Including Tomato, Eggplant and Peppers. *Encycl. Food Health* **2016**, 24–32.

Paolo, D.; Blanchi, G.; Scalzo, R. L.; Morelli, C. F.; Rabuffetti, M.; Speranza, G. The Chemistry Behind Tomato Quality. *Nat. Prod. Commun.* **2018**, *13*(9), 1225–1232.

Parmar, M.; Sonia, J.; Rajput, H.; Bhat, J. L. Quality Attributes, Biochemical Profile and Calorific Status of Functional RTS Drink from a Blend of Mango and Tomato. *Int. J. Food Ferment. Technol.* **2019**, *9*(2), 1–8.

Pascale, S. D.; Maggio, A.; Fogliano, V.; Ambrosino, P.; Ritieni, A. Irrigation with Saline Water Improves Carotenoid Content and Antioxidant Activity of Tomato. *J. Hortic. Sci. Biotech.* **2015**, *76*, 447–453.

Perveen, R.; Suleria, H. A. R.; Anjum, F. M.; et al. Tomato (*Solanum lycopersicum*) Carotenoids and Lycopene Chemistry, Metabolism, Absorption, Nutrition and Allied Health Claims: A Comprehensive Review. *Crit. Rev. Food Sci. Nutr.* **2015**, *55*, 919–929.

Pietta, P. G. Flavonoids as Antioxidants. *J. Nat. Prod.* **2000**, *63*, 1035–1042.

Prasad, N. R.; Karthikeyan, A.; Subburagan, K.; Reddy, B. V. Inhibitory Effect of Caffeic Acid on Cancer Cell Proliferation by Oxidative Mechanism in Human HT-1080 Fibrosarcoma Cell Line. *Mol. Cell. Biochem.* **2011**, *349*(1–2), 11–19.

Preedy, V. R.; Watson, R. R. *Lycopene: Nutritional, Medicinal and Therapeutic Properties*; CRC Press Science Publishers, 2008.

Prochazkova, D.; Bousova, I.; Wilhelmova, N. Antioxidant and Prooxidant Properties of Flavonoids. *Fitoterapia* **2011**, *82*(4), 513–523.

Przybylska, S. Lycopene - a Bioactive Carotenoid Offering Multiple Health Benefits: A Review. *Int. J. Food Sci. Tech.* **2020**, *5*, 11–32.

Rajoria, A.; Kumar, J.; Chauhan, A. K. Anti-Oxidative and Anti-Carcinogenic Role of Lycopene in Human Health: A Review. *J. Dairy. Foods Home Sci.* **2010**, *29*(3–4), 157–165.

Rao, A. V.; Fleshner, N.; Agarwal, S. Serum and Tissue Lycopene and Biomarkers of oxidation in Prostate Cancer Patients: A Case-Control Study. *Nutr. Cancer* **1999,** *33*(2), 159–164.

Rahman, M. A.; Rhim, H. Therapeutic Implication of Autophagy in Neurodegenerative Disease. *BMM Rep.* **2017,** *50*, 345–354.

Roldan-Gutierrez, R. J. M.; De Castro, M. D. L. Lycopene: The Need for Better Methods for Characterization and Determination. *Trends Anal. Chem.* **2007,** *26*(2), 163–170.

Rowles, J. L.; Ranard, K. M.; Applegate, C. C.; Jeon, S.; An, R.; Erdman, J. W. Processed and Raw Tomato Consumption and Risk Of Prostate Cancers : A Systematic Review and Dose-Response Meta-Analysis. *Prostate Cancer Prostatic Dis.* **2018,** *21*, 319–336.

Sahni, S.; Hannan, M. T.; Blumberg, J.; et al. Protective Effect of Total Carotenoid and Lycopene Intake on the Risk of Hip Fracture: A 17 Year Follow Up from the Framingham Osteoporosis Study. *J. Bone Miner. Res.* **2009,** *24*(6), 1086–1094.

Salles, C.; Nicklaus, S.; Septier, C. Determination and Gustatory Properties of Taste-Active Compounds in Tomato Juice. *Food Chem.* **2003,** *81*, 395–402.

Sesso, H. D.; Buring, J. E.; Norkus, E. P.; Gaziano, J. M. Plasma Lycopene, Other Carotenoids and Retinol and the Risk of Cardiovascular Disease in Women. *Am J. Clin. Nutr.* **2004,** *79*(1), 47–53.

Shi, J.; Maguer, M. L. Lycopene in Tomatoes: Chemical and Physical Properties Affected by Food Processing. *Crit. Rev. Food Sci. Nutr.* **2000,** *40*(1), 1–42.

Silaste, M. L.; Alfthan, G.; Aro, A. Tomato Juice Decreases LDL Cholesterol Levels and Increases LDL Resistance to Oxidation. *Br. J. Nutr.* **2007,** *98*(6), 1251–1258.

Silva, M.; Santos, M.; Caroco, G.; Rocha, R.; Justino, G.; Mira, L. Structure-Antioxidant Activity Relationships of Flavonoids: A Re-Examination. *Free Radic. Res.* **2002,** *3*, 1219–1227.

Slimestad, R.; Fossen, T.; Verheul, M. J. The Flavonoids of Tomatoes. *J. Sci. Food Agric.* **2008,** *5*, 436–2441.

Souci, S. W.; Fachmann, W.; Kraut, H. *Food Composition and Nutrient Tables*; Wissen-schaftliche verlagsgesellschaft: Stuttgart, 1996.

Stahl, W.; Sies, H. Antioxidant Activity of Carotenoids. *Mol. Aspects Med.* **2003,** *24*, 345–351.

Stevens, M. A.; Kader, V. L.; Albright, M. Potential for Increasing Tomato Flavor via Increased Sugar and Acid Content. *J. Am. Soc. Hortic. Sci.* **1979,** *104*(1), 40–42.

Tan, H.; Thomas-Ahner, J. M.; Grainger, E. M.; et al. Tomato Based Food Products for Prostrate Cancer Prevention: What Have We Learned. *Cancer Metasis Rev.* **2010,** *29*(3), 533–568.

Tonucci, L. H.; Holden, J. M.; Beecher, G. R.; Khachik, F.; Davis, C. S.; Mulokozi, G. Carotenoid Content of Thermally Processed Tomato-Based Food Products. *J. Agric. Food Chem.* **1995,** *43*, 579–586.

Toor, R. K.; Savage, G. P. Effect of Semi Drying on the Antioxidant Components of Tomatoes. *Food Chem.* **2005,** *94*, 90–97

Toor, R. K.; Savage, G. P. Antioxidant Activity in Different Fractions of Tomatoes. *Food Res. Int.* **2005,** *38*(5), 487–494.

Traber, M. G.; Atkinson, J. Vitamin E, Antioxidant and Nothing More. *Free Radical Biol. Med.* **2007,** *43*(1), 4–15.

Upritchard, J. E.; Sutherland, W.; Mann, J. L. Effect of Supplementation with Tomato Juice, Vitamin E, and Vitamin C on LDL Oxidation and Products of Inflammatory Activity in type 2 Diabetes. *Diabet. Care* **2000,** *23*(6), 733–738.

Urbonaviciene, D.; Viskelis, P.; Viskelis, J.; Bobinas, C. Stability of Tomato Lycopene Under Thermal and Light Irradiation Treatments in an Oil Based Model System. *Zemdirbyste-Agric.* **2015**, *102*(2), 185–192.

USDA (United States Department of Agriculture). Food Composition Databases (USDA, 2016).

Van Het Hof, K. H.; West, C. E.; Weststrate, J. A.; Hautvast, J. G. Dietary Factors that Affect the Bioavailability of Carotenoids. *J. Nutr.* **2000**, *130*(3), 503–506.

Viskelis, P.; Vilkauskaite, G.; Noreika, R. K. Chemical Composition, Functional Properties and Consumption of Tomatoes. *Sodininkyste ir Darzininkyste* **2005**, *24*(4), 182–189.

Watada, A. E.; Aljlenbach, B. B.; Worthington, J. T. Vitamins A and C in Ripe Tomatoes as Effected by Stages of Ripeness at Harvest and by Supplementary Ethylene. *J. Food Sci.* **1976**, *41*(4), 856–858.

Zhao, J.; Xu, Y.; Ding, Q.; et al. Association Mapping of Main Tomato Fruit Sugars and Organic Acids. *Front. Plant Sci.* **2016**, *7*, 1286.

Index

For Product Safety Concerns and Information please contact our EU
representative GPSR@taylorandfrancis.com
Taylor & Francis Verlag GmbH, Kaufingerstraße 24, 80331 München, Germany

www.ingramcontent.com/pod-product-compliance
Lightning Source LLC
Chambersburg PA
CBHW060341220326
41598CB00023B/2776

* 9 7 8 1 7 7 4 6 3 9 0 9 2 *